Grant Writing Handbook for Nurses

Second Edition

Barbara J. Holtzclaw, PhD, RN, FAAN
Professor Graduate Program/Nurse Scientist
College of Nursing, University of Oklahoma Health Sciences Center
Oklahoma City, Oklahoma
Professor Emeritus and Former Associate Dean for Research
University of Texas Health Science Center at San Antonio

Carole Kenner, DNS, RNC, FAAN
Dean/Professor
College of Nursing, University of Oklahoma Health Sciences Center
Oklahoma City, Oklahoma
President
Council of International Neonatal Nurses, Edmond, Oklahoma

Marlene Walden, PhD, RNC, NNP, CCNS
Neonatal Nurse Practitioner/Nurse Scientist
Texas Children's Hospital
Houston, Texas

JONES AND BARTLETT PUBLISHERS
Sudbury, Massachusetts
BOSTON   TORONTO   LONDON   SINGAPORE

World Headquarters
Jones and Bartlett Publishers
40 Tall Pine Drive
Sudbury, MA 01776
978-443-5000
info@jbpub.com
www.jbpub.com

Jones and Bartlett Publishers
Canada
6339 Ormindale Way
Mississauga, Ontario L5V 1J2
Canada

Jones and Bartlett Publishers
International
Barb House, Barb Mews
London W6 7PA
United Kingdom

Jones and Bartlett's books and products are available through most bookstores and online booksellers. To contact Jones and Bartlett Publishers directly, call 800-832-0034, fax 978-443-8000, or visit our website, www.jbpub.com.

Substantial discounts on bulk quantities of Jones and Bartlett's publications are available to corporations, professional associations, and other qualified organizations. For details and specific discount information, contact the special sales department at Jones and Bartlett via the above contact information or send an email to specialsales@jbpub.com.

The authors, editor, and publisher have made every effort to provide accurate information. However, they are not responsible for errors, omissions, or for any outcomes related to the use of the contents of this book and take no responsibility for the use of the products and procedures described. Treatments and side effects described in this book may not be applicable to all people; likewise, some people may require a dose or experience a side effect that is not described herein. Drugs and medical devices are discussed that may have limited availability controlled by the Food and Drug Administration (FDA) for use only in a research study or clinical trial. Research, clinical practice, and government regulations often change the accepted standard in this field. When consideration is being given to use of any drug in the clinical setting, the health care provider or reader is responsible for determining FDA status of the drug, reading the package insert, and reviewing prescribing information for the most up-to-date recommendations on dose, precautions, and contraindications, and determining the appropriate usage for the product. This is especially important in the case of drugs that are new or seldom used.

Production Credits
Publisher: Kevin Sullivan
Aquisitions Editor: Emily Ekle
Aquisitions Editor: Amy Sibley
Editorial Assistant: Patricia Donnelly
Editorial Assistant: Rachel Shuster
Associate Production Editor: Amanda Clerkin
Associate Marketing Manager: Rebecca Wasley

Manufacturing and Inventory Control Supervisor:
    Amy Bacus
Composition: Shepherd, Inc.
Cover Design: Brian Moore
Cover Image Credit: © Olga Shelego/ShutterStock, Inc.
Printing and Binding: Malloy, Inc.
Cover Printing: Malloy, Inc.

Library of Congress Cataloging-in-Publication Data
Holtzclaw, Barbara J.
    Grant writing handbook for nurses / Barbara Holtzclaw, Carole Kenner, and Marlene Walden. — 2nd ed.
        p. ; cm.
    Rev. ed. of: Grant writing tips for nurses and other health professionals / Carole Kenner, Marlene Walden. c2001.
    Includes bibliographical references and index.
    ISBN-13: 978-0-7637-5602-4 (alk. paper)
    ISBN-10: 0-7637-5602-4 (alk. paper)
    1. Nursing—Research grants. 2. Proposal writing for grants. 3. Proposal writing in medicine. I. Kenner, Carole.
II. Walden, Marlene, 1956- III. Kenner, Carole. Grant writing tips for nurses and other health professionals. IV. Title.
    [DNLM: 1. Nursing Research. 2. Research Support as Topic. 3. Fellowships and Scholarships—standards.
4. Writing. WY 20.5 H758g 2009]
    RT73.K46 2009
    610.73'079—dc22
                2008003029

6048

Printed in the United States of America
12 11 10 09 08   10 9 8 7 6 5 4 3 2 1

Contents

CHAPTER 3: WHAT TYPE OF GRANT DO YOU WANT?

CHAPTER 4: IT TAKES A VILLAGE (AND THE VILLAGE HAS A SYSTEM!)

CHAPTER 5: WRITING THE RESEARCH PROPOSAL

CHAPTER 6: CHECK YOUR PARACHUTE! A FEW MORE HOOPS TO JUMP THROUGH

CHAPTER 7: THE ELECTRONIC FLIGHT PLAN FOR GRANT SUBMISSION

CHAPTER 8: GAUGING PROGRESS AND REVIEWER FEEDBACK

CHAPTER 9: SO NOW YOU'VE BEEN FUNDED

CHAPTER 10: DISSEMINATION OF GRANT FINDINGS

Acknowledgments

We would like to thank Kevin Sullivan at Jones and Bartlett for supporting this second edition. The original project grew out of a presentation done by Drs. Carole Kenner and Marlene Walden at a National Association of Neonatal Nurses conference. This second edition includes content from grantsmanship workshops presented by Dr. Barbara Holtzclaw at national and regional conferences and for nursing and interdisciplinary faculty development programs in Texas, Oklahoma, Alabama, and North Carolina.

Preface

Few nurses enter the profession thinking they will ever write a grant. Yet many of the goals and realities of a meaningful nursing career require nurses to request funding for projects that focus on education, clinical practice, research, or a combination. Grant writing is an essential skill for nurses today, but one we receive little training for, even in advanced graduate programs. So where do you start? Where do you look for guidance? Where do you find foundations or agencies that fund enterprises like yours? These questions tend to be of first concern to most new grant writers. However, as you sit at the keyboard to actually write the grant, you may feel somewhat intimidated by unfamiliar terminology, puzzling forms, and a variety of submission formats required by funding agencies. This process is more frustrating if you are unfamiliar with the structure, conventions, and essential elements of grant preparation. This grant-writing monograph is a very informal conversation about the art of proposing and the process of how to write grants with minimal frustration. At least we hope we accomplish that goal! Each of the authors is an experienced grant writer, grant reviewer, and grantsmanship consultant. Examples include tips from their grant-writing workshops and experiences from their own projects. The book is formatted to follow the basic steps of grant writing. We've written this in first person to get the reader involved in the process. You will find other books on writing fundable grants that are very detailed, grant-specific, and devoid of real-life experiences. We attempted to cut to the chase and give you bare bones strategies and quick tips that a busy nurse—a would-be grant writer—needs for this adventure.

Grant writing can be exciting and even profitable given the right tools. This book is one of the "right tools." Happy grant writing!

Barbara J. Holtzclaw, PhD, RN, FAAN
Carole Kenner, DNS, RNC, FAAN
Marlene Walden, PhD, RNC, NNP, CCNS

CHAPTER 1

Why Grant-Writing Skills Are Needed Now and in the Future

Perhaps your incentive to write a grant may have come from a deep-seated desire to be a grant writer. If so, you are unusual and have an interesting life's work cut out for you. However, for the rest of us, and the majority of health professionals, the motivation to write a grant comes from a need to finance a project, a study, or an educational program. If that is where you are beginning, it is worthwhile to resist the "means to an end" view of looking for expediency rather than a good fit with an idea and a potential funding agency. Also, if unfamiliarity with grantsmanship makes grant writing seem overwhelming and intimidating, remember that grant writing is a *learned skill* and one that draws on your existing abilities and talents. Taking the long view of grant proposal writing involves realizing these skills can be used again and again. Acquaintance with today's rapidly changing professional demands and economic conditions emphasizes the urgency for prospective strategies and skills for successful grant writing. This chapter addresses a few of the important demands and constraints that make strategic grantsmanship essential.

Increasingly, many faculty or project coordinators in healthcare settings find job security depends on the art of grant writing. Therefore, grant writing is not a skill for the select few who seek this as their life's work; it is an essential form of communication for healthcare professionals across a diverse spectrum of positions. It is to be taken seriously as something you can add to your already-developed set of communication skills. Acquiring solid grant-writing knowledge means learning some new language, conventions, processes, and skills that will enable you to be successful in an increasingly competitive funding market.

NATIONAL TRENDS DRIVE NEED AND BOOST COMPETITION FOR FUNDING

Competition for grant funds has increased appreciably in response to several national trends that go beyond the expected rise and fall of economic conditions. Below are a few trends that directly drive the need for grant funding but, at the same time, tend to make competition for funds stiffer.

1

The NIH Roadmap

A major funding initiative began in 2002 when the director of the National Institutes of Health (NIH) convened leaders in academia, industry, government, and the public to chart a plan for medical research in the 21st century. The initiative came from growing recognition that individual disciplines and single NIH institutes could not tackle major opportunities and gaps in biomedical research alone. A plan emerged to engage all of the NIH entities in the process of transforming and translating new and developing scientific knowledge more quickly into "tangible benefits" for the health of people (NIH, 2006). This meant moving research findings from bench to bedside more quickly, but it also meant forming new relationships across disciplines, including nursing. The three areas of emphasis included new pathways to discovery, research teams of the future, and re-engineering the clinical research enterprise. *Translational research* became the goal of training efforts, collaborative studies, and coordination activities. Although the goals and outcomes of the plan, termed the *NIH Roadmap*, were easily embraced, its implementation offered new challenges and a need for scientists to interact differently. The NIH recognized the need for broad re-engineering to bring about a new discipline of clinical and translational science. The Clinical and Translational Science Awards (CTSA) Consortium was launched in 2006, and initially 12 academic health centers were funded with competitive CTSA awards. Other institutions competed for planning grants. The influence of the NIH Roadmap and translational research remains evident in the National Institute for Nursing Research agenda and initiatives. Priorities for translational research are addressed in NIH application instructions for research and training grants. Whereas this trend offers new hope for faster translation of science into action and greater interdisciplinary, transdisciplinary, and cross-disciplinary research, it also introduces a variety of new complexities in shared support, subcontracts, budgets, contractual obligations and oversight; all of these are discussed in later chapters.

The Magnet Hospital Movement

As the name suggests, the *magnet hospital* is one that can attract and retain nurses to work in the setting. During the staffing crisis of the early 1980s, the American Academy of Nursing found that hospitals with the best record of staffing were those that met a common set of criteria that exemplified quality care. The magnet hospital movement was developed a decade later in 1994 by the American Nurses Credentialing Center. This initiative recognizes healthcare organizations that provide nursing excellence. To compete for excellent staff and recognition of excellence, nurse administrators are engaging in research efforts to measure nurse-sensitive indicators of quality in their agency. Nurse administrators, in turn, are also encouraging bedside nurses to carry out unit-based research and evidence-based practice (EBP) studies and to apply for seed grants from foundations or practice organizations. The process of validating the effectiveness of current nursing and medical therapies became a concern of clinical staff as well as the academicians in health science centers and nursing organizations.

Quests for Funding to Demonstrate Nurse-Sensitive Quality Care

In 1994, the American Nurses Association (ANA) launched a safety and quality initiative seeking links between nursing care and patient outcomes that led to several competitive requests for proposals, or invitations to submit grants. Early outcomes of the ANA's initiative were publication of the *Nursing Care Report Card for Acute Care* and development of the *National Database of Nursing Quality Indicators*. In 2001 the Midwest Research Institute and the University of Kansas School of Nursing were awarded the management contract for the ANA's National Database for Nursing Quality Indicators (NDNQI). NDNQI funded early pilot studies from 1997 to 2000 to test nurse-sensitive quality indicators and established a system to collect and provide comparative information to healthcare facilities for use in quality improvement activities. In 2001 the NDNQI developed a fee-based process of data submission and comparison reports.

Today, more than 1000 hospitals subscribe to NDNQI's program and contribute data to a growing national database available to qualified researchers to study the relationship between nurse staffing and patient outcomes. This trend has not only engaged hospitals in the process of seeking best practices, but it has generated a movement toward testing new interventions to improve nurse-sensitive quality outcomes. Tied to this trend is the move to EBP.

Evidence-Based Practice Movement

Interest and funding activity increases around development and testing of research-based protocols because of the EBP movement. EBP has stimulated organizations and hospitals to offer seed grants for unit-based studies that test best-practice nursing intervention protocols. The movement to base clinical nursing practice on research findings causes many to confuse EBP with "research utilization" (RU). While they both embrace some of the same philosophic underpinnings, EBP goes beyond the review, critique, and application of scientific research that characterizes RU. Sackett and colleagues (1996) define EBP as "the conscientious, explicit, and judicious use of current best evidence in making decisions about the care of individual patients." The quality-filtering aspect of seeking best evidence requires expertise on the part of clinicians and researchers to find and review relevant literature, weigh its merit to provide best evidence, and finally to consider the patient's preferences and values to guide patient care. The EBP movement has engaged nearly every health profession, and each group struggles with issues of integrating newly emerging discoveries into practice decisions. Preparing nurses to participate fully in the quality-filtering enterprise requires many to receive additional training. Still other nurses rely on evidence-based medicine databases, such as the Cochrane Reviews, or best nursing practice information sheets, such as those provided by the Joanna Briggs Institute. These well-developed databases provide evidence reports that are based on rigorous, comprehensive syntheses and analyses of the scientific literature.

There is a level of excitement about EBP among nurses who found their research course in nursing school difficult or boring. Some view EBP as a way to improve clinical practice without engaging in the rigor or preparation to conduct research. However, all should realize that nursing research is still the basis for providing the scientific basis for the *evidence* in EBP. Finding nursing research on a specific problem or intervention and weighing its merit is only possible if such research evidence exists. Mitchell challenges the profession to improve the culture for nurturing well-prepared research-active practitioners (2006). Although well-planned research investigations are increasing the knowledge base, there remains a significant gap in providing sufficient evidence to meet our present and future needs.

Rapid Move to Electronic Extramural Grant Submission

The electronic age has made an unusual impact on the grant-writing enterprise. The movement to Web-based electronic grant proposal submission requires not only a remarkable increase in computer skills for grant writers and secretarial support; it requires a competent infrastructure in support services and personnel from universities, hospitals, and organizations. While these changes are most evident in the grant application process of the NIH and other federal funding agencies, even small practice and professional organizations are moving to electronic submissions. Electronic submission processes will be discussed more fully in later chapters.

Quests for Extramural Funding for Conference Support

The need for support for large conferences, summits, and think tanks has grown as nursing has increased in absolute numbers and its consciousness of the profession's role and power to exert widespread change. The costs for large meetings of this sort can be beyond a single institution or group's capability, so many turn to extramural funding to pay for meeting sites, speakers, and in some cases, travel for attendees. Foundations, such as the American Nurses Foundation, or agencies, such as the Agency for Healthcare Research and Quality (AHRQ), have funded grants for such meetings. Other agencies fund conferences that disseminate important information. For example, Substance Abuse and Mental Health Services Administration (SAMHSA) Center for Mental Health Services, Center for Substance Abuse Prevention, and Center for Substance Abuse Treatment fund grants to disseminate knowledge about mental health and substance abuse prevention and treatment.

RISING LEVEL OF PREPARATION FOR CLINICAL NURSE LEADERS COMPETING FOR GRANTS

Advance practice nurses and nurse administrators in clinical settings soon realize that grant writing is not just an activity for their colleagues in the ivory tower of nursing research and education. They find grant-writing skills are a necessity as health care moves toward implementing EBP and nurse-sensitive quality evaluation. Managed care contracts emphasize evidence of cost-effective, outcome-based care through standardization of clinical protocols and treatment plans. Care maps have become benchmark processes in the care of specific patient populations. As hospital-based nurses face these rigorous challenges to validate standards of care, they lack the personnel or financial resources to do so. Clinical nurse leaders are realizing the necessity for advanced preparation in writing proposals and designing projects with measurable outcomes. Several nursing organizations have responded to their members' need for skills in grantsmanship and offered workshops on proposal writing. Doctoral programs that prepare nursing administrators have begun to include grant writing as part of their career training. Hospitals have engaged faculty from academic institutions to provide consultation to their nurse leaders as they write grants to support important clinical practice priorities. A growing trend is for hospitals and clinical agencies to employ nurse scientists with research training who can provide assistance in setting up well-designed projects and evaluation plans.

NURSING SHORTAGE HEIGHTENS NEED FOR EDUCATORS AS FUNDS DWINDLE

Several economic trends have affected the need to seek external funding for educational training programs and research. As money becomes scarcer for agencies and institutions, positions and programs are threatened. Training and demonstration grants have traditionally been resources that keep important programs afloat until better times. However, widespread economic deficits have spread these grant funds thin. At the same time, nationwide cuts in general employment tend to increase numbers of applicants to healthcare programs, as laid-off workers return to school seeking second careers. While the applicant pools swell, there has been a trickle-down effect of the need to raise funds to sustain the educational programs and hire faculty to teach. Faculty, in turn, must maintain a program of research and scholarship to be seriously considered for promotion and tenure. Institutions that once may have granted these attributes to good teachers without programs of research have raised the bar. Grant writing is an expectation to fund the research or demonstration project that will yield publications and demonstrate scholarly merit. Funding agencies and granting foundations have dealt with the tremendous increase in grant applications they receive in a fair, but highly competitive, manner. They too have raised the bar by requiring applicants to meet stiffer criteria and engaging experts in the field to review grant proposals.

RAPID PROLIFERATION OF DOCTORAL PROGRAMS REQUIRING PROGRAM AND TRAINING SUPPORT

The need for more nursing faculty at all levels has stimulated the proliferation of doctoral programs. Yet, it is surprising how little instruction is spent on grantsmanship in an educational program to prepare nursing faculty. Even with the advance of nursing science and the growing numbers of nurses involved in research, they tend to receive little training on seeking funding for their work. Yet, in university settings, faculty members soon become aware that successful grantsmanship is a valued step toward promotion, tenure status, and/or continued employment at a particular academic or clinical institution. Faculty are under great pressure to write research grants to develop, revise, or expand their own programs of research and to write program training grants to meet changing student, institutional, or managed care demands that affect educational programs.

CONSTRAINTS IN FEDERAL FUNDING FOR RESEARCH VS. INCREASED DEMANDS FOR FUNDS

No funding agency has felt the economic pinch more than the U.S. federal government. Funds allocated by Congress are lobbied for competitively by each of its institutes, centers, and divisions. The U.S. Public Health Service houses several of the major competitors for federal funds. These include the Administration for Children and Families, Administration on Aging, AHRQ, Agency for Toxic Substances and Disease Registry, Centers for Disease Control and Prevention, Centers for

Medicare and Medicaid Services, Food and Drug Administration, Health Resources and Services Administration, Indian Health Service, NIH, and SAMHSA. The NIH, a major funding agency for nursing research, has seen a decline in federal research spending as national priorities of defense and biodefense take precedent. Despite the rising need for research funds, 2005 saw the smallest percentage funding increase in decades. By 2007, the NIH appropriation was barely keeping up with inflation, leaving the agency with a real-terms deficit of 3% lower than its 2004 level (AAAS, 2007). Reports on these latest appropriations hinted that increases in funding were likely for the Nurse Faculty Loan Program and the Loan Repayment and Scholarship Programs because of the nursing shortage. Nursing research remains a low funding priority despite evidence of outstanding contributions, particularly in the area of women's health and geriatric research. Although this may seem distant from your early efforts in grant writing, all citizens have a voice in encouraging support of federal funding for nursing research. The Friends of the National Institute for Nursing Research is an active effort on the part of nursing to raise funds to lobby Congress to increase funding in this area.

NEED FOR INCREASED COMPETENCIES AND NEW GRANT-WRITING INFRASTRUCTURE

The days of liberal funding are over, and as waning funds boost competition for grant funds, the bar for acceptable quality of grant proposals is raised. No longer can nursing deans and administrators casually expect of their employees, "While you're up, get me a grant!" Instead, thoughtful nurse leaders are recognizing the need to provide support and training to new faculty and key clinical leaders. Some nursing schools are implementing "nurse scholars" programs with light teaching loads for selected faculty who are being trained in grantsmanship by the institution's research dean and designates. Others encourage faculty to seek postdoctoral training and career awards to improve competencies in research and grantsmanship. Finally, the complexity of maintaining a "well-oiled machine" for providing support and consultation to faculty or nursing staff who submit grants has led many institutions to create a grant-writing infrastructure with writing, statistical, and budgetary consultation.

CONCLUSION

Grant writing is an activity that crosses the boundaries from clinical to academe. It requires as much skill as everything else we master in our professional lives. The next chapters will illustrate the steps required to succeed in the grant-writing process.

CHAPTER 2

So You Want to Write a Grant! Where to Begin?

Like any worthwhile endeavor, the process of grant writing is time consuming. At times it may feel all-encompassing, with a life of its own. However, getting a grant funded is also doable, given the right idea and some basic grant-writing skills. Breaking down the project into manageable pieces is often the key to success. This chapter focuses on developing the approach to or "art" of proposing, finding sources by which to generate fundable ideas, and finally, how to know if you are asking the right question. Although many types of grants are available, three of the most common include *research*, *program/training*, and *special projects/demonstration* grants. Examples in this chapter primarily address the research grant, although the majority of grant-writing principles may apply to the other types of grants.

THE FINE ART OF PROPOSING

There is an art to requesting someone to give something of value to you. There should be something inherently desirable that you can offer to the party you are requesting funds from. A proposal is a formal kind of request, whether it is for someone's hand in marriage or for funds for a research or training grant. If the marriage comparison seems a little absurd to you, remember that both situations involve requests to convince a person or persons to form a relationship and both require commitments and outcomes in return for the exchange. Acknowledging these similarities can help you to recognize the need to make abundantly clear the following points in your proposal:

- Is the relationship relevant?
- Is the partner capable?
- Is the partner reliable?
- Can the partner be trusted with money?
- Does the partner present a neat, attractive, or positive image?
- Does the partner pay attention to schedules and time agreements?

Specifically, each element of a successful proposal must convincingly present and justify your desirability as a partner to your funding agency. Grant reviewers will be looking at different aspects of your grant proposal to determine how well your plan, your training and experience, and your overall presentation reflect these points. A successful research proposal will accomplish the following four objectives:

1. Ask a meaningful question that is relevant to the funding agency.
2. Employ good science to answer the question.
3. Pay careful attention to the application.
4. Demonstrate that the applicant is qualified to carry out the project.

Table 2-1 explains how the elements of a successful proposal relate to the types of information that must be included.

Table 2-1   Elements of a Successful Proposal

The Meaningful Question	
Articulates the following:	Supported by these characteristics
• What will we learn from your research? • Why is it important to have the answer? • Is there a reasonable expectation that we will get the answer? • Why is the answer important to the funding agency?	• Clear sense of long-term scientific objectives. • Rationale for need clearly linked to current state of the science. • Evidence of thorough understanding of current research and literature. • Relevance to the funding agency's priorities and congruence with its philosophies.
Good Science	
Articulates the following:	Supported by these characteristics
• Thorough planning • Rationale for selected methods • Adequate description of methods	• Conceptual and methodological links between each section are clear. • Every approach, method, instrument, and analytic step is clearly justified. • Complex or new procedures, protocols, devices, and instruments are clarified with description, citations, and schematics.

• Clearly stated assumptions and limitations • Identified problems and anticipated solutions • Power calculations	• Assumptions, potential biases, and study limitations are clearly articulated. • Potential problems and factors affecting recruitment, retention, and protocol are acknowledged with possible solutions. • Sample size is based on statistically sound power calculations with postulated effect size estimated from relevant pilot data or previous research (Birkett & Day, 1994).

Careful Attention to the Application

Articulates the following:	Supported by these characteristics
• Compliance with instructions • Clear, lucid writing style • Neat appearance • Grammatically and typographically correct • Proper type size • Appropriate use of appendices	• Proposal submitted with proper format, supporting documents, and on time. • Proposal is written in clear, active voice, jargon-free style, no run-on sentences. • Orderly and consistent organization of text, graphics, and tables. • Careful proofreading, grammar and spell-checking of proposal and references. • Careful attention to font type and size. • Compliance with number and indexing of appendices in proposal.

Qualified Applicant

Articulates the following:	Supported by these characteristics
• Showing your familiarity with the topic • Showing understanding of the methods • Demonstrating ability to carry out the planned study	• Prior research and publications reflect interest in and familiarity with topic. • Methods are justified in detail to explain testing for outcomes. • Biosketch, pilot, and preliminary work reflect knowledge of research skill, previous funding, and research partners.

Source: Primary elements adapted from a presentation by Dr. June Lunney, NINR/NIH at Southern Nursing Research Society Annual Conference, 11th Annual Research Conference, February 1997, Norfolk, VA.

THE MEANINGFUL QUESTION

A meaningful question has relevance to something of importance to the funding agency. Few funding sources will be anxious to provide support to fill a gap in knowledge just because it is empty. In fact, many organizations or agencies offering grants have specific initiatives or priorities that must be addressed in your proposal's purpose and aims. Therefore, you should *clearly conceptualize* the question or knowledge gap you are proposing to address by your project. Articulate the outcomes of your project in the form of *clearly stated aims*. Write your study aims in specific, measurable terms (that is why they are called *specific aims*) and avoid using the "shotgun" approach of using generalities.

Grant reviewers look for a "flow" in proposals—not just a grammatical flow, but also one between your work as a scientist and how the proposed study fits with your future plans. Reviewers will find helpful a statement clarifying links between your proposed project and your past and future program of research and scholarship. Likewise, a logical flow between your proposed project and the funding organization's priorities helps to establish relevance of the project. Tables or outlines can also help demonstrate links between the project's broad goals, the narrower purpose or purposes, and the specific aims and related questions or hypotheses. As you develop the proposal, your description of the sampling frame, methods chosen, and plan for analysis or evaluation must follow a logical progression to measure how well the aims are achieved. For quantitative research proposals, the proposal usually includes plans to demonstrate achievement of specific aims through tests of hypotheses, analyses of costs and benefits, and clear descriptions of previously unknown phenomena. Qualitative research studies have expected outcomes also, but the nature of the inquiry, methodology, and data collection produces outcomes that are inductively analyzed for meaning, categorizations, and description. A qualitative research proposal can stay true to its inductive roots but have a higher likelihood of meeting funding priorities if you can (1) justify how the information you will gain can achieve the specific aims, and (2) state how it will help to meet the broad goals of the study.

EMPLOYING GOOD SCIENCE

We have established that writing a proposal that is scientifically sound requires sufficient knowledge about a topic to ask meaningful questions. But it is just as important to write a convincing proposal that shows that you are likely to get meaningful answers to these questions. This process involves the science of research. First of all, your research design deserves thought and consultation from an expert. Getting outside help to confirm or suggest alternatives to your design is time and possible expense that may save you considerable rearranging and distress later. The design should be selected and justified to show a reviewer that the approach you have selected is the best possible approach to answer the specific question and achieve the specific aim. Finding support for a particular approach in the literature is often excellent rationale to be included (and cited) in the proposal. You will need to follow the process of justifying each different question and aim, which may or may not, have a similar rationale or approach.

Justify Measurement Instruments and Devices

Describing the choice of instruments or measurement devices may also require some help from experts or colleagues who have access to or familiarity with your selected method. For instruments with psychometric properties, getting reliability and validity estimates on similar types of research participants may be possible from the literature or directly from the author or developer. If you plan to use the instrument to measure variables in a study with a different type, age, or situational group, your proposal will be strengthened by testing it on a sample from your proposed group. Particular attention should be given to estimating the feasibility, validity, and reliability of instruments when using them with persons who do not have English as their first language and in persons with temporary or progressive cognitive impairment. Many psychosocial instruments were normed from tests done with college-age students, so you should seek documentation or demonstrate that the instrument is relevant to the age or developmental capabilities of your study subjects.

Justify Biological Measures

Measurement devices, medical instruments, biological assays, and tissue samples are being incorporated more often in nursing care studies. Although they may be mystifying and appear to have a scientific objectivity to the lay public, funding agencies usually engage reviewers with the background to know or easily find out the sensitivity, precision, accuracy, reliability, and appropriateness of such measures. Therefore, it is a measure of "good science" to articulate and justify the ability and the limits of the biological test you intend to use. In some cases, you may need to justify the use of a new assay that replaces a previously unreliable one. Consider including a brief "mini-tutorial" in your justification to help you pose and resolve an objection before the reviewer does.

Figure 2-1   Using a Diagram to Explain a Complex Design

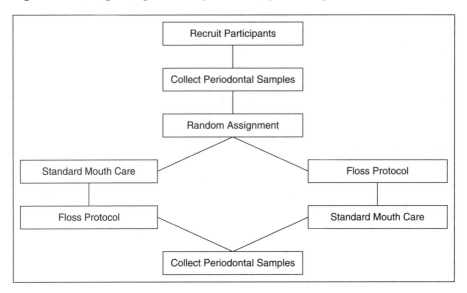

Justify Steps for Data Collection

Procedures and protocols can get complicated, particularly if you are using one design to test one specific aim and a different design to test another aim. Using a diagram is helpful to reviewers to show the variations in a complex protocol. Figure 2-1 is an example of a diagram depicting a comparison of persons infected with human immunodeficiency virus (HIV) to determine if an established flossing protocol done before or after mouth care was associated with less residual debris in periodontal pockets.

Justify Statistical Approaches

Determining the appropriate statistics to use is always a concern in proposal development. Here is another place where expert consultation is not only desirable but often essential. If you have clearly mapped out your design, identified your measurement variables, and know the nature of the data your instruments or measures will yield, the chore for you and your statistical consultant will be much easier. You will save considerable time with your consultant if you will get specific with *what*, *when*, and to *what degree of precision* you wish to measure each variable. Simply generalizing that you want to use blood pressure to measure stress or use hemoglobin

A1c (HbA1c) to measure glucose control during pregnancy is a plan that is neither precise nor manageable enough to plan a statistical approach. Blood pressure measurements raise the questions, which ones (diastolic or systolic; standing or sitting; time of measurement)? Also, at what points during pregnancy will these variables be measured? HbA1c use raises similar questions about which measurements will be used and whether you want to know exact levels, whether the levels will be meaningful without serial measures, or simply whether the patient was normoglycemic. If the latter is the case, you could possibly convert the numerical interval-level values of the variable HbA1c to ordinal-level variables of hypoglycemic, normoglycemic, or hyperglycemic. The choice depends on the question, the design, and the availability of relational data. However, making a global statement such as "appropriate statistical tests" or "univariate and multivariate approaches" to explain data analyses leaves reviewers guessing if you actually understand what answers are possible from your planned analytic procedures.

Justify Sample Size

Seek consultation if you are unclear about how to justify your sample size. This is true of both qualitative and quantitative studies. Each approach has different guidelines underlying the choice. To show your familiarity with "good science," include the rationale for your choice.

Qualitative Sample Justification

There is an erroneous misconception among those less familiar with qualitative methods that sample size justification in qualitative studies is not important. According to Sandelowski, the sufficiency of a sample size for qualitative research has more to do with its adequacy to perform the study's goal (1995). In general, the quality rather than the quantity has been used in the past to justify and sometimes dodge the issue of sample size. Sandelowski's article points out that having too small or too large a sample can undermine a study. Knowledgeable grant reviewers understand this concept and expect you to justify a qualitative sample size. Although a relatively small sample of 10 might be adequate for homogeneous or critical case sampling, it would be too small to provide the variation needed to gather characteristics of a complex phenomenon. It would also be too small to develop theory. On the other hand, more is not always better, depending again on the study purpose. An extremely large sample is neither feasible nor desirable for conducting certain types of narrative analysis. Therefore, it is important to discuss and document the rationale for your choice.

Quantitative Sample Justification

The issues involved in justifying adequacy of a sample size in quantitative research are aimed at (1) gaining a representative sample, and (2) avoiding error. In general, a sample will be more representative of a population if it contains more members. This makes sense because the smaller the sample, the greater the likelihood that you have missed members with various characteristics. The closer you get in size to the entire population, the less likelihood of missing members. However, it is usually not economically feasible or even necessary to include an entire population in a study. On the other hand, if the sample is too small, you may fail to detect a significant relationship (type II error). In justifying the sample size for a grant proposal, reviewers will want to know the factors you have considered in arriving at that number. The gold standard for estimating the ability of a statistical test to detect a difference, if one exists, is a *power analysis*. Cohen (1988) developed the most frequently used method that uses three parameters to calculate the power estimate. These include the *level of significance*, the *desired power*, and the *expected effect size*. The formula is not difficult, and the fact that power analyses can be readily done with certain computer programs has led many to simply choose arbitrary estimates of effect size, plug in the numbers, and "crunch" out a seemingly acceptable number for a power estimate. This is where a statistical consultant comes in handy to help you with the fine-tuning of the process. While the first two parameters can be set by the investigator to avoid chances for error, the third parameter, the expected effect size, is determined by the "degree to which the phenomenon exists," as best you can determine (Cohen, 1988, p. 4). This is not just a wild guess or a desired level, but rather an estimate based on preliminary data, pilot work, or existing studies found in the literature. According to Cohen, the degree of effect can be measured in a variety of ways that include "mean differences (raw or standardized), correlations and squared correlation of all kinds, odds ratios, kappas—whatever conveys the magnitude of the phenomenon of interest appropriate to the research context" (Cohen, 1990, p. 1310). Failing to estimate an accurate effect size might lead to incorrect conclusions about a study hypothesis because you might have a variable with such a small effect that a larger sample would be required to detect it. To make it clear to grant reviewers how you arrived at the effect size, indicate its source. Effect size is often misunderstood and one of the most often ignored aspects of sample selection, yet its role in establishing your sample size is critical. Grant reviewers also want to know that you have considered *each proposed statistical test* in arriving in estimating the power. Different tables exist for estimating power, depending on the particular analysis, the numbers of groups, and whether or not it is a directional or nondirectional hypothesis (the latter takes more subjects). The sample size required to obtain the desired power will be different.

CAREFUL ATTENTION TO THE APPLICATION

The instructions for applying for a grant vary across funding agencies and organizations to the extent that nothing should be taken for granted. A useful exercise is to gather the application instructions from a printed or computer-generated source and begin marking it up with a colored highlighter marker. Highlight important facts that you will need to comply with to get your grant submitted in a timely, appropriately packaged form. For easy reference, it helps if you look for and highlight information related to the following:

- Submission deadline, review, and award dates (include whether submission date is the postmark date or the date of receipt by the agency).
- Name and address (or in some cases the e-mail address) to which the proposal is to be sent.
- If paper copies are required, the number and type of collation or binding required.
- Page and space limitations per section as well as for the total grant proposal.
- Type font size, margins, pagination, and reference style requirements.
- Acceptability and limits on tables, figures, and appendices.
- Budget page forms, budgetary limits, indirect cost limits, and modular requirements.
- Acceptable categories or positions for key personnel, consultants, and services.
- Limitations on salary for key personnel, consultants, and research assistants.
- Limitations on travel, lodging, and support services.
- Allowable expenses for equipment and supplies.
- Requirements for biographical sketches, consultant information, and clinical agency clearances. For research training grants, required clearances from supervisors or sponsors.
- Requirements for institutional review board clearance prior to or after funding.

The above list will vary depending on if you are applying for a small seed grant versus an extramural federal grant. However, the principles of carefully reviewing each and every requirement are essential in either case. Too often grants are submitted in improper format, without proper documentation, or too late because the researcher failed to read the instructions closely. Nothing turns off a grant reviewer more than a sloppily organized grant proposal, full of grammatical and spelling errors, and with improperly cited references. Presenting a neat and attractive image is one of the least difficult ways to propose that you know how to organize your work. Writing in a clear, logically arranged sequence will make reviewing your proposal a pleasure. Making your figures, tables, and information easy to locate will gain you favor as well.

A tip about space allocations (beyond the simple fact that using extraneous words quickly uses up your allowed space) is to reduce the need to write lengthy paragraphs by using "bullets," lists, tables, or figures. Avoid the temptation to put important details in the appendix, hoping the reviewers will seek it there. If it is important, state it briefly in the text of the proposal. In National Institutes of Health (NIH) reviews, the appendices are given only to the 3–4 main reviewers and not the entire review committee.

A second tip that will save you considerable space, if the application allows it, is to use the numbered reference format for citing references instead of the author/year format. It is easy to see how a string of eight cited references might take an entire line of text, while a numbered reference format would simply list the range of numbers (e.g., 1–8). Using superscripts (as in the style of the *Journal of the American Medical Association*) saves space because the numbers are small and compact, which makes this style a favorite among NIH submissions. Be sure to check if there are no stipulations for using American Psychological Association (APA) format or other styles mentioned in your grant application guidelines.

SHOWING YOU'RE A QUALIFIED APPLICANT

Your qualifications for carrying out a grant can be found in several places in your proposal. These include your (1) biographical sketch of education, experience, research, and publications; (2) preliminary studies section that explains your prior work relevant to the proposed grant; (3) letters of support and agreements; and (4) your selection of collaborators. Holtzclaw in her "Six P's of Funding Qualifications" presents some general principles of demonstrating these qualifications to help you build this capacity (2007). The list includes the following:

1. Program of research
2. Publications
3. Pilot or preliminary work
4. Previous funding support
5. Partners
6. Passion

Program of Research

A *program of research* shows that your proposed research "fits" with your previous history of scholarship (dissertation and/or thesis, pilot work, projects, courses, publications, and future goals). Your future goals may be the most important item if you are a new graduate or if you are changing your area of interest. Not everyone who gets research funding fulfills each qualification, but the list is helpful in preparing for and writing the sections of your proposal that reveal your qualifications. This characteristic of your background assures grant reviewers that you not only have familiarity with the proposed topic and methods but that you intend on developing this further in the future. Developing a program of research lets you build on each succeeding step rather than going in many directions.

Publications

Publications are your retrievable milestones of research productivity and scholarship. They are included in your grant biographical sketch to give reviewers a quick indication of the types, topics, and numbers of publications you have produced. Scanning the dates of publication also reveals something about the consistency and continuity of your scholarly activity. Scanning the topics reveals how focused you have been.

Pilot or Preliminary Work

Pilot or preliminary work is included as a section in many grant application forms. This refers to *your* work and not to work found in the literature. Ideally, preliminary work includes findings that led you to the present study. This is a place where a program of research is highly beneficial in reflecting careful exploration of a topic, from small pilot work to more preliminary studies leading to the present proposal. If the proposed study is a pilot study and you have no preliminary work, include an explanatory statement ("there is no preliminary or pilot work" or "the proposed study is the initial pilot for a future study of . . . "). Applicants sometimes include previous work on someone else's research study if they have gained expertise or experience with the methods or population related to the proposed study. The idea is to show how your previous research relates to the grant proposal.

Previous Funding Support

Previous funding support shows reviewers that you have successfully traveled this road before. You were entrusted with prior funding because you showed capability. It implies that you were able to manage these funds. The frosting on the cake is when you have a publication to show for each of your prior grants. Previous grants with no published findings raise a red flag of suspicion that funding has yielded no results. So a word of caution is in order to publish your results or at very least lessons learned.

Partners

Partners, meaning a research team and collaborators in research, are hallmarks of research capacity. Granted, research for your thesis or dissertation was probably a solitary activity. Beyond that, however, the ability to demonstrate that you have an established team of colleagues that offer expertise and commitment and collaborate on publications and previous research is a major strength in research qualifications. Partners also include community or agency partners granting you entrée to their facility, excellent consultation, and advisory committees to projects.

Passion

Passion for your topic and program of research is reflected in prior scholarship. Your work roles, community and professional contributions, prior research, and publications reflect your choices of topics and commitment. If they are consistent with the present proposal, it tells reviewers that the present topic is not a passing interest. Although you will not likely find *passion* on a grant reviewer's checklist, you will find statements evaluating your commitment to a particular research goal or topic.

ESTABLISHING THE NEED FOR YOUR PROPOSAL

Identifying the Need

Need is usually in the eye of the beholder, yet a successful grant application attempts to convince the funding agency that the statement of need expressed in the proposal is congruent with the funding agency's goals or missions. If there is not a good fit between your grant and the funding institution, it is unlikely you will get funded through that particular group. Perhaps your need for grant funding may be as simple as the need to evaluate and justify outcomes in a competitive managed healthcare environment. More commonly, however, grants are written for the purpose of funding one's own program of research and gaining release time from clinical or classroom teaching responsibilities for scholarly activities. Academicians often seek training grants to expand or significantly revise the curriculum within a college or university while keeping costs down by hiring program faculty specifically on the grant monies. This strategy allows the school to demonstrate the self-sufficiency and success of the program during the first three years (program grants are usually three to five years in length) before assuming the total costs involved in a new program. A special projects or demonstration grant is sometimes used to facilitate the development of an educational or clinical program where no similar programs exist in a particular geographic area. Funds must often be obtained to demonstrate the efficacy of the program before the community will embrace the idea. For example, this strategy was used for the first school-based, nurse-run health clinics. Each of these situations reflects applicant-specific needs with aims that must be articulated in outcome-oriented language consistent with the funding organization's perception of need. Research needs must go beyond your own personal need to achieve tenure, complete a dissertation, or get published. The need your funding agency is interested in is why the *research*, not the funding, is necessary. The need should emerge clearly in the problem statement and the proposed study outcomes that address the need.

Recognizing Your Investment in the Process

The need for writing a grant may be a professional choice on your part, or it may be dictated by the employing institution. In either circumstance, writing a grant can often be very stressful for the individual involved. Having the self-determination and personal energy reserves necessary to survive the grueling parts of the grant-writing process depends in large part on the commitment one has to the grant, the passion felt for the answer to the question, and the resources to assist in the process. One cannot and should not downplay the many sacrifices that are necessary to get a grant ready for a timely submission to an external funding agency. The sheer pressure of tight timelines and competing responsibilities of grant writing has turned many "angelic" Dr. Jekyll colleagues into grant-writing "terrors" resembling Mr. Hyde. It is unpleasant to discover these hidden personalities when individuals turn unpleasant in the midst of the grant-writing process. On the flip side are colleagues who thrive on the academic challenge of taking an idea and turning it into a fundable project. These are the colleagues that help to form excellent collaborative teams that you will treasure and find helpful in the future. Those finding themselves in the survival mode during the grant-writing process are less likely to be successful in their efforts and certainly will make themselves, and perhaps others, miserable in the process. When not given a choice about writing the grant, the process becomes arduous and the person slips into survival mode. By contrast, the person approaching grant writing in the "thrival" mode views the future possibilities and opportunities provided by the experience; the potentially burdensome task of writing becomes an exciting intellectual adventure. The grant is the opportunity to answer that nagging clinical question or to develop a program or clinical project to meet an aggregate need. Not only is that personally exciting, but you are contributing to the body of scientific and theoretical knowledge.

This excitement overcomes the dread of the journey and creates the energy and focus needed to sustain the process of grant writing. The choice to survive or thrive in writing a grant is a personal one. Although jobs often depend on the task of grant writing, the individual has the option to view it as an arduous task or to be challenged about the opportunities and possibilities that the future holds for the successful grant writer.

Formulating a Fundable Idea

Developing a fundable idea takes ingenuity on the part of the grant writer as well as skill in turning the idea into a meaningful question. Ideas may come from a number of sources, both clinically and professionally. Some of the best ideas often arise from clinical practice. This clinical base has been a rich resource of fundable research ideas. When Marlene Walden entered neonatal nursing in the late 1970s, healthcare professionals in the neonatal intensive care unit (NICU) did not believe that preterm infants had the autonomic or functional capacity to perceive pain because of their immature central nervous systems. Walden's clinical observations told her otherwise. After seeing the hurt and hearing the cries of infants during painful procedures, she questioned the current thinking about neonatal pain. This early professional observation was the source for her program of research and grant-writing efforts. She could not, however, just go out and study neonatal pain. She needed equipment and personal resources. Writing a grant fit into her research plans.

Regardless of which clinical area one practices, evaluating the research base of that practice is a source of many fundable ideas. Gaps in the literature or conflicting results from previous studies provide another source of ideas for research and meaningful questions for a grant proposal. Questions that the literature leaves unresolved are great avenues for future research and, depending on the research priorities of the various funding agencies, are also great venues for external funding.

Professional conferences are other excellent sources for generating research ideas. One usually becomes energized at a conference and believes the world is conquerable. The power of networking with researchers in the field and talking with other healthcare professionals from around the country cannot be underestimated. Many researchers are anxious to replicate their studies in another setting or for their instruments to be retested. Both of these strategies add to their own database and research credibility. This replication provides novices a chance to use already developed and tested methods and data collection instruments. Use of nationally known experts on grants as project team members or consultants increases the credibility of the grant application. Staying in touch with experts and engaging in conference networking allows one to become knowledgeable about what others are doing in a particular field, avoid duplicating current work, and avoid replicating errors. It allows the researcher to focus on a grant angle that has the potential for generating new knowledge or adding depth to existing knowledge. Furthermore, networking may also help to form collaborative relationships between individuals with similar interests. These interactions may help to strengthen an idea or may lead to ideas not previously considered.

Identifying mentors in your topic area, whether for a research, training, or special projects grants, has many advantages. Involving mentors not only allows the grant writer to utilize his or her expertise to develop the grant proposal, but it may also set the stage for future collaborations. If these individuals are considered the experts in the field, they are likely to be scientists of the caliber the funding agency will use to review your proposal. Learning from the "master" as you shape your own ideas and educational or research program will be invaluable as will the relationship you establish.

Although strong attention to literature and colleagues within your own area of interest may lead to a plausible grant idea, pushing the interdisciplinary envelope by exploring other related fields may produce novel ideas. For example, Medoff-Cooper and colleagues (2000) wished to study neurobehavioral development in preterm infants by observing their suck, swallow, and breathe coordination. Her collaboration with a biomedical engineer who developed a sucking device that would measure sucking pressure, amount of fluid delivered, and the suck-swallow-breathe patterns (Kron & Litt, 1971) led to a Small Business Innovative Research grant. The device was useful in several other studies that followed and to other researchers needing to measure these variables (Medoff-Cooper, McGrath, & Bilker, 2000).

Keeping abreast of advances in other fields can often gives new insights into research questions. A still unanswered question about pain in neonates will likely be answered by molecular neurobiology. Parents of children who were former preterm infants, often report high pain thresholds in their infants; for example, "My child does not exhibit the same level of pain as other children do when they fall down or touch a hot stove." These anecdotal reports by parents were substantiated in at least one study where the researchers report decreased pain sensitivity among former preterm infants who were now at a corrected age of 18 months (Grunau et al., 1994). Such observations, coupled with preliminary research findings, may stimulate the grant writer to draw on new and emerging concepts within the field of molecular neurobiology. These complex findings could possibly offer plausible rationale for generating hypotheses for why these children have higher pain thresholds than healthy infants born at term. Subsequent studies could then explore and compare outcomes of effective interventions to minimize the long-term effects of chronic, repeated pain in critically ill preterm infants. Along the same lines, journal clubs may be a source of ideas for future research questions. These meetings often point to differences in care practices between healthcare providers from different institutions. They may also lead to the realization that the current research base is insufficient to support a current therapeutic regimen and thus support the need for further research in this area.

Making Room for Writing

Whatever the strategy you find helpful in generating ideas, it will be important at some point in this process to set aside time to think about all the information that you have gathered. One of the hindrances to the success of grant writers is busy schedules and other demands. In today's work setting, everyone is asked to work harder, often with fewer resources. Many times, by the end of the workday, you may feel exhausted. Yet the work does not end there. Working at this level consistently promotes professional burnout and stifles creativity in your grant writing. Successful grant writers and researchers often emphasize the need to selfishly protect sufficient time for scholarship. This dedicated time must fit your own work schedule and your knowledge of how you best function. One day a week or even a few hours each day are two variations of dedicated writing time. The schedule is up to you. You determine whatever works for you. But whatever it is—do it!

Tips for Dedicated Time

Try the following tricks of the trade:

- If you find yourself spending too much time figuring out where you left off when the writing is done in shorter work sessions, you might increase your productivity by scheduling longer sessions.
- If you find yourself spending too much time before writing sessions finding materials, reference books, prior drafts, or computer supplies, try creating a "portable office" by keeping these materials together in a briefcase, box, or suitcase.
- You need to determine what kind of environment increases your personal productivity. For some, it is a quiet environment free from distractions; for others, it might be the library.

Asking the Right Question

Determining whether your question is the "right question" involves considerable thought. Ideally, the right question is one that is congruent with your own research interests. Your passion for the topic will help you persevere in your pursuit through the long, tedious grant-writing process.

Your passion alone is not enough to gain research funding. It must also be of critical interest to others. The competitive nature of external funding requires that your area of interest be broad enough to appeal to a sufficient target population to warrant a grant award. This does not mean you need to give up your original passion for a topic, but rather that you tailor your proposal to fit one of the funding priorities or initiatives available. Funding agencies often set broad research funding priorities, with many using *Healthy People 2010* objectives. (See Appendix C for a list of *Healthy People 2010* objectives.) Some funding priorities are more narrow, such as those dealing with a certain disease or symptom. You need to examine each of the potential funding agencies, determine their funding priorities, determine their individual rules for obtaining funds (such as using your professional association membership to access members-only funds or having certain credentials), and choose the best match for your particular area of interest.

While you consider targeting a specific priority or a broad focus, give your idea a unique slant. In fact, finding a novel or innovative angle to studying a problem is one of the areas that improve a grant reviewer's score. Many times the specific slant of your question will need to be tailored more directly to the funding priorities identified. For example, the National Institute of Nursing Research (NINR) has an ongoing call out for proposals for health promotion among racial and ethnic minority males. The NINR goal of funding grants that develop and test culturally and linguistically appropriate health-promoting interventions designed to reduce health disparities among racially and ethnically diverse males is broad enough to accommodate a variety of specific questions and research approaches from individual and group studies to health services research. Likewise, the initiative is broad enough to cover health behavioral studies as well as biologically based research.

CONCLUSION

Writing a great proposal starts with a great idea. Before starting to write any grant proposal, systematically review the literature, talk with experts in the field, and obtain consultations as necessary. Identify a question that is relevant, one that has the potential to generate new knowledge, solve a clinical management problem, or produce a new type of educational program. In addition, be sure your question is broad enough to be of interest to a significant portion of the funding source's population. By taking the time to do your homework and finding a match between your area of research and current funding options, you will substantially increase your success at obtaining grant monies.

CHAPTER 3

What Type of Grant Do You Want?

IS YOUR IDEA A MATCH?

There are many types of grants available to healthcare professionals, but finding a match between your idea and the granting agency is an absolute necessity for funding success. Well-written proposals and superb ideas won't likely be funded if an agency is not interested in the project. For this reason, you should always acquaint yourself with your funding source's goal and mission. If the match is possible, but not overtly obvious, then establishing the connection between your idea and the funding agency's goals becomes a priority in your grant proposal. If you're still unable to see a fit, move on! There are many more sources of funds.

HOW MUCH FUNDING DO YOU NEED?

Where you seek funding may be, in part, dictated by the amount of financial support your project needs. If you need "seed" money to support pilot work, a small conference, or a short-term survey, you may find a small grant sufficient. Foundations, practice and research organizations, universities, hospitals, institutions, and agencies are potential sources of small grants. Small grants are defined differently by different organizations, but they are typically under $50,000 and include no salary support. Very small seed grants may be as small as $100. Although the National Institutes of Health (NIH) sponsors a Small Grant Program (R03) that offers $50,000 per year for up to two years and includes salary support, this is not typical of small grants in general. NIH Small Grants are discussed under the section on federal funding.

Major or "large" grants, like smaller grants, are designated as such by those that award them. One typical feature that sets large grants apart is the support of salary, support personnel, major equipment, and institutional indirect costs. As in any grant submission choice, the decision to apply for a major grant should rest with your need and readiness to carry out a major project. Readiness for major funding, even for "new investigator" awards, generally involves some preliminary pilot work and evidence or capability.

Some sources of grant funding are limited by geographic region, membership in a professional organization, place of employment, or career level. Primarily these grants fall into six categories: foundation grants, hospital-based or institutional grants, professional association grants, corporate partnerships, pre- and postdoctoral research training fellowships, and federal grants.

FOUNDATION GRANTS

Foundation grants are nongovernmental awards that support the mission and goals of specific philanthropic societies, corporate or organizational foundations, or charitable groups. They may or may not have a specific funding cycle. Some foundations review grants when they are submitted. Others have timelines and guidelines for application. Certain health maintenance organizations and managed care groups now have foundations that support community projects in order to increase visibility of their organization. Professional association foundations, created to support their members, or company-sponsored foundations that support charitable causes, are separate corporate entities from the parent organization. A professional association may require membership as a criterion for grant eligibility. Foundation grants may have a definite application deadline or a rolling deadline, which means they review grants whenever one is received. Foundations sometime require a letter of intent (see Appendix D for a sample). This letter of intent describes in just a very few pages what the focus of the project will be. It allows the foundation reviewers to determine if in fact the project is within the scope of the foundation's mission. Then if the project is acceptable to the mission, the grant seeker will be asked to submit a full proposal according to specified guidelines. This "pre-proposal" offers an opportunity for the foundation to examine the match between your idea and their goals as well as gauging their interest in learning more about it. For the applicant, it saves the lengthy process of writing the full foundation proposal and waiting for the peer review. The foundation grant process is usually less intimidating and often provides a quicker turnaround time for an answer to whether or not the project is fundable. A word of caution—the very brevity of a foundation grant can be a challenge. The human tendency is to give a lot of information instead of a concise presentation. Therefore, in many respects short grants for a small award can require as much thought and more careful editing than a lengthier grant for major funding.

Foundation grants are a nice way to start your attempts at funding. For most foundations, the submission process is fairly straightforward and brief compared to federal grants. They tend to provide small sums of money for very specific focus areas. These funds are excellent sources of seed money to start projects. For example, Carole Kenner saw a request for proposals from the Purdue Friedrick Foundation in a foundation's newsletter. Their areas of interest were perinatal health care. She submitted a brief proposal for a qualitative research study "Transition from Hospital to

Home for Mothers and Babies." The grant was awarded within three months of submission and was used to fund her dissertation. This seed money then gave her a good start to seek more funding for her next project that again focused on research on transitions. Barbara Holtzclaw needed a small grant to pilot her intervention study "Control of Shaking Chills During Amphotericin B Therapy: A Pilot," during her postdoctoral work at the University of Pennsylvania. She submitted a proposal for an institutionally managed grant and was funded by the Mabel Pew Myrin Trust. This small award of $2,000 helped Holtzclaw to gain the preliminary evidence needed to launch a program of research and two major federally funded grant awards. The ability to successfully write a foundation grant gave us confidence that we could go on for other foundation monies as well as federal grants.

A larger grant was awarded to Professor Kenner by the March of Dimes Birth Defects Foundation of Greater Cincinnati. She sought funds for a professional educational component of her Centers for Disease Control and Prevention (CDC)-funded Perinatal Alcohol Users grant. Foundation funds were to support an educational intervention aimed at increasing the awareness of health professionals about the harmful effect of perinatal alcohol use at any stage of the pregnancy. As a clinician, she and other members of her research team felt they were seeing more women delivering alcohol-exposed babies than the report rates reflected in their prenatal clinics. The aim of the research to include health professional education about potential harmful birth defects from perinatal alcohol exposure fit with the March of Dimes Birth Defects Foundation's goals. The first step in the application process was a letter of intent to ensure there was a match between the project's specific aims and the foundation's mission. The March of Dime's Birth Defects Foundation's request for proposal (RFP) was sent about two weeks following submission of their letter of intent. (See Appendix D.) She then submitted a full proposal. A positive funding decision arrived about eight weeks after the proposal submission.

Professor Kenner found other foundations helpful as her career developed. The University of Cincinnati Colleges of Medicine and Nursing sent a joint proposal to the Gates Foundation requesting support for education of faculty in Honduras in medicine and nursing. The proposed project was directed at providing faculty exchanges and eventually student exchanges. This was consistent with the Gates Foundation's search for projects designed to increase the general educational level, not just that of health professionals, in developing countries. The application was very brief and required a concise synthesis of the project. Trimming the ideas down to a meaningful short version was more challenging than writing a longer proposal, although the process itself seemed less awesome.

The following are examples of foundations that provide grant opportunities:

- W.K. Kellogg Foundation
- Robert Wood Johnson Foundation
- John A. Hartford Foundation

- Choice Care Foundation of Cincinnati, Ohio
- Pew Charitable Trusts Foundation
- March of Dimes Birth Defects Foundation
- Rockefeller Foundation
- Gates Foundation

These foundations change their focus or shift their priorities from time to time so it is always best to consult their Web sites for current funding initiatives. Foundations that are associated with professional associations are discussed below.

A comprehensive resource on foundations, *The Foundation Center*, is accessible on the World Wide Web at http://foundationcenter.org. The Foundation Center was established in 1956 and supports more than 600 foundations. It is a leading authority on philanthropy with a mission to strengthen the nonprofit sector by advancing knowledge about U.S. philanthropy. The center maintains a comprehensive database on U.S. grant makers, provides several free search options, and makes its *Foundation Directory Online* available for a subscription fee.

HOSPITAL-BASED OR INSTITUTIONAL GRANTS

Hospitals, universities, school systems, and other institutions often offer grants that are generally offered only to employees of their organizations. The institution may request proposals for certain projects that it wishes to see started. In the past, hospital or university grants were most likely to go to physicians or established scientists, simply because other health professionals did not know they existed. These grants support small budgets, and they act as seed money for preliminary work or phases of an existing project. A wealthy donor may tie the funds to a specific type of research related to an institutional endowment. Other funds may be administered through a hospital foundation with the express purpose of furthering any research that addresses a specific disease or enhances the health care of individuals served by the hospital.

A particularly positive aspect of partnering with a hospital is access to the patient population, especially if that is important in accomplishing the research. The clinical agency may have a need to provide sound clinical or quality assurance outcomes, but it may lack the available expertise or time to set up a research protocol. Magnet hospitals have promoted considerable activity in both of these areas and may welcome your proposal and willingness to carry out their desired work. This is an excellent opportunity for academicians who may have the personal desire as well as pressure from tenure and promotion committees to do research but who lack access to the clinical setting. The "marriage" of the academic and clinical institutions can benefit both parties.

A good example of a local hospital-based grant is a grant that came to the attention of Professor Kenner's master's student in Cincinnati. The hospital sought to increase the customer satisfaction of their inpatient obstetric patients. Extending the previously mentioned research in the area of "Transition from Hospital to Home for Mothers and Babies," the student wanted to do an extension of Kenner's transition research as her thesis. Professor and student approached a maternal/child clinical nurse specialist (CNS) who worked at an area level II nursery. The specialist was most anxious to make changes in the nursery's follow-up care for mothers and babies, but she needed evidence to support the need for more coordinated follow-up and teaching after discharge. After talking with her about the proposed project, she told of the funds her hospital provided for research. Within two months, the student wrote a proposal that served three purposes: extended Kenner's research to a new setting, gave her a master's thesis, and gave the CNS an opportunity to gain support for her clinical ideas. Another aspect of this process was that all of them were gaining experience in grant writing. The proposal was very short and easy to write. The project was funded in a few weeks. The master's student came out with a thesis and her first grant. She finished her study with a positive feeling toward research. For the hospital, the project provided the basis for what would eventually become a home follow-up program that netted a profit and good public relations.

PROFESSIONAL ASSOCIATION GRANTS

Many professional associations offer grant opportunities to their members. These grants are either directly administered by the association or through an auxiliary foundation. Corporate sponsors of the association sometimes partner with the professional society to offer educational scholarships or research grants. For example, equipment companies that exhibit their wares at medical conferences will also allocate monies to an association for the express purpose of a research protocol that tests their equipment. This type of grant would be a focused or targeted grant. Practice-focused associations, such as the Oncology Nurses Society, have associated foundations that give seed monies once per year to grantees who want to conduct research in the areas targeted by the association. Foundation grants linked with nursing specialty associations will generally support research in the area of specialty focus. As the nursing shortage has increased, so has the number of scholarships or foundation grants that are aimed at education. Educational endeavors are aimed at increasing the level of education of nurses in the specialty focus. A benefit to the foundation is that such grants attract members to their parent association. Organizational research grant recipients are often required to present their research findings at the organization's national or regional conference. Membership in the association is usually a prerequisite to the application process.

The American Nurses Foundation (ANF) is the philanthropic arm of the American Nurses Association (ANA) and a good example of a foundation that supports research and special projects across nursing specialties. The foundation awards a number of small research grants to nurses at both the beginning and experienced researcher levels ranging from $3,500 to $25,000. Some ANF grants are generated internally by ANF endowment funds, while others receive annual external support from contributions to the ANF Nursing Research Grants Program by nursing organizations such as Sigma Theta Tau International; the regional research groups: Western Institute of Nursing, Midwest Nursing Research Society, Southern Nursing Research Society, and Eastern Research in Nursing Association; and the Council for the Advancement of Nursing Science. Other external contributions come from ANA's Presidential Scholar Fund, the Commissions on Graduates of Foreign Nursing Schools, and corporate foundations. Because some of the funding streams for ANF grants vary each year, applicants should examine closely the availability, eligibility, and level of funding for these grants in the specific year they wish to apply. Although ANA membership is not required to apply for ANF grants, those that are sponsored by nursing organizations and regional research groups require membership in their specific group. Several of the ANF grants are specifically targeted at a special topic or individuals with a designated level of preparation, while others are without restrictions. A recent survey of ANF research grant recipients over its 50-year history demonstrated the long-range impact on nursing science made by these small grants (Holtzclaw, 2006). Recipients include many of today's top nurse scientists who credited the initial boost of their program of research to the ANF funding of their pilot work.

Professional association grants represent nearly every nursing specialty, and many are distributed directly from the association itself. The following are just a few examples:

- Society of Pediatric Nurses awards a $1,000 Corrine Barnes Research Grant.
- International Society of Nurses in Genetics Nursing Research Small Grant Program supports research related to genetic nursing practice or that which contributes to the development of genetic nursing science.
- American Cancer Society Targeted Grants for Research Directed at Poor and Underserved Populations are designed to support research that addresses the disparity in cancer morbidity and mortality in poor and underserved populations. This initiative includes research that addresses a variety of clinical, cancer control, behavioral, epidemiologic, health policy, health services, and basic science questions.
- The American Association of Critical-Care Nurses offers a variety of grants for research that is relevant to acute critical care nursing practice.

- The National Association of Pediatric Nurse Associates and Practitioners (NAPNAP) Foundation offers grants for nursing research that contribute to the improvement of quality of life for children and their families.
- The Association of Perioperative Registered Nurses supports the development of nurse researchers to contribute to the scientific knowledge related to perioperative nursing practice.
- The NAPNAP Graduate Student Research Award was developed to support child and family research among graduate students.

CORPORATE PARTNERSHIPS

Corporate partnerships often award grants for research, product development, implementation, or evaluation. These partnerships or strategic alliances are forged directly with a researcher/educator, an academic institution, or as described above with a professional association. These grants are viewed with skepticism by some professionals out of concern that researchers might be pressured to change study findings or not report them if they do not support the company's view. Although there is always an element of pressure from companies seeking to disassociate their "good name" from negative press, the responsibility rests with the researcher or grant seeker to clearly investigate the parameters of ownership before signing on the bottom line. Among the information needed are the steps that must be followed for reporting, presenting, and publishing the data. In other words, who owns the data and who has the right to manipulate it? These are important up-front questions that must be answered before any partnerships are forged.

A researcher seeking a certain type of equipment or protocol that is to be used may seek corporate partnership grants from companies that produce these products. Seeking support from that company can make good sense for this type of partnership and can be a win-win arrangement for both parties as long as each party is clear about expectations of the research and the dissemination of the findings. If a researcher is interested in this type of relationship, then either the local sales representative for the company or the research and development department of the company is an appropriate contact. Many larger companies have at least one person if not a whole department of people responsible for clinical research. Some even have "loan closets" where small devices and equipment may be borrowed by responsible researchers. Often the researcher can help the company gain entry to a clinical or academic setting that otherwise would be closed to it. Corporate grants can open up possibilities to do international, multisite studies that in the past were difficult to perform unless the researcher had the right connections. Today, with the globalization of industry, the corporate world provides opportunities to use already established markets for their products as research sites.

Examples of corporate partnership grants include the following:

- Children's Medical Ventures funds developmental care research, not just studies using their products.
- MedImmune funds research regarding pharmacologic intervention with respiratory syncytial virus.
- Roche U.S. Pharmaceuticals funds studies based on genomics (study of encoded information in DNA) that examines the sequence of infectious pathogens and drugs to combat them.
- Parke-Davis along with the Canadian Pain Society funds chronic pain research.

FELLOWSHIPS FOR PRE- AND POSTDOCTORAL RESEARCH TRAINING

Pre- and postdoctoral fellowships are expressly for career development and training of professionals interested in specializing in a focused area of research or education. Most of these fellowships support part if not all the academic costs associated with moving into a higher level of education or research sophistication. Foundations, associations, or the federal government offer these grants.

A *predoctoral fellowship* focuses on gaining further education and training for a person who has not attained a doctoral degree but who is committed to seek further research and education. These fellowships pay for tuition and a stipend for the grantee's doctoral education. Most predoctoral fellowships include research training and experience with mentors to give the professional a new skill set to conduct research and apply competitively for research grants. It is one way that academic institutions can groom professionals for academic life that includes an active research career.

Postdoctoral grants are aimed at perfecting and honing already existing research skills. Generally, grants in these highly specialized areas of expertise are offered for 1 to 2 years of in-depth studies. Today, many of these are focused on laboratory or clinical science research in the areas of pain, the human genome, and cancer treatments. Other hot topics are ethics, workplace analysis, health policy, and interdisciplinary research programs.

The purpose of pre- and postdoctoral fellowships is to create a cadre of scholars across disciplines that will lead the health profession into the next millennium. The rapid growth of technology has made it essential to have experts who can set the direction and give vision to the profession. Predoctoral training is designed to move the postbaccalaureate scholar toward the doctorate. Many doctoral programs in nursing with significant NIH funding are recruiting BSN graduates to their doctoral program trajectory. A postdoctoral scholar is defined by NIH and the National Science Foundation as "An individual who has received a doctoral degree (or equivalent) and is engaged in a temporary and defined period of mentored advanced training to enhance the professional skills and research independence needed to pursue his or her chosen career path." (Bravo & Olsen, 2007) Excellent tips for applying for NIH National Research Service Award (NRSA) fellowship grants are provided in an article by Parker and Steeves (2005). Examples of pre- and post-doctoral fellowship grants include the following:

- Pfizer Postdoctoral Fellowship Program in Biological Psychiatry
- NRSA Training Grants and Fellowships that include:
  - Ruth L. Kirschstein NRSA Institutional Predoctoral Fellowships (T32) are awarded to university units with a significant number of existing federally funded studies in a focused topic area (topics vary from palliative care to biobehavioral research). Students are usually funded two to three years.
  - Ruth L. Kirschstein NRSA Individual Predoctoral Fellowships (F31) are awarded to individuals submitting high-quality proposals and demonstrating a match with significantly funded research mentors in institutions with suitable resources to support the work.
  - NRSA Individual Postdoctoral (F32) Fellowships are awarded to individuals seeking a defined period of mentored advanced training who submit high-quality proposals and demonstrate a match with significantly funded research mentors in institutions with suitable resources to further the applicant's previous work. Students are usually funded two to four years.
- NIH NRSA Individual Predoctoral Fellowships for Minority Students (F31) provide up to five years of support for research training leading to the doctorate. Fellowships are designed to enhance the racial and ethnic diversity of the biomedical, behavioral, and health services research labor force in the United States.
- NIH NRSA Predoctoral Fellowships for Students with Disabilities (F31) provide up to five years of support for research training leading to the doctorate and are designed to encourage students with disabilities to seek graduate degrees and increase the number of scientists with disabilities prepared to pursue careers in biomedical and behavioral research.

FEDERAL GRANTS

Federal funding offers some of the largest grants and best-administered research funding in the nation. Much of the funding for health care is administered through the U.S. Department of Health and Human Services (DHHS), which oversees the U.S. Public Health Service agencies below:

- NIH
- Agency for Healthcare Research and Quality (AHRQ)
- CDC
- Indian Health Services (IHS)

Federal Mechanisms and Codes

Different levels of federal funding are categorized by a *funding mechanism*. Familiarizing yourself with the various funding mechanisms and codes assigned to each will make it easier to locate grants that are appropriate for your experience and interests. You will find each NIH funding mechanism designated with a three-digit code consisting of a letter and number (e.g., F32, K12, P01, R01, T32, etc.). The letters preceding the mechanism code indicate the general category of the grant and include:

- F—Fellowships
- K—Career development awards
- N—Research contracts
- P—Program project and research center grants
- R—Research project grants
- S—Research-related programs
- T—Training grants
- U—Cooperative agreements
- Y—Interagency agreements

The numbers that follow indicate the activity code and are specific to the level of funding and activity to which the award can be made. Research mechanisms most commonly used by the National Institute of Nursing Research (NINR) include the following:

R 01   **Research Project:** To support a discrete, specified, circumscribed project to be performed by the named investigator(s) in an area representing his or her specific interest and competencies.

R 03   **Small Research Grant:** To provide research support specifically limited in time and amount for studies in categorical program areas. Small grants provide flexibility for initiating studies that are generally for preliminary short-term projects and are nonrenewable.

R 15 **Academic Research Enhancement Awards (AREA):** To support small-scale research projects conducted by faculty in primarily baccalaureate degree-granting domestic institutions.

R 21 **Exploratory/Developmental Grants:** To encourage the development of new research activities in categorical program areas (generally restricted in level of support and in time).

R 25 **Education Program Grants:** To support the development and implementation of curriculum-dependent programs that focus on educational activities before, during, or after the completion of a terminal doctoral degree. They must address a need that is not funded by another NIH mechanism.

K 01 **Research Scientist Development Award—Research and Training:** To support a scientist, committed to research, in need of both advanced research training and additional experience. Other K awards (e.g., K02, K05, K06, ranging to K99) are designed for advanced levels of research, training, and/or mentorship and have specific targeted activities assigned to each.

K 02 **Research Scientist Development Award—Research:** To support a scientist, committed to research, in need of additional experience.

New mechanisms and activity codes continue to evolve in NIH funding. For this reason, it is important to use the latest updated information from the NIH Web site at http://www.nih.gov when selecting a mechanism.

National Institutes of Health

The NIH began as a laboratory for hygiene in 1887. It has grown into 25 separate institutes and centers. The mission is to uncover new knowledge for the betterment of health. It is one of eight health agencies under the Public Health Services, a part of the DHHS. NIH sets research priorities in each of the institutes and publicizes them on their Web site. About 10% of the research dollars goes to intramural research programs; the remaining percentage goes toward extramural research. The intramural projects are those conducted within the confines of the NIH campus, and extramural projects can be anywhere in the world. The current institutes and centers are as follows:

- National Cancer Institute
- National Center for Complementary and Alternative Medicine
- National Center for Research Resources

- National Eye Institute
- National Heart, Lung, and Blood Institute
- National Human Genome Research Institute
- National Institute of Diabetes and Digestive and Kidney Diseases
- National Institute on Drug Abuse
- National Institute of Environmental Health Sciences
- National Institute of General Medical Sciences
- National Institute of Mental Health
- National Institute of Neurological Disorders and Stroke
- NINR
- National Library of Medicine
- National Institute on Alcohol Abuse and Alcoholism
- National Institute of Allergy and Infectious Diseases
- National Institute of Arthritis and Musculoskeletal and Skin Diseases
- National Institute of Child Health and Human Development
- National Institute on Deafness and Other Communication Disorders
- National Institute of Dental and Craniofacial Research
- Center for Information Technology
- Center for Scientific Review
- John E. Fogarty International Center
- Warren Grant Magnuson Clinical Center

NIH funds health professionals and scientists across disciplines. Most grants are competitive, and the requests for proposals or applications are available through its Web site (http://www.nih.gov) or the national library system. The dates or cycles of funding as well as the priorities are listed. The main source of information is through the NIH Guide to Grants and Contracts. The contact person at NIH is included in all postings about grants, and it is this person's job to assist with grant preparation. Use his or her expertise when preparing your grant to guide you in the process of putting a grant together. Remember the contact person is there to help potential grantees submit the best possible grant. All NIH agencies (including NINR, CDC, DHHS, and AHRQ) use similar application processes and the PHS-398 form unless otherwise specified.

National Institute of Nursing Research

The NINR is but one of the NIH institutes. It will be discussed separately because many nurses apply for its grant monies. In 1985, the NINR first was established as the National Center for Nursing Research. In 1986, the center moved under the auspices of NIH. Finally in 1993 the Center was changed to an Institute, opening a portion of the NIH funds to its services. The structure and function of NINR changed: Becoming an institute gave it an equal status with the other institutes of health. Fund allocations now came from the general NIH budget. This placed nursing research (even though nonnurses can apply) on par with other disciplines at a federal level.

The National Advisory Council for Nursing Research, primarily composed of nurses, provides a second-level review of grants. The council recommends to the director of NINR which grants should be funded. Each grant that is submitted receives a priority score, but only a certain percentage of the grants are awarded funding. The grants are judged on scientific merit and the relevance of the proposed project to NINR's funding priorities.

NINR also supports the training of nurse researchers for expanding the cadre of nurse researchers. Thus almost 10% of the 1999 budget was focused on pre- and post-doctoral training grants; less than 7% was for career development grants and core centers in specialized areas of research; 3% was for intramural programs; and the remaining funds were used for extramural research programs. NINR participates in joint research programs with DHHS, the Health Resources and Services Administration (HRSA), AHRQ, and the CDC.

The current NIH funding priorities are the following:

- Chronic illnesses
- Quality and cost-effectiveness of care
- Health promotion and disease prevention
- Management of symptoms
- Adaptation to new technologies
- Health disparities (differences in health among age, social, or ethnic groups)
- Palliative care at the end of life

The emphasis in these areas is on clinical research involving direct patient contact or basic science linked directly to patient problems.

The mission of NINR is to establish a scientific basis for health care across the life span. Multidisciplinary or collaborative research remains a thrust of intramural projects. The NINR goals for 2006–2010 are the following:

- Integrate biological and behavioral science for better health.
- Adopt, adapt, and generate new technologies for better health care.
- Improve methods for future scientific discoveries.
- Develop scientists for today and tomorrow.

Areas of research emphasized by NINR include:

- Promoting health and preventing disease
- Improving quality of life
- Eliminating health disparities
- Setting directions for end-of-life research

Centers for Disease Control and Prevention (CDC)

The CDC is one of eight federal public health agencies. The CDC's mission is to promote health and the quality of life by disease, injury, and disability control and prevention. The CDC includes 11 centers, institutes, and offices:

- National Center for Chronic Disease Prevention and Health Promotion
- National Center for Environmental Health
- National Center for Health Statistics
- National Center for HIV, STD, and TB Prevention
- National Center for Infectious Diseases
- National Center for Injury Prevention and Control
- National Immunization Program
- National Institute for Occupational Safety and Health
- Office of Genetics and Disease Prevention
- Office of Global Health
- Public Health Practice Program Office

The CDC funds public health conferences. This agency also forms cooperative agreements (through competitive grants) in the following areas:

- AIDS/HIV
- Chronic disease prevention and health promotion
- Diabetes control and disability
- Emerging infections
- Environmental health
- Immunization, injury, and violence prevention and control
- Minority health/health promotion
- Occupational safety and health
- Sexually transmitted diseases
- Tuberculosis

The RFP and request for applications forms are available on their Web site (http://www.cdc.gov) or in the national library system.

The CDC is very active in global health initiatives. Health education in the form of distance-based graduate degree programs in public health in developing countries is another fundable area.

Department of Health and Human Services Training Grants

The DHHS is the largest grant-making agency in the federal government. The department contains the:

- Administration for Children and Families
- Health Care Financing Administration

- CDC
- Agency for Toxic Substances and Disease Registry (ATSDR)
- Food and Drug Administration (FDA)
- HRSA
- IHS
- NIH
- Substance Abuse and Mental Health Services Administration

The mission is to enhance the health and well-being of Americans through support of effective health and human services. The DHHS goals focus on improving quality of care through health services and education. One of the core values is to form partnerships among government, universities, and the private sector to improve quality of care. The DHHS challenges that affect quality of care are the following:

- Managed care transformation
- Rising number of uninsured Americans
- Changes in the composition of the American family
- Aging of America
- Rising costs associated with chronic illness
- Need for collaborative healthcare partnerships; patients need care coordination among specialists attending their health needs
- Genetic breakthroughs
- Threats of bioterrorism
- Privacy of healthcare information
- Emerging and reemerging infectious diseases
- Changing role of the government in health care (DHHS, 2004)

The DHHS administers approximately 300 different grant programs. The Catalog of Federal Domestic Assistance (CFDA) is the official listing of these grants and is available through GrantsNet on line (http://www.grantsnet.org). *Who's Who in Federal Grants Management* is a quick resource for all federal grant agencies and their management offices.

DHHS provides funding opportunities for educational grants. Some are very specific to a disease entity such as cancer education, whereas others are for basic or advanced education. Beginning in fiscal year 2000, Advanced Education Nursing Traineeship Grants that were previously funded require recipients to reapply. Only one grant application from an institution is recommended for grants that are similar in content. For example, a primary care women's health nurse practitioner grant and a pediatric nurse practitioner training grant from the same institution could be combined to simplify panel review and allow each grant to compete against one another. If the grants, however, are from different areas or there is a compelling need for each grant, then the institution may choose to submit more than one grant during a funding cycle. These changes are part of the Nursing Education and Practice Improvement Act of 1998 (HRSA, 1998).

Training grants are well known to most educators. They provide the monies to support nursing programs, especially at the advanced practice level. These grants are part of Title VIII of the Public Health Service Act, programs administered by the HRSA, Bureau of Health Professions, Division of Nursing. The purpose of these grants is to support education with the long-term outcome of improving healthcare delivery. The funding cycle is generally once or twice per year but depends on the particular grant. Grants are reviewed on the merits of the curriculum, availability of faculty, faculty expertise and credentials, and media resources, as well as the potential to draw a population of students. The request for proposals or applications can be found along with other federal grants at the HRSA Web site (http://www.hrsa.dhhs.gov/grants.htm).

Examples of these training grants are numerous, and include the following:

- Academic Administrative Units in Primary Care
- Predoctoral Training in Primary Care
- Physician Assistants Training in Primary Care
- Residency Training in Primary Care
- Faculty Development in Primary Care
- Podiatric Residency in Primary Care
- Model State-Supported Area Health Education Center (AHEC)
- Geriatric Education Centers
- Geriatric Training Regarding Physicians and Dentists
- Allied Health Special Projects, Public Health Training Centers
- Health Administration Traineeships and Special Projects
- Health Careers Opportunity Program
- Centers of Excellence
- Basic Nurse Education and Practice
- Advanced Education Nursing
- Nursing Workforce Diversity
- Advanced Education Nursing Traineeships
- Advanced Education Nursing—Nurse Anesthetist Traineeships
- Public Health Experience in State and Local Health Departments for Baccalaureate Nursing Programs

During this time of a critical nursing shortage, training grants are an important aspect of recruitment and retention of faculty positions. Undergraduate and graduate student enrollments have significantly dropped over the last five years. DHHS has funds available to schools that are interested in recruiting minority students and faculty and then retaining them. DHHS places a high priority in getting junior high and high school students excited about a health services career. Thus, a part of the undergraduate or special projects grants contains an element of Kids into Health Careers, a program aimed at marketing the positive aspects of health careers.

Schools must include how they are going to implement this form of marketing. A major debate has arisen over the past few years about whether the training grant is able to demonstrate retention as well as strong recruitment strategies. Recruitment costs are high and not profitable to the nursing profession if they are not successful in retaining the students.

Training grants at the advanced practice level are more likely to have a community-based focus and some component of distance learning. Some grants have demonstrated the need for a specific specialty program within a geographic area. The institutions, however, may lack the faculty expertise or dollars to support a freestanding program. For example, the University of Kansas, University of Missouri, and Wichita State University formed a consortium program for neonatal nurse practitioners, and the University of Cincinnati College of Nursing and Ohio State University started a joint nurse midwifery program. The latter was funded at the state rather than federal level. But in each of these examples, the partnership meant bringing together competitors to sit at the table and work out a joint curriculum or neither program would be able to start. Are these joint programs difficult? Yes, at times, but it is a successful strategy for receiving federal funds.

Many schools are also recognizing that at the graduate level they cannot be all things to all people; thus, Centers of Excellence are being established. An institution will build a reputation for a certain type of graduate education such as oncology nursing or substance abuse. The center concept provides a strong support component for resources when other grant funds for specific education are sought. Center grants are also available through various governmental agencies. Center grant writing is beyond the scope of this chapter, but it is important to remember that they exist and remain a potential source of funding in certain well-established research academic or healthcare centers. The Center Training Grant may provide a tangible commitment on the part of the institution to support specific, focused training.

Agency for Healthcare Research and Quality (AHRQ)

The AHRQ (formerly the Agency for Health Care Policy and Research) has gained a good deal of recognition over the last five years. It was started in 1989 to bridge the gap between biomedical research knowledge and the delivery of health care. The focus of AHRQ research is to find answers to questions about the population served, the costs involved, and what form of delivery system works best (Jones, Tulman, & Clancy, 1999). This agency supports both intramural and extramural research. Special emphasis is on minority health care, women's and children's health, international health, ethical issues in health care, and analyses of cost-effectiveness of delivery systems (Jones et al., 1999). Extramural research may be supported through grant applications or cooperative agreements and contracts. RFPs or applications are available at the AHRQ Web site (http://www.ahrq.gov/fund/98049.htm). The time cycle is included in the information found at this site.

Some grants are only given annually, while others are rolling (submission is not time dependent). Project officers are ready and willing to help the potential grantee write a successful grant. They encourage calls early in the grant-writing process. AHRQ suggests that a 3- to 7-page concept paper be submitted first for critique rather than waiting to submit an entire grant. This concept paper is not required (see Appendix D for a sample abbreviated concept paper). Four study sections conduct grant reviews. They are Health Systems Research, Health Care Quality and Effectiveness Research, Health Care Technology and Decision Sciences, and Health Research Dissemination and Implementation (Jones et al., 1999).

Grants are reviewed for scientific and technical merit and how well they fit with the priorities of the agency. This agency looks at grants as to their policy relevance or impact on policy making. Use of a multidisciplinary team is favored in research grants. A population or aggregate focus is also suggested. The project officer may contact the principal investigator after the first-level review for clarification of certain areas of the grant (Jones et al., 1999). This practice is generally not done by other federal agencies. As with the other federal agencies, AHRQ funds R01 (research grants that meet priority areas), R03 (small grants, which are often pilots ˋ or dissertation grants), R13 (conference grants), and F32 grants (individual postdoctoral research training grants) (Jones et al., 1999).

CORPORATE OR SMALL BUSINESS GRANTS

Corporate or small business grants may be awarded by specific corporations or foundations, as well as through the small business grant office at the federal level, primarily through the Office of Extramural Research of the NIH. The NIH offers Small Business Innovation Research (SBIR) grants and Small Business Technology Transfer (STTR) grants. The SBIR program's aim is to support small businesses that have the potential for commercializing research. Biomedical and behavioral research are two of the priority funding areas. The STTR program is a cooperative agreement between a small business and a research institution. Innovation and commercialization of research are two of the major criteria for these grants. On the Web site (http://www.grants.nih.gov/grants/funding/sbir.htm) there is a link to previously funded SBIR and STTR awards, which provides an abstract of successful grants and contact information on the project directors. This Web site also has two links to help small businesses develop. They are the National Venture Capital Association and the National Association of Small Business Investment Companies.

Funding is also available from venture capitalists who are independent contractors or associated with larger parent companies. For the venture capitalist, the return may be a percentage of the business, or they may offer to buy the company if it supports other corporations that they own. The list of potential companies is endless. There are online services such as Liberty Online and Federal Money Retriever that will match a business with a potential financial backer. State departments of commerce are another good resource. For example, the State of Illinois has an initiative to advance Illinois technology. Funds are available to support science and technology projects, university commercialization centers, and technology transfer activities. Other resources are universities themselves; West Texas A&M University, University of Cincinnati, and Indiana University have all supported special projects including small businesses.

Recently, small business grants have emphasized start-up monies for women attempting to start their own businesses. These businesses can be for-profit or not-for-profit companies. The grant applications are clear about what will or will not be covered in such grants. Like all other grants, the funding priorities are available.

Examples of resources for small business grants beside those listed above include professional organizations and magazines. They include *Entrepreneur Magazine*, National Association for Female Executives, National Association for Women Business Owners, and Service Corps of Retired Executives.

SPECIAL PROJECTS OF REGIONAL AND NATIONAL SIGNIFICANCE

Special Projects of Regional and National Significance (SPRANS) grants are special projects or demonstration programs that are funded through the Maternal Child Health Board (MCHB) and other federal agencies such as HRSA. The thrust is to support innovative programs, training, and research in maternal and child health. For example, the Cincinnati Center for Developmental Disorders and Children's Hospital Adolescent Clinic identified a need for more training in adolescent health issues for physicians and nurses. The director of nursing at the adolescent clinic spearheaded the writing of several SPRANS grants to support educational activities. A few of these SPRANS projects evolved into nursing electives for the University of Cincinnati's undergraduate and graduate students. Traineeships for health professionals that desired training in the area of adolescent health were also made available through SPRANS support.

Demonstration projects highlight changes in healthcare delivery or in the communities' healthcare needs. The rationale for these programs is to determine the feasibility of providing a service or expanding an educational program such as adolescent health education. If the pilot project is successful, other funding sources or the parent organization, such as a university, takes over the continuing costs. These projects generally provide strong positive public relations for the institution because they serve a community need. These grants can be a win-win situation. The downside is that when the funding dries up, these programs end, returning a population of patients to having no services again. This situation has happened many times when substance abuse clinics have been started, run well for the funding cycle, and then closed once the funds were gone. Reassurances are supposed to be made to the funding source that programs will continue at least for a time after the project's end, but in these tight financial times that is not always possible.

Another example is Georgetown University's National Center for Education in Maternal Child Health. This program represents a SPRANS Synthesis Project to bring together information and data derived from SPRANS programs across the country. These data are used to support needs for other grants or to change practice services. Healthy Tomorrows Partnership for Children Program (HTPCP) Analysis and Synthesis Project—Georgetown University is an example of a grant that is impacting practice. This project includes support from the American Academy of Pediatrics for the purpose of blending public health resources with professional pediatric expertise. The synthesis aspect of this program includes data from 107 nationwide projects. These are but two examples of special projects. The Web site http://www.ncemch.org/spr/default.html provides links to other projects.

CONCLUSION

Many resources exist for funding. Some of these monies are awarded only for research, whereas others are for clearly educational and demonstration projects. The latter grant category helps to support new innovative clinical programs or expansion of existing programs to meet community healthcare needs. The entrepreneur also has resources within the federal government and private sector to "grow" a small business. Today these small businesses provide services to healthcare professionals or their patients that otherwise might not be available.

CHAPTER 4

It Takes a Village
(and the Village Has a System!)

Writing a grant cannot be effectively done in isolation. Even if you are writing a grant for a thesis or dissertation (which is expected to be an independent scholarly work), your request for funding is going to involve other individuals beyond you and your supervisory committee. These persons may include study subjects or participants, consultants, institutional review committees, clinical site authorities and personnel, clerical or technical services, and administrative research office personnel. If your grant is not being requested to support your graduate work, it will be an *expectation* that your project itself will involve a team. How well you choose and assemble a competent experienced team is the mark of a knowledgeable grant writer and is part of the criteria by which your application will be scored. Selecting and asking for entrée to conduct your study in a clinical or community study site also involves negotiation with the appropriate personnel. Understanding the importance of these interpersonal links in the grant process will not only make the grant submission process less bumpy, but it will also ensure a smoother journey throughout the entire pre- and post-award period of your study. Understanding the system by which each group of individuals operates will allow you to plan for the time and procedures ahead.

YOUR GRANT CONSTRUCTION TEAM AND SYSTEM

Your grant construction team can take on a variety of configurations. It may be a dissertation or thesis committee, a research team you build from nursing or interdisciplinary colleagues, or in some instances a team put together with input from the funding agency.

Dissertation or Thesis Committees

If you are writing a small seed grant, you will likely write the scientific research plan yourself, or perhaps with the supervision of a thesis or dissertation chair, consultant, or statistical advisor. Usually, the largest hurdles in this process are getting the time and help you need from assisting individuals when your grant submission date is growing close. This may have to be orchestrated around receiving institutional review board (IRB) approval from one or more institutions. For example, Professor Kenner had to have her proposal reviewed and approved by her doctoral committee (taking three weeks) as well as the associate dean for research where she was on faculty (taking two weeks). The IRB for the University Medical Center where she was a student, though not actually collecting data there, reviewed her proposal (taking four weeks), and finally the hospital IRB where the data were collected had to approve the proposal (taking four weeks). The process took three to four months. She found it helpful to submit each previous letter of approval to the next IRB. Planning ahead, getting firm commitment for appointments, and preparing your agenda and questions prior to each of your meetings with these members will keep your relationships strong and move you ahead.

Larger Grants: More Complex Systems

For larger grants, particularly those with interdisciplinary partners, your grant writing will be similar to joint authorship of any kind. The literary give-and-take must eventually produce a readable plan for meeting the aims and objectives of the grant application. Meeting first to discuss your overall plan will get you all in the same conceptual ballpark. If you, as principal investigator (PI), have specific aims and a short background of the problem, you can ask co-investigators to write parts of the background and significance section for you to include in the grant application. This will help you incorporate additional items in the specific aims section, and your discussion may lead you to add or modify one or more of your aims. At some point, the input of your research site authority, your expert topical consultants, your statistical scientist, and your institutional financial office will shape the final grant proposal. As PI, your ultimate challenge will be to make this plan understandable, cohesive, and acceptable to these individuals as well as to your funding agency.

Other members of your grant construction team include any secretarial and financial office assistance you plan to use. Remembering that your grant is likely not the only task they are responsible for, give them your grant submission timeline and allow sufficient lead time for them to respond to your requests. Maintaining excellent relationships with your financial office will help keep communication lines open in the planning and later administration of your grant funds. If available, use your institutional accountant to help you with your budget pages. You must first come up with what you need: personnel and percent effort, equipment type and specifications, types and amounts of supplies, travel, and other technical or episodic services. In large institutions, such as universities, health science centers, and military installations, your grant must be submitted to an institutional office of research administration (sometimes termed "grants and contracts") to have its budget reviewed and signed off by the institution. Find out before you begin your grant writing what timeline this office requires to sign off on your grant. As institutions across the country have become more research active, the time they require to sign off has lengthened. Some require several days, while others require a week or more.

If your project will include human subjects, another part of your grant construction team is your institution's human research participant protection office, or IRB. Developing a continuing relationship with an IRB spokesman is important in determining the type of IRB review you wish to request and for dealing with future questions that arise during your review. For animal studies, your institution's institutional animal care and use committee (IACUC) will serve a similar purpose. In both cases, the IRB and IACUC will inform you of any training or preliminary steps that must be taken in using either humans or animals in your study. Know how often these committees meet and what their review cycles are well in advance so these times can be built into the timeline of grant writing.

Last, but certainly not least, keep your dean, director, or supervisor aware of your employment time and institutional resources committed in your proposal. Your employment home is crucial to housing you and your project. Early involvement of your supervisor can avoid snags in the application process or later disappointments if your release time or uses of resources are refused. Know the informal and formal politics of who should be notified that a grant is being submitted. For example, most department heads do not like to find out, after the fact, that a grant is being submitted by a departmental faculty member without their knowledge. This is not a control issue, but rather a workforce issue. If faculty release time is needed in the grant, supervisors must anticipate the possibility of replacing that person. If a key personnel member is employed outside your institution and has agreed to work on your grant, you should get assurance that they have received internal support for their time commitment as well. If an "expert" in your institution might feel your grant is in competition with his or her area or research, consider engaging that person in your project or in an advisory capacity. Even having him or her write a letter of support for the grant would show your respect for that individual's expertise. It is better to find out where you stand on competitive issues before the grant is submitted than to have problems surface when it is funded.

A potential barrier during the summer months, or December holidays, is the unavailability of persons to sign off on grants or to agree to serve on grants. Again, anticipate these scheduling problems early. Check vacation schedules and fit them into the grant. Sometimes this is not possible if a grant opportunity suddenly arises, but in those rare cases there is usually a designated person who has signature authority.

BUILDING A RESEARCH TEAM

Choosing your co-workers for a research study or project is serious business. Aside from choosing people with expertise, you are looking for a cooperative team. A cooperative team is one that will work well under your leadership. There is a line of authority and responsibility in a funded research study that is often overlooked by groups that wish to be democratic and supportive to each member of the team. This resides in the fact that the PI is the person that is ultimately responsible for the conduct of a study, no matter how large or small the size of the team. Even when there are co-investigators on a project, you have administrative authority over selection of the other team members, assignment and supervision of their work, and in making sure that the budgeted award is spent correctly and on time. Again, the responsibility rests with the PI to answer scientifically and fiscally to the funding agency.

As PI, you are the leader of the project team. Selecting the key personnel for your grant is like recruiting a winning lineup for a competitive challenge. All persons designated as grant personnel must be justified in terms of their role, their preparation for the role, and the amount of time they will spend in that role. In these times of shrinking grant funds and growing competition, these aspects of the grant proposal are scrutinized closely. Two primary places where role competency and time commitment show up in the grant are in the list of key personnel, which includes the percent effort and in the budget justification. A statement in the budget justification tells reviewers precisely the role that the person will play on the project. A person's preparation for the role appears in the biographical sketches for key personnel, which usually follow those of the PI. If the person has any significant research findings that lay groundwork for the proposed work, this also demonstrates competency and appears in the preliminary studies section of the proposal.

Be sure to acquaint all members of the research team with what their role will be, how much time commitment is involved, and how much, if any, of the grant funds will be used to pay for their time or offset their salary. This seems like an obvious requirement, but it is surprising how many people forget this information by the time a grant is funded. Some even sign up for other grants and find they are 100% committed elsewhere by the time you are ready to begin your study. Others mistakenly believe they are funded on your grant when in fact they have committed their "in-kind" participation at no cost. If salary or a large time commitment is necessary, this will require negotiation between the team member and his or her employer. A sign-off from a department head or agency is one of the documents that your research administration office will require before submitting a grant requiring salary. If the appropriate people have not signed off for in-kind donation of time and the grant gets forwarded to the office of research administration in the university or hospital, it will more than likely be sent back to the PI. If by chance the grant goes to the funding agency without proper sign-off, they also may send it back or just not review the proposal. This is not a time to beg forgiveness later because it can spell disaster for the grant. In some cases, your co-investigator or collaborator may be in a different institution that requires a subcontract. Be sure your key personnel have reviewed and have copies of these documents and review them when your grant is funded.

Key Personnel

Key personnel include the PI, co-investigators, collaborators, research assistants, technicians, data collectors, data managers, and a variety of persons who play an ongoing part on your grant project. In grants that provide salary support, the percent effort and fringe benefits are calculated into the annual budget in detail. Personnel who play an episodic part, such as consultants, transcriptionists, or offsite data analysts are often paid by the visit or by the hours engaged in the project. As such, they are contracted for the work and paid episodically. It is both a function of the pattern of work as much as the type of job that determines this. For example, a graduate research assistant may be a key personnel member assigned the work of data entry or data transcription, depending on their research training or desire for experience. In some cases, an onsite clinical expert may play a small, but continuing role in the project while serving as consultant. In other cases, these tasks may be allocated to a contracted person by the job.

Co-investigators and Collaborators

Co-investigators and collaborators should represent significant roles on the project, either in intellectual contribution to the scientific endeavor or in oversight of portions of the work. They are often interdisciplinary scientists that offer a valuable insight and source of expertise to the conduct of the study and interpretation of findings. Having interdisciplinary partners is recognized as a strength by the National Institutes of Health (NIH) as they seek applications "to facilitate an interdisciplinary research approach that brings together the biological, behavioral, and social sciences to tackle our most pressing health problems" (NIH, 2007).

The title "Co-Principal Investigator" (Co-PI) is often used inaccurately to reflect a co-investigator or collaborator. NIH has never formally recognized a Co-PI designation, and this policy will continue even though they have recently designated grants that can be awarded to "multiple principal investigators." This decision is under a trial run at present and was instituted to maximize the potential of "team science" efforts and the need for formal recognition of PIs. A request for applications was issued in 2006 for a selected group of multiple PI model proposals to be funded (NIH, 2005). However, such grants must justify a compelling rationale for multiple PIs, and a Leadership Plan must be included to show the exact scope of appropriate authority and responsibility. The leadership plan includes the governance and organizational structure of the research project, with communication plans and procedures for resolving conflicts. In addition, the administrative, technical, and scientific responsibilities for each specific aim or activity should be delineated for the PIs and other members of the scientific team.

Project Director (PD)

Project director is a second-level position that is often necessary for a large funded study with salary support. For smaller studies, the role of PD is often taken on by the PI. This is the PI's "right-hand person" in the sense that the role includes supervision of many of the day-to-day tasks. In some cases, the PD will recruit and train the research assistants, set up meetings for the team, make rounds to recruit subjects for a clinical study, or be responsible for gathering and managing data collection forms. The variety of tasks involved with a larger project can involve a large percent of effort, so that a PD might be hired as a full-time member of the team.

Graduate Research Assistants

Graduate research assistants (GRAs) and nonstudent research assistants are important members of your team. They are listed as personnel if they have an ongoing time commitment for a significant portion of your grant. A GRA can be named in the listing of key personnel. However, if you are not sure which specific students will fill these roles, you may need to put "To be announced" in the space where a name would go. Hiring research assistants after the grant is funded may require checking with your institutional human resource department. Some of the best GRAs for your project may come from students you have mentored or those that apply because they are interested in your research. While some applicants for research assistant positions may apply because they need part-time work, those who develop an interest in the project will ultimately be the best team members. Students can generally be hired with institutions with little preliminary advertisement beyond posting a "help wanted" sign. However, nonstudent research assistants usually require placement through your institution's human resource office. Good relationships with research assistants make your project run smoothly. The research assistants deserve good training, good communication channels with the PI, and continued feedback on their performance and contribution.

Consultants

Consultants are a quality check on the scientific conduct of your study. Although previous research and publications help to demonstrate the expertise of the research team, consultants can be used to contribute specialized expertise to the project and enhance the overall quality of the proposal. For example, if an infant researcher's expertise is in pain and the proposal is to examine the interface between pain and sleep, adding a consultant with national recognition in infant sleep may strengthen the credibility of the project and enhance its ability to successfully compete for funding. Another example is a study concerning cancer rehabilitation and exercise physiology. For this study consultants who are expert oncologists coupled with ones who are exercise physiologists are good additions to an academic center grant where no such expertise is on site. Statistical consultants may give your team added strength in data analysis and interpretation as well as helping you with design sensitivity in your initial planning. Consultants can contribute to the project in a variety of ways, including conceptualization of the study design, selection of research instruments, implementation issues, and data analysis and interpretation. Although consultant costs may vary, provide a detailed description of the consultation services to be rendered, number of days anticipated for consultation, the expected rate of compensation, and travel, per diem, and other related costs. Most grants, including NIH applications, require a letter from the consultant confirming their willingness to provide the service. It is important that this letter include the type of service they will provide.

Specialized Team Members

Specialized team members are persons who can be key personnel if they are serving a continuing role on the projector, or if they are working only episodically, they can be listed in the "other" category. These might include data transcriptionists, translators, laboratory technicians, medical device engineers, instrumentation or software trainers, and other experts that are necessary for the conduct of your project.

CARE AND FEEDING OF YOUR RESEARCH TEAM

Open communication is the key to caring for your research team. Up-front understanding of each member's responsibilities and chain of communication is crucial. Whereas most of the attention to your team will come after the project is funded, clearly stated expectations should be outlined before a team member is included in your grant application.

Once the grant is funded, you should outline early the expectations for GRAs and other data collectors to attend training sessions and carry out study procedures. Give the entire team telephone, pager, or cell phone numbers to contact a supervisory project person when they are unable to fulfill their work schedule or responsibilities. Transmitting the importance of their contracted participation is essential, particularly for students, who may not realize the seriousness of lost data collection opportunities that occur when personnel are missing. A communication book is sometimes helpful if there are overlapping shifts of grant personnel working around the clock. In a study of fever in human immunodeficiency virus (HIV) patients, personnel made rounds on each shift to seek participants who had temperature elevations. Each person made notes about potential cases and reported any messages about the study to the next person coming on. The PD checked each day to validate something was done about any requests. Regular meetings, at least monthly, with all personnel will keep everyone in touch with the study progress, updates in procedures, and problems that need solving. Mutual respect between every member of the team reinforces his or her value to the study's success. Celebrations and parties help to form a collaborative spirit. Taking team members to research conferences makes them feel more a part of the study. We have found that allowing GRAs or other team members to present portions of the study methodology in symposia helped to groom them for their own scientific careers. At least three of our GRAs discovered spin-off ideas for their own dissertations from involvement with our study.

Every research team needs training to the specifics of your project. In many cases this involves training data collectors and PDs to the instrumentation, whether it includes medical devices or test administration. Plan to hold training/demonstrations of how to approach a participant as well as how to administer a procedure, test, or intervention. Role playing sometimes helps a beginning research assistant. Give constructive feedback with support for areas of weakness and praise for accomplishments.

Make it clear to all participants that the collected data belong to the grant and cannot be used for any other purpose. If delineating the publication plans for your project is not done early in your planning and orientation, you will deal with sticky issues after the fact. Co-investigators can expect to be a co-author in publications arising from a grant project, although this varies across studies. Responsible conduct of research principles call for authorship to be limited to persons who make a major contribution to concept, design, analysis and/or interpretation of the work (APA, 2001; ICMJE, 2006). This includes participation in drafting the article, revising it critically for important content, and having a voice in its final draft. The PI must decide whether collaborators, experts, and research assistants, or consultants are included as co-authors, and their authorship should responsibly be based on their contribution to the project and manuscript.

Data collection may require varying amounts of training, and this time should be considered in setting up the timeline of your grant. Recognize that gaining intra-rater reliability can take considerable practice and trials before measurement skills are honed and ready for data collection. For example, in a study of drug-induced shivering, we wished to determine if skin-fold thickness might be an intervening variable that would influence neural perception of discrepancies between environmental temperature and a rising thermoregulatory set point. An unplanned delay in readying our data collection was our unawareness of how difficult it was to get precision in skin-fold thickness, even with good instruments. It took approximately 100 trials before our PD gained acceptable intra-rater reliability within her own measurements. In that same study, we found it necessary to train GRAs in proper measurement of tympanic membrane temperatures by first teaching them to use an otoscope to visualize a tympanic membrane. When otoscope visualization was mastered, this in turn rapidly improved their inter-rater reliability in measurement of tympanic membrane temperatures.

Another area of training that should not be overlooked involves scientific integrity and the importance of maintaining the integrity of the study design. For GRAs and new investigators, impressing them with the importance of finding the *truth* rather than *proving the hypothesis* is essential. Most institutions require that any research personnel be trained by their IRB office and take training in the protection of human research subjects from a recognized service, such as the Collaborative Institutional Training Initiative (CITI) online program, found at https://www.citiprogram .org/default.asp. However, the training in scientific integrity and guarding against fraudulent misconduct in research requires constant reinforcement. Research assistants and colleagues, eager to help their PI succeed, must understand that success is in *finding the truthful answers* to research questions, not in proving you were right in your hypothetical test.

DEMONSTRATING LINKS WITH COMMUNITY, AGENCY, OR INSTITUTIONAL RESOURCES

Gaining Access

A hallmark of an experienced and competent researcher is the ability to build networks, not only of a strong research team, but of cooperating community or study site partners. This is not simply a description on paper, but a living breathing network that takes planning, negotiation, and respect for the requested resources. It starts with a request for entrée (power, permission, or liberty to enter). In many situations starting at the top is essential to gain authorization to conduct a study in a hospital or clinical agency, but recognizing that the persons you may need cooperation from are at the midlevel or service-level providers. It is important to build relationships with those individuals while you wait for formal permissions. Permission to access a military or Veterans Administration facility requires special steps that are formalized with applications, credentialing, and chains of command. Approaching a Native American tribal affiliation also requires meeting with and approval from their governing body as well as from any local agency or site. Recognizing that one cannot expect rapid access when asking for permission to study a group you are not already a part of, successful researchers spend considerable time building relationships with key groups and involving them in participatory roles on the study.

Many successful liaisons are built by having clinical or agency people serve on your study as agency coordinators, inpatient or outpatient clinical site coordinators, or facilitators. Most will agree to serve in this role at no cost, since their duties are limited to making sure your study does not conflict with the daily schedule of the clinical unit or agency. It gives the agency person, often a head nurse or unit manager, close contact with the operations of the study so they can explain it to other personnel.

Watch Out for Crowds!

As research activity grows in clinical sites, the numbers of studies competing for the same participants grows. Some clinical sites and agencies monitor this and keep the number low to avoid interfering with their operations. Others either do not monitor or are glad for any added interest in their site. One problem with competition for subjects emerged at a public welfare clinic for mothers and infants, currently being used by a nurse researcher with small grant funding. The clinic wrote a support letter for a second researcher employed by the same university as the first, welcoming the project to the site to conduct the study without regard to the study currently taking place. Unfortunately, the second PI also failed to check and discuss the availability of subjects with the first nurse researcher, and when a large NIH proposal was funded, it encroached on the existing study. Bad feelings resulted all around and affected relationships between the PIs, the agency, and university research administration. Because there may be no oversight committee at your research site monitoring the use of clients, students, patients, or attendees as research subjects, you should try and find out if other studies are going on and determine if conflicts are likely.

Remembering Where You Are

The research site, whether it is a hospital, clinic, senior center, church, tribal center, or school, is hosting your project and you are the guest. As such, PIs should treat this gift with the respect and consideration it deserves. A spirit of cooperation between others working and studying in the site is far more productive than becoming adversarial over factors that might affect your access. If you anticipate that another study PI is seeking the same type of participants in a different study, try to work this out in a straightforward, but amicable, way. For example, we discovered that a physician was seeking bone-marrow transplant patients to study the lymphatic effects of the same drug that caused the drug-induced shivering we were studying. We found it was helpful to include him as an expert in our advisory committee. We also found he was more than cooperative to alternate with us in acquiring study participants. In fact, our PD contacted him with participants when it was his turn to accept the next study subject. Whether or not your study is a nursing study, recognizing the interface between medicine, pharmacy, nursing, and agency administration should alert you to be respectful and considerate to all who are linked to the patient's care.

Once the grant is funded and procedures begin, the site coordinator can facilitate a time when you can present the study goals to the staff. Keep the staff informed about any changes in your project that would affect your presence, coming and going, from the study site. Be sure that GRAs and on-site grant personnel are introduced to the agency staff. Always be available by phone or pager to the research site, in case there are problems or questions arising about the study or study participants. Expressions of gratitude to cooperative clinical staff are much appreciated. For example, on Christmas holidays, the study team treated each of the clinical research study sites used for the HIV fever study and the drug-induced shivering study with a colorful basket of red delicious apples. Study personnel delivered them to the hospital units and labeled a basket for each shift. Staff also appreciated feeling included in the study by our presentations of study progress and problem solving.

Navigating the Internal Grant Submission System

Each grant writer must determine the internal mechanism for submitting grants, no matter what type of grant it is. This statement may seem simpleminded, but it is an essential early step in the grant-writing process. Many offices and people must sign off on a grant before it is submitted to an IRB or a funding agency. A timeline is needed for staying on target and getting these sign-offs early in the grant-writing process.

Some people find creating a flow sheet or a project timeline helpful. Whatever tool is used, determine what steps are necessary before getting too far into the grant-writing process. Find out if there are restrictions on how many grants may be submitted in the category in which you are applying. For example, no more than one training grant may be applied for by any institution from the Department of Health and Human Services in a single funding cycle. Therefore, a clearinghouse in the institution for grant development must make sure this rule is followed. This clearinghouse may be a center for nursing research, a department-level committee or chair, or the dean's office.

Next, find out who must approve the grant submission and when. Does the project require submission of a concept paper to a department? A training grant may require that the department or curriculum committee see the proposal before any grant is submitted. If approval by the curriculum committee is necessary, find out how often and when they meet, and how long it will take for final approval. Also carefully read the request for proposals; it may state that a grant must have curriculum, college, or IRB approval prior to submission. For example, the NIH requires that, once the researchers are notified that their grant is within the fundable range, IRB approval must be sought. The NIH regulations further state that no grant award funds are to be released until NIH receives in writing that IRB approval has been obtained.

Early in the grant-writing process, determine whether a research office or grants office must oversee or approve the project. If so, this office may have staff and support services that would facilitate the grant-writing process. In addition to providing assistance, the grants office often serves as the final check of the grant before submission. Remember too, it is important to know who, outside the college or institution, must sign off before submission. If the project is a cooperative agreement or if subcontracts must be drawn up for outside personnel to be hired, determine who does this, how long this process takes, and what the procedure is. An external agency that is to supply personnel as well as the college or grant writer's own institution often has their own indirect cost rates and financial reviews that produce additional budget pages for your grant. Most will wish to review a grant before submission.

CONCLUSION

The "village" analogy is highly relevant to the grant-writing, submission, and conduct processes. The diversity of backgrounds, cultures, and competencies are especially heterogeneous in this group. Therefore, communication, respect, and clarity of expectations are keys to successful relationships among its members. Choose your team carefully, and take exceptional care of them. They will make you proud! Planning is the name of the game when it comes to internal institutional grant submission procedures and processes. Find out the steps in this process and adhere to them. Always assume the internal review steps are going to take twice as long as you expect. These steps are important to getting your grant out the door, so don't try to rush them. Finally, remember that your activities aren't the only ones in the village. Avoid traffic jams by planning each step in the submission process ahead of your journey.

CHAPTER 5

Writing the Research Proposal

THE GRANT FORMAT

Beginning grant writers often fall "victim to the dictum" of the required headings in specific grant instructions and formats. Because a grant announcement usually includes a format of headings, the novice tends to believe that it is a type of questionnaire, and all one has to do is fill in the blanks. Reviewers can spot this inexperience immediately when the specific aims section of a grant comes in with nothing in the section but a list of aims and other sections seem disconnected from the aims. Explaining this point is a little like trying to understand physiology from anatomical relationships alone. If you will consider the grant *format* as a sequence or order of presentation (anatomical relationships), you will see that the format alone does not provide the logical links (interactive relationships) that explain how the sections support and justify one another. Figure 5-1 shows the general anatomy and format of most grant proposal formats. Each arrow shows the order each element follows and what is to be included in a particular section, but it does not emphasize the need to show how one link explains the other.

Figure 5-2, by contrast, shows how each section explains and justifies each of the following important essentials of a successful grant:

- Meaningful question
- Good sciences
- Careful attention to the application
- Qualified applicant

The above elements are not headings in a format, but all grant reviewers will be looking for these characteristics as they evaluate your grant.

FLESHING OUT THE BLUEPRINT OF A RESEARCH GRANT

Once you have examined the guidelines and format for your intended grant application, you will need to begin constructing your proposal in a well-justified,

Figure 5-1 Anatomy of a Grant Proposal

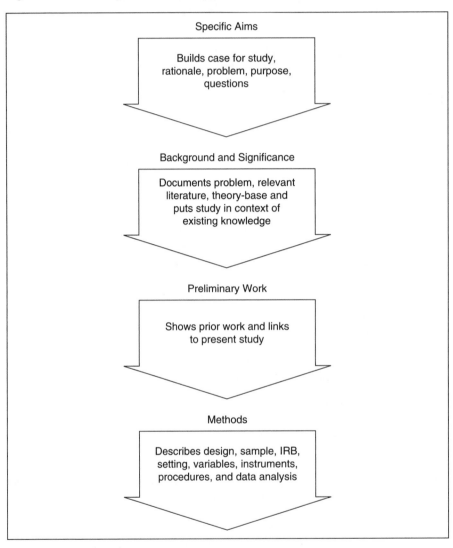

Figure 5-2 Interacting Parts of the Grant Proposal

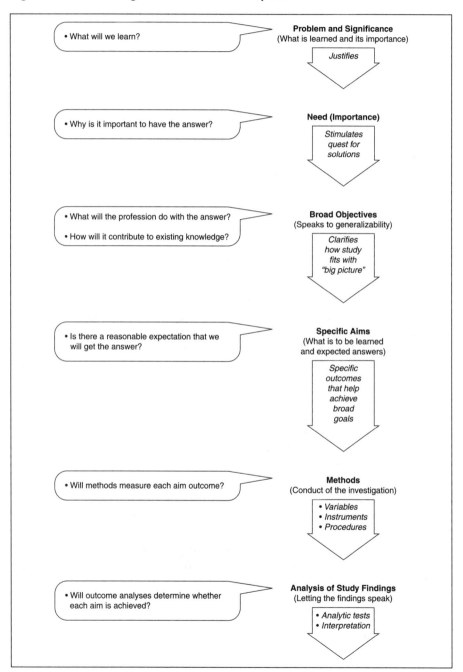

convincing way. Following is a typical format required by many funding agencies.

- Abstract
- Research plan
- Specific aims
- Background and significance
- Preliminary studies
- Research design and methods
  - Setting and sample
  - Intervention
  - Instruments
  - Data collection procedures
  - Data analysis
- Timeline
- Literature cited
- Budget
- Human subjects considerations: review type and reviewing board
- Appendices

Clarity and consistency within the grant is one of the major challenges that a grant writer must address. Constructing a research grant application is much like using building blocks: The specific aims form the foundation and structure for the research proposal. From the specific aims emerge testable questions or hypotheses. The research design and methods are then chosen to answer the identified research questions or hypotheses. Appropriate analyses are selected to statistically test hypotheses or systematically answer qualitative questions. One of the ways to promote clarity between hypotheses, variables, instruments, and data analyses is to use consistent vocabulary and terminology between the specific aims, questions/hypotheses, and analytic procedures. Avoid calling a variable by more than one term (e.g., "core temperature," and "central temperature"). Organize each section of the research proposal so that the specific aims are in the same order and sequence as their related questions/hypotheses and plans for analytic procedures. Variables should also be listed in the same sequence in the specific aims, research questions, and hypotheses. The funding agency's application guidelines should include instructions about using special font styles. If the funding agency allows use of special font styles (e.g., bold, underline, or italics), use this feature to highlight key variables throughout each grant section. Finally, well-designed tables and figures can greatly enhance the presentation of materials related to research design and methods.

COMPONENTS SPECIFIC TO ALL GRANTS

The major components of a research grant application include the following:

- Abstract
- Research plan
- References
- Budget
- Curriculum vitae or biographical sketch
- Past and ongoing research support
- Institutional resources
- Institutional review board approvals
- Appendices

The components are not necessarily arranged in this order. Several grant application formats, including those from the National Institutes of Health (NIH), have the budget and justification pages, biographical sketches, and administrative information in the front. Newer NIH biographical sketches now include research support, which eliminates the older "other support" pages. Although the research grant has been used as the exemplar for this chapter, all elements described here are generally the same with any grant application, including training and special projects, discussed later in the book. Instead of a research plan, demonstration grants or other project grants may use the terms *plan and implementation, project plan,* or *methodology.*

Even if your grant guidelines allow grant proposals to include appendices, do not put information that is critical to understanding your grant into an appendix. First of all, it is annoying to a grant reviewer to flip back and forth between the main body of the proposal and appendices. Secondly, you cannot assume that all reviewers who discuss your proposal will receive the appendices in the review process. Only the three or four assigned principal NIH grant reviewers for each proposal receive the appendices for their grants. Therefore, include all the critical information needed to evaluate the quality of the proposal in the Research Plan section of the proposal. Space is a premium and usually limited to a specific number of pages. The challenge then is to present concise yet detailed plans. Although the format for the research plan may vary depending on the funding source, most research plans include the following sections: Abstract, Specific Aims; Background and Significance; Preliminary Studies; and Methods. The individual sections of a research grant will be discussed below.

Abstract

Proposals often begin with a short summary of the proposed research. However, writing the abstract is usually one of the last parts of the proposal you write. A good reason for writing the abstract last is to ensure that any changes that evolve, while writing the body of the grant, are reflected in the abstract. The abstract briefly introduces the research problem and then summarizes the specific aims, background and significance, and research design and methods sections. The greatest challenge to writing this section is adhering to the word limit. An editor can be extremely useful by helping you cut out unnecessary words and phrases. Remember, too, the abstract sets the stage for the remainder of the proposal. Write the abstract with care because, as the introduction to your proposal, any flaws will raise questions about your scholarship and set up the proposal for a more critical review. Consistency between the abstract and the remainder of the proposal and your attention to detail help to show your capability as well as "selling" the grant's idea.

Specific Aims

The section called Specific Aims requires a brief introductory explanation describing the study purpose(s), why it is important to do the study, the potential usefulness of the findings, what the research intends to accomplish, and the study's relationship to long-term goals. There is no required order for how the Specific Aims page is written, but proposals in nursing, successfully funded by the National Institute for Nursing, tend to follow a favored format. Instead of starting right off the bat with a list of aims, the elegant Specific Aims page begins with a brief reasoned argument that (1) poses a problem of relevance to the funding agency, (2) briefly discusses the inadequacy of existing knowledge to address the problem, and (3) sells the need for the proposed research to help fill the knowledge gap. The introductory information helps to "sell" your study idea, and the line of reasoned discussion leads logically into a *statement of the purpose*. The purpose statement should be a concise, clear statement of the study's goal that comes from the study's research problem. It usually includes the relationships sought between the key study variables, as well as the population and setting for the study (Burns & Grove, 2005, p. 71). In fact, if the introductory discussion is compelling enough, you can begin the statement of the purpose with the words "Therefore, the purpose of the study is . . ." An example of this approach appears below.

In a funded proposal to study human immunodeficiency virus (HIV) symptom management of HIV-related fever, the introductory paragraph focused on the study problem and factors relevant to fever in HIV infection as follows:

Fever is one of the most common responses associated with human immunodeficiency virus (HIV) infection, acquired immunodeficiency syndrome (AIDS), and the opportunistic infections accompanying these conditions. Persons living with AIDS (PLWA) experience predictable symptoms with fever episodes, regardless of the infectious agent. Symptoms result from nonspecific and antigen-specific host mechanisms that combat invading microorganisms by activating antibacterial chemical secretion and neutrophil migration. Although T-cell and host immune functions are deranged by HIV infection, proinflammatory responses are activated through alternative complement pathways. Whether the cytokine-modulated effects related to fever hold immunostimulant benefits for PLWAs is controversial, but the negative effects are well recognized. Pyrogens stimulate hypermetabolic and proteolytic processes that expend oxygen, calories, and body water. In AIDS, these catabolic effects often affect an already compromised nutritional state. Fever is the highest predictor for malnutrition among risk factors in HIV disease. Subjectively fever symptoms are distressful, interfering with rest, comfort, and functional ability. While medical fever management is understandably concerned with control of the underlying infection with drugs, nursing fever management is directed at symptomatology, regardless of etiology. Goals are to maintain body temperature within a safe range, maintain and restore fluid balance, conserve energy, avoid fatigue, and promote thermal comfort during fever.

Following the introductory statement, the study problem is discussed in light of existing knowledge as follows:

Although nurses devote hundreds of hours daily to treatment and palliation of fever, methods of care have changed little over the past century. Nurses tend to monitor fever progress and follow pharmaceutical prescriptions strictly, while resorting to poorly justified nursing activities to cool the patient. Cooling sponge baths or fans are implemented without regard for expected physiologic responses. Effects of environmental temperature, patient hydration, and physical activity on febrile responses are seldom considered. Only recently have specific interventions for fever management been tested, and these have yet to find their way into nursing textbooks. Efforts to aggressively cool febrile patients by convective heat-exchange blankets and ice packs are counterproductive because they stimulate shivering and vasoconstriction. Compensatory warming responses generate and conserve heat, while increasing oxygen consumption 3–5 fold. Anemic, weak, and cachectic patients tolerate exertion of febrile shivering poorly, as respiratory rate, heart rate, and blood pressure rise to meet oxygen demands. Fatigue, dyspnea, and aching muscles follow shaking chills in febrile immunosuppressed cancer patients.

The next part of the paragraph emphasizes the *need* for the study and the proposed solution:

Interventions are needed that (1) promote heat loss, without inducing compensatory warming mechanisms; (2) promote energy conservation and restoration through rest and control of shivering, and (3) restabilize hypothalamic thermostatic control functions through rehydration and antipyretic drug therapy. Therefore, this study will test effectiveness of a structured protocol to modify thermoregulatory responses during various phases (chill, plateau, or defervescence) of the febrile episode by use of (1) nonpharmacological, scientifically based interventions to control chills and febrile shivering at the onset of temperature spikes and during warranted cooling procedures, (2) warmth, insulation, and convection control to reduce reactivation of chills during the "warm" phases of the febrile episode, and (3) a regimen of nonsteroidal antipyretic therapy and fluid restoration during the febrile episode.

Finally, the intent of the proposal becomes highly focused and specific as it ends with the aims. Each aim is elaborated with the appropriate hypothesis relating to it. The accepted abbreviation for hypothesis H is used with a subscript of its number:

Specific aims are to test the efficacy of a structured protocol during acute febrile episodes in PLWAs to:

1. Reduce frequency, severity, duration, and reactivation of shivering during fever episodes.
   H_1 **Febrile shivering episodes are less frequent, severe, and of shorter duration with extremity wraps than without.**
2. Reduce distress, chill perception, and fatigue associated with the chill phase of fever.
   H_2 **VAS distress, chill, and fatigue perceptions during chill phase of fever are less with extremity wraps than without.**
3. Influence cardiorespiratory indicators of exertion during febrile episodes.
   H_3 **Elevations of BP, RPP, and respiratory rate during febrile episodes are less with extremity wraps than without.**
4. Influence body temperature patterns and variability during febrile episodes.
   H_4 **Body temperature elevations are less severe and shorter with extremity wraps than without.**
5. Control shivering when aggressive cooling treatments are warranted.
   H_5 **Shivering activity is less frequent or severe during surface cooling with use of extremity wraps than without.**
6. Maintain body hydration during febrile episodes.
   H_6 **Skin and mucous membrane hydration and daily body weight are more stable with a fluid protocol than without.**

By leading into the purpose statement with your persuasive introduction, your reviewers will find it easier to see the logical link between the need and the solution (your proposal). This also means that the last thing they will read before leaving the page is the list of specific aims, their related hypotheses, and questions. All of the cited examples should appear on one page, which can be seen in Table 5-1.

Table 5-1 Example of an NIH Specific Aims Page

Specific Aims: Fever is one of the most common responses associated with human immunodeficiency virus (HIV) infection, acquired immunodeficiency syndrome (AIDS), and the opportunistic infections accompanying these conditions. Persons living with AIDS (PLWA) experience predictable symptoms with fever episodes, regardless of the infectious agent. Symptoms result from nonspecific and antigen-specific host mechanisms that combat invading microorganisms by activating antibacterial chemical secretion and neutrophil migration. Although T-cell and host immune functions are deranged by HIV infection, proinflammatory responses are activated through alternative complement pathways. Whether the cytokine-modulated effects related to fever hold immunostimulant benefits for PLWAs is controversial, but the negative effects are well recognized. Pyrogens stimulate hypermetabolic and proteolytic processes that expend oxygen, calories, and body water. In AIDS, these catabolic effects often affect an already compromised nutritional state. Fever is the highest predictor for malnutrition among risk factors in HIV disease. Subjectively fever symptoms are distressful, interfering with rest, comfort, and functional ability. While medical fever management is understandably concerned with control of the underlying infection with drugs, nursing fever management is directed at symptomatology, regardless of etiology. Goals are to maintain body temperature within a safe range, maintain and restore fluid balance, conserve energy, avoid fatigue, and promote thermal comfort during fever. Although nurses devote hundreds of hours daily to treatment and palliation of fever, methods of care have changed little over the past century. Nurses tend to monitor fever progress and follow pharmaceutical prescriptions strictly, while resorting to poorly justified nursing activities to cool the patient. Cooling sponge baths or fans are implemented without regard for expected physiologic responses. Effects of environmental temperature, patient hydration, and physical activity on febrile responses are seldom considered. Only recently have specific interventions for fever management been tested, and these have yet to find their way into nursing textbooks. Efforts to aggressively cool febrile patients by convective heat-exchange blankets and ice packs are counterproductive because they stimulate shivering and vasoconstriction. Compensatory warming responses generate and conserve heat, while increasing oxygen consumption 3–5 fold. Anemic, weak, and cachectic patients tolerate exertion of febrile shivering poorly, as respiratory rate, heart rate, and blood pressure rise to meet oxygen demands. Fatigue, dyspnea, and aching muscles follow shaking chills in febrile immunosuppressed cancer patients. Interventions are needed that 1) promote heat loss, without inducing compensatory warming mechanisms; 2) promote energy conservation and restoration through rest and control of shivering, and 3) restabilize hypothalamic thermostatic control functions through rehydration and antipyretic drug therapy. Therefore, this study will test effectiveness of a structured protocol to modify thermoregulatory responses during various phases (chill, plateau, or defervescence) of the febrile episode by use of 1) nonpharmacological, scientifically based interventions to control chills and febrile shivering at the onset of temperature spikes and during warranted cooling procedures, 2) warmth, insulation, and convection control to reduce reactivation of chills during the "warm" phases of the febrile episode, and 3) a regimen of nonsteroidal antipyretic therapy and fluid restoration during the febrile episode. Specific aims are to test the efficacy of a structured protocol during acute febrile episodes in PLWAs to:

1. reduce frequency, severity, duration, and reactivation of shivering during fever episodes.
   H_1 **Febrile shivering episodes are less frequent, severe, and of shorter duration with extremity wraps than without.**
2. reduce distress, chill perception, and fatigue associated with the chill phase of fever.
   H_2 **VAS distress, chill, and fatigue perceptions during chill phase of fever are less with extremity wraps than without.**
3. influence cardiorespiratory indicators of exertion during febrile episodes.
   H_3 **Elevations of BP, RPP, and respiratory rate during febrile episodes are less with extremity wraps than without.**
4. influence body temperature patterns and variability during febrile episodes.
   H_4 **Body temperature elevations are less severe and shorter with extremity wraps than without.**
5. control shivering when aggressive cooling treatments are warranted.
   H_5 **Shivering activity is less frequent or severe during surface cooling with use of extremity wraps than without.**
6. maintain body hydration during febrile episodes.
   H_6 **Skin and mucous membrane hydration and daily body weight are more stable with a fluid protocol than without.**

Source: Holtzclaw, 1994.

67

In summary, the goals of the research proposal should be of major significance in terms of the health of the people of the United States of America. Well-developed specific aims should logically follow your study goals and purpose and be clear, concise, attainable, and distinct from one another. A well-written Specific Aims section is crucial and should guide the research design and methods.

Background and Significance

The Background and Significance section connects your proposed study to what is known about the problem. It familiarizes the reviewer with the documented research findings about the problem and discusses your study in light of the existing knowledge. This is another area where logical flow is extremely important because the significance of your research will be determined by how it will confirm, refute, or fill a gap in what is currently known. It is important to convince the readers that this study is the next logical step based on the state of the science. It is also important to show how this research addresses a widespread or significant health concern. Linking your proposed research to national health objectives such as *Healthy People 2010* (see Appendix C) or a professional organization's research priorities will strengthen the likelihood of funding for the proposed research.

The Background and Significance section in NIH grants is where the review of *relevant literature* appears, including the conceptual or theoretical framework. Even if another grant application format calls for a section titled "Literature Review," this section should be written carefully to display the strengths or weaknesses of the existing knowledge. The review should be balanced, revealing evidence that both supports and disputes your proposed hypotheses. Be assured, that at least one of your grant reviewers will be familiar enough with the literature to find any existing evidence you might overlook. A well-written Background and Significance section displays your familiarity of the area and its underlying scientific base. Proposals use the review of relevant literature about the study's phenomenon of interest (e.g., pain) to inform the reviewer of how existing knowledge supports the study design, methods, or approach.

With today's emphasis on evidence-based practice, integrated reviews on specific topics lend support to a proposed area of study, intervention, or educational program. Systematic or integrated reviews available on the Internet include such databases as the Cochrane Collaborative, Vermont Oxford Database, or specific topic reviews such as the Joanna Briggs Institute for Evidence-Based Nursing and Midwifery. These databases are repositories for findings and reviews of different levels of research, but primarily contain randomized clinical control trials. The information available from these integrated reviews provides a strong foundation for your study's question, research plan, and Background and Significance sections of your grant application. You may find that your own search and integrated review of literature provides you a better tailor-made explanation of your study phenomenon. In either case, the literature reviewed to support your proposal should be both relevant and current. Move beyond simply summarizing the literature to critically evaluating existing knowledge and identifying gaps in the scientific evidence. After all, if the existing literature is complete and has no gaps or controversies, you will have a more difficult time justifying why your study is needed. Likewise, if you present only literature that supports your view, your reviewers may decide you are either biased or uninformed.

Conceptual Basis of the Research

All grant proposals must be defended by sound rationale. Reviewers will look for your study's scientific or conceptual underpinnings. Even theory-generating, qualitative, or naturalistic research is *informed* by the investigator's ideas or by the context in which it is studied in order to determine what, and under what conditions, is to be studied. In quantitative research, the conceptual links between variables, even the variables themselves, originate in the context of existing knowledge. If the study is quantitative with descriptive or manipulated variables, the idea for why you should be collecting them is driven by observed or theoretical connections. Conceptual frameworks may be highly formalized and "named," or they may be constructed logically from commonly accepted principles of psychology, physiology, physics, or other sciences. In any case, the conceptual basis for your proposed research should be stated clearly and identified and accompany the review of relevant literature. Once you have identified a conceptual model or theoretical basis for your questions, these concepts must be connected to your research plan. Grant reviewers will be looking for how the framework of your study drives or explains the relationships you are studying. Explain and clarify how the relevant concepts are empirically evidenced in your study. If a conceptual framework is used, it should be clearly tied to the present study but also well mapped to other parts of the application. A diagram of a conceptual framework is a visual way of demonstrating relationships that are known and relationships that have not been investigated and may be the focus of your study. Finally, the Background and Significance section should clearly support the specific aims of the study. The Background and Significance section is a reasoned argument that builds on your specific aims to justify the need and importance of your study. For example, if your study's conceptual framework is based on the Whole Person Suffering Model, each of the four areas (physical, psychological, spiritual, and social) should be addressed in the review of relevant literature.

Preliminary Studies

Depending on the specific format of your selected funding agency, you may not always have a specific section that allows you to showcase explicit evidence of your qualifications in the proposal itself. However, for NIH grant applications, the Preliminary Studies sections allows you to build a case that your earlier research and any preliminary findings have led you to the present investigation. Even if your grant format does not have a Preliminary Studies section, you can usually describe the contribution of earlier work to the proposed study by describing it in the background section or in justifying the methodology. Be sure to include any relevant information that highlights your qualifications to carry out the proposed study in your biographical sketch. Tailor your biographical sketch to highlight relevant accomplishments. These may not always be the same depending on the funding agency. Remember too that the grant proposal is a marketing piece to showcase how good you are and how you are the perfect person or team to carry out the work. This is not the time to be modest.

Research Design and Methods

The research plan is actually the "meat" of a research proposal and the Research Design and Methods section includes the methodological portion of the proposal. As such, it is the most critical component of the proposal. The research plan should be clear, concise, and cogent while at the same time containing sufficient information to evaluate the proposal. In NIH grants, the Research Design and Methods section includes the following subheadings:

- Design
- Setting and Sample (including inclusion/exclusion criteria and sample size justification)
- Intervention Protocols or Experimental Conditions (if relevant)
- Variables, Measurements, and Instruments
- Data Collection Procedures
- Data Analysis
- Study Timeline

These elements are discussed below.

Design

The research design is the "blueprint" or strategic plan that the researcher uses to accomplish the specific aims and answer or test the research questions and hypotheses. Research proposals should explicitly describe the design to be used. Depending on how complicated your plans are, your description may entail using a different approach for each of your specific aims.

There are several ways to categorize research design. In the past, most research methodology was categorized as either quantitative or qualitative. However, these terms are very nonspecific and primarily refer to the type of data rather than the actual research design. Tripp-Reimer and Kelley assert that the more accurate terms are *naturalistic* and *positivistic* designs in which qualitative or quantitative data are collected (2006). As new design strategies developed to meet unique research needs, textbooks and researchers began to use the terms *quantitative* and *qualitative* as *approaches* rather than designs.

In each global category (naturalistic, positivistic, qualitative, quantitative) there are more specific terms that fine-tune the approach and more completely inform the grant reviewer of the type of design you plan to use. In some situations, you will wish to examine a cross section of the population, correlating one variable with another to test one specific aim. In the same study you may wish to collect repeated measures of a variable over time to test another specific aim. Sometimes a researcher may wish to examine a phenomenon both quantitatively and qualitatively to meet the needs of a particular research study.

Quantitative Data

Quantitative data are analyzed using statistical methodology that focuses on counting or quantifying data by defining, measuring, and analyzing it. The research questions answered by this method are concerned with describing quantifiable attributes, finding relationships, causality between variables, and predicting outcomes. Statistics are used to summarize data, determine sampling error that could influence the findings, and to test hypotheses (Levine, 2006). The study design using quantitative data can be further classified by the terms *descriptive* or *observational, case, time sequenced* or *longitudinal, prospective, retrospective, experimental,* or *quasi-experimental*. The gold standard for experimental studies remains the randomized controlled trial (RCT), but in reality, most clinical studies use quasi-experimental designs, because the clinical situation makes it difficult to meet the three criteria for experimental research: (1) manipulation, (2) randomization, and (3) control. Quasi-experimental research may often lack a control group, random selection, random assignment, or active manipulation (Abraham & Wasserbauer, 2006). The fact that research subjects are free to refuse or withdraw from participation in a study limits randomization considerably.

Qualitative Data

Qualitative data collected by naturalistic approaches are used to describe the nature or meaning of "what is" according to the person or phenomenon being studied. Six characteristics characterize the work of qualitative researchers:

(1) a belief in multiple realities; (2) a commitment to identifying an approach to understanding that supports the phenomenon studied; (3) a commitment to the participant's

point of view; (4) the conduct of inquiry in a way that limits disruption of the natural context of the phenomena of interest; (5) acknowledged participation of the researcher in the research process; and (6) the reporting of the data in a literary style rich with participant commentaries (Speziale & Carpenter, 2007, p. 21).

The most often used approaches to collecting qualitative data include ethnography, grounded theory, and phenomenology. However, case study methods, hermeneutics, oral histories, and critical, philosophical, and historical approaches to inquiry are emerging, along with their own set of undergirding philosophies, theoretical perspectives, and approaches for collecting and analyzing data (Tripp-Reimer & Kelley, 2006). Naturalistic research seeks an in-depth understanding of a phenomenon that pays particular attention to its contextual nature. The *inductive* characteristics of this type of research often yield rich data that inform science about the meaning of a situation. A comparison of characteristics of studies dealing with quantitative and qualitative data is seen in Table 5-2.

It is beyond the scope of this book to provide detailed descriptions of design methodologies. Each design has a different goal, and the best design for your study is the one that flows logically from the problem statement, literature review, theoretical framework, and research question or hypothesis. The choice of a research design is a major research decision because each requires familiarity and skills with its unique data collection, data management, and analytic approaches. With these ideas in mind, the strongest research design feasible should be used to maximize the credibility and dependability of the study findings. In addition, the selection of cred-

Table 5-2   Comparison of Qualitative and Quantitative Research Methods

Quantitative	Qualitative
Objective	Subjectivity value
One reality	Multiple realities
Reduction, control, prediction	Discovery, description, understanding
Measurable	Interpretive
Mechanistic	Organismic
Parts equal the whole	Whole is greater than the parts
Report statistical analyses	Report rich narrative
Researcher separate	Researcher part of research process
Subjects	Participants
Context free	Context dependent

Source: Speziale and Carpenter, 2007. Reproduced by permission from Lippincott, Williams & Wilkins.

ible and capable consultants to help you navigate your chosen research design will strengthen the research grant proposal.

Examples of both qualitative and quantitative research data were used in Kenner's study "Transition to Home." She first wanted to find out, "What was it like for a mother taking a baby home from a neonatal unit?" "What concerns or problems did the mothers have during the first and fourth weeks at home with the baby?" and finally "What could we have done differently at the hospital to ease the transition to home?" She used a phenomenological approach to gather these data, gathering qualitative data in three different settings. From these data she developed a transition questionnaire based on the five categories of concern that evolved from the qualitative studies. The transition questionnaire was a quantifiable tool used to measure the phenomenon of transition. While she was still concerned with the three original research questions, Kenner then used the transition questionnaire to quantify the mothers' responses.

Once the research design is chosen, the researcher should clearly describe the design and methods as well as the rationale for selection. In many studies, a quasi-experimental design is chosen over a stronger true experimental design because of the inability to physically or ethically manipulate certain variables. These variables include such elements as overall environmental lighting, the heating level within an incubator, or responses to prescribed medications.

The researcher should articulate other designs that were considered and the rationale for why the proposed research design is superior to alternate designs. For example, instead of a clinical trial with an experimental and control group, a repeated measures design, where patients serve as their own control, may be justified by the ability to control for possible contamination by variability between participants. In use of a crossover design, this same justification is used, but with the added benefit of controlling for *order effects* by having half the subjects exposed to an intervention and half in the control group, then switching the groups to the opposite condition (treatment/control). If a third trial is used, the groups are switched back to the original condition. In a study of the efficacy of wrapping extremities to prevent drug-induced febrile shivering, Holtzclaw used a crossover model (see Figure 5-3). Although the strength of this model was the control for subject variability between treatment and control conditions and the control for order effects, the design was not without limitations. This design required a 10-day "washout" period to remove any carryover effects of the intervention and involved the participation of each participant in the study for a longer period of time. Each of these limitations was anticipated and justified in the proposal.

Clearly state the assumptions and limitations of the proposed research. If problems are anticipated, possible solutions or strategies should be discussed to minimize their occurrence. For example, in longitudinal studies, subject attrition is expected, and the principal investigator should include a discussion of strategies to maintain subject participation over time.

Figure 5-3   Crossover Design

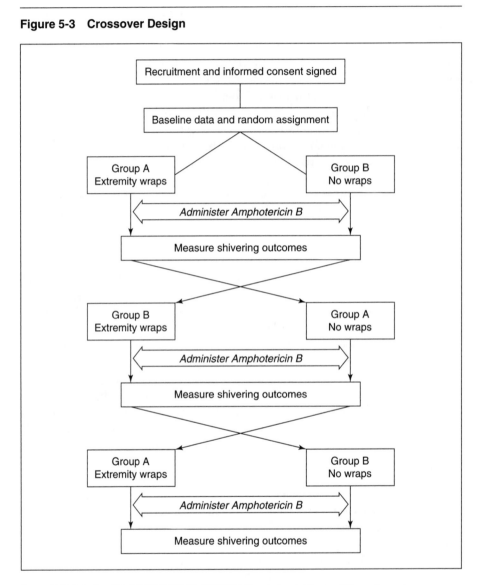

Source: B. J. Holtzclaw, P.I., NIH/NCNR R01 NR01890. Drug induced shivering: Effects of a nursing measure.

Setting and Sample

Provide a description of the setting chosen for the study along with the rationale for its selection. Describe in detail the type of setting, location, and typical patient population. Selection of this particular setting over other possible ones must be specifically stated and convincing. Furthermore, if you select a distant site instead of a local site, it is important that you provide a rationale for that decision. Address how distance will affect data collection and quality of data collection methods. For instance, the grant writer may describe a plan for the selection of a site coordinator employed by the clinical agency or one who lives close to the site as a strategy to handle the issue of distance. The proposal must also address plans for ensuring appropriate training and reliability of research assistants, and it must address plans to monitor the site to ensure the integrity of data collection methods. Finally, the researcher must document that the research site is willing to provide the researcher with access to subjects. This is usually best accomplished by submitting letters of support from key personnel at the study site such as the medical director, nursing director, or other applicable administrative personnel. If you have chosen a study site in a hospital, clinic, educational institution, or organizational setting, you should anticipate the need to show entrée, access, or permission to use that site. In many grant proposals, including NIH applications, reviewers will be looking for letters of agreement or approval to conduct the study in these sites.

Clearly describe the criteria for inclusion and exclusion of subjects in the study (see example in Appendix D). Depending on the space available in the grant application, the grant writer must describe more fully why these criteria were selected and how they help control for threats to external validity. In addition, the researcher has an obligation to convince the reviewer of the adequacy of the site to produce a sufficient number of subjects based on inclusion and exclusion criteria. To address this issue, include in narrative text or table format the number of subjects available per month or year for study at the data collection site who meet the inclusion criteria. In addition to the number of subjects, federal grants now require that the principal investigator address the recruitment of special populations, including gender and racial and ethnic groups as well as women and children. Federal grants also require a completed Targeted/Planned Enrollment Table (see "Inclusion of Women, Children, and Minorities" section below).

The sample size of the proposed study is also important to emphasize. As we discussed in Chapter 2, a power analysis should be performed to justify the proposed sample size. The power estimate will justify the sample size needed to avoid drawing a conclusion with findings that occurred by chance alone. For a grant proposal, reviewers will want to know the factors you have considered in arriving at that number. That is, you must make clear the *level of significance*, the *desired power*, and the *expected effect size* used in the power analysis. Because the calculated *p* value of your findings reflects the probability that a significant finding occurred by chance *alone*, the level of significance (*p* value) is usually set at less than .05 (the lower the *p* value, the lower the likelihood the finding happened by chance). The power estimate and significance criterion is set a priori (before beginning the study). Base the sample size on the most conservative number needed to answer the research question or hypothesis being proposed. For example, if you plan to use both hierarchical regression and repeated measures ANOVA statistical analyses in your study, base your sample size on the number needed to achieve the desired power for *each* of the analyses. The researcher should also discuss how sample size is adjusted to account for subject attrition. For example, in a previous pilot study, if 15% attrition was noted due to mortality of subjects, the sampling plan was adjusted to oversample by 15%.

Sample selection strategies and group assignment protocols should be explained. Two groups of sampling techniques used in nursing research are probability (random) sampling and nonprobability (nonrandom) sampling. Random sampling techniques are preferred and result in more representative samples; nonprobability sampling techniques are more feasible, practical, and economical. Variations on *simple random sampling* include *stratified random sampling, cluster sampling,* and *systematic sampling.* All of these strategies depend on having access to all members of a given population from which the sample will be drawn. Although random sampling is difficult to achieve in clinical settings, *random assignment* to groups is often easily accomplished. Subjects can be randomly assigned to treatment conditions by using such methods as flipping a coin, pulling slips from a hat, or more commonly, a table of random numbers.

Nonprobability sampling is frequently used in beginning studies because individuals are found in the situation or location that is accessible. The *convenience sample,* also called *accidental* or *incidental sample,* is an example where participants are included because they happen to be there and because there is generally less cost involved in finding them. The biases possible with such sampling should be recognized, and any anticipated influence on study outcomes acknowledged. For example, possible biases influencing an intervention study may be linked to the likelihood of greater motivation among people who volunteer for studies.

Intervention Protocols or Experimental Conditions

If an intervention or experimental study is proposed, the grant proposal should clearly describe the intervention protocol and the rationale supporting the expected outcome. Describe how the intervention is administered in detail. Include how the treatment condition differs from the control or comparison group. For major grants, pilot testing of the intervention is expected prior to the grant. All NIH grants will expect some preliminary work supporting an intervention, even for a pilot study. However, some foundations and granting agencies accept proposals for early pilot work if sufficient evidence from the literature or observations shows a strong possibility an intervention might be effective. Once the pilot is completed, the data form the foundation for larger, more competitive grants. If your research proposal does not involve an intervention protocol, this section is omitted.

An example of an intervention protocol is found in Holtzclaw's HIV symptom management study testing the efficacy of extremity wraps to prevent febrile shivering:

Intervention Protocol: The treatment condition for this study involves the use of warmth, insulation, and protection from sensed heat loss throughout the febrile period, while allowing heat excesses to be lost from areas that do not trigger warming responses. All subjects have documented HIV infection and abrupt temperature elevations indicating fever "spike" (> 1°C within 1 hour). The control group is monitored without the extremity wraps. Wraps are applied to the treatment group according to the following protocol:

1. Apply monitoring electrodes, blood pressure cuff, and temperature probes prior to wrapping procedures.
2. Place three bath towels lengthwise under each arm. Bring up lateral edges of towels to form a seam. Secure with plastic clips along seam. Allow intravenous lines, monitor leads, and blood pressure tubing to exit along seam. Roll up excess toweling at fingertips to form a "mitten." Secure with tape.
3. Place three bath towels lengthwise under each leg. Bring up lateral edges of towels to form a seam. Secure with plastic clips along seam. Allowing monitor leads to exit along seam. Roll up excess toweling at toes to form a "boot." Secure with tape.
4. Take care to avoid overlapping excess toweling against extremity in order to maintain consistency of insulation.
5. Do not allow towels to remain damp. If sweating is excessive or towels become damp, replace quickly with warmed towels causing as little exposure or air movement as possible. Note time and length of exposure on the record.

Variables, Measurements, and Instruments

The researcher should provide operational definitions for each of the independent and dependent variables within the proposed study. Study variables can also be clarified in a table format that matches each of the independent and dependent variables to a particular instrument or subscale on an instrument. For pen and pencil questionnaires, describe the population, method of administration, reliability, and validity for each instrument used. For scientific devices, provide information as to the accuracy, precision, range, and reliability. Specialized devices and laboratory assays may have specific qualities, such as collection condition, temperature, and linearity requirements. *Variables* are logically associated with the *instruments* used to measure them in a research study. If space is at a premium in your grant application, it may be to your advantage to deal with them together by stating the variable, its measurement modality, and the company or author of the instrument. However, if specifications of the instruments are complex, you may need to operationalize each variable, ascribing its measurement modality, but follow with a detailed separate section called Instruments.

The following example uses separate variable and instrument sections:

Variables: The following independent variables are under study: The *independent variable* in each case is the study protocol implemented at the fever onset. Contained in the protocol are: (1) *documented fever spike* measured by a $\geq 1°C$ rise in temperature within 1 hour, (2) *insulative extremity wraps* to protect dominant heat loss skin sensors in arms, legs, hands and feet (see Tables 1 and 2), and (3) *warm liquids* given in metered amounts, in insulated cups, and (4) *acetaminophen* 650 mg given every 4 hours for temperature > 39°C. The *dependent variables* to be measured are: (1) *shivering* measured for onset by prototypic phasic masseter EMG signals, for *severity* by an ordinal scale 0–4, and actigraph signal on the multichannel monitor indicating extremity involvement, and *duration* by timing from onset to end with a stopwatch. *Chill perception* and *thermal distress* will be measured on two separate visual analog scales measuring these related, but different subjective responses to sensed changes in temperature. *Fatigue* will also be measured by visual analog scale. *Heart rate* will be monitored by the multi-channel monitor, as will *skin temperatures* and *aural canal* temperatures. *Blood pressure* will be measured by battery-powered automatic self-inflating blood pressure cuff and recorded by the observer. *Respiratory rate* will also be a variable observed by the data collector. *Core temperature* will be measured from the tympanic membrane by a handheld infrared light reflectance thermometer by the data collector. *Water loss* will be measured by 24 hours *weight loss*, by *observed sweating severity* on an ordinal scale, and by *dehydration severity* on an ordinal scale.

Instruments and Data Collection Procedures: Shivering stages will be measured on an ordinal *severity scale* of 0–4, with each stage representing extension of shivering to progressively larger muscle groups. Based on work by Hemingway, that demonstrated shivering follows a cephalad to caudal progression, with earliest hard-to-detect tremors beginning in the masseters, and most violent shivering including the extremities, a scale has been refined by Abbey and adapted for nursing studies. In the inpatient setting, stages will be verified by the following:

0 = No shivering activity. Absence of phasic bursts on EMG and no palpable or visible muscle fasciculation found by nurse observer.
1 = Masseter contractions measured by EMG and nursing observations. Light touch over mandibular angle reveals vibration to fingertips of examiner. This hard-to-detect tremor precedes shivering and any significant effects on oxygen consumption.
2 = Face and neck contractions observed by investigator. In clinical studies, this stage was accompanied by significant increases in metabolic rate and oxygen consumption.

3 = Pectoral contractions extend to abdomen, palpation of abdomen reveals involvement of lower trunk, extremity movement is *passive* (assessed by grasping elbow and wrist).

4 = Generalized shivering, measured by nursing observations of generalized rigor and bed shaking contractions, teeth chattering. Signaled by actigraph on the multichannel monitor. Described as the highest muscle involvement in shivering. Extremities *actively* contract.

Electromyogram (EMG): Nursing observations and EMG monitoring will be continuous. Onset and stage 1 will be verified by masseter EMG activity. Although implanted needle electrodes are more sensitive, they are rejected for use with immunosuppressed patients because they penetrate skin and subject patients to infection and/or bleeding. Disadvantages of surface electrodes include lack of discrimination between muscles and lack of sensitivity in measuring activity levels in deep or small muscles. Interference from electrical environment is also problematic. Surface measurements are satisfactory, however, when general information about onset and severity of shivering is required, particularly when the patient is under bedclothes. For maximum sensitivity, electrodes will be placed as close as possible to the middle of the muscle belly. Shivering activity has been noted to differ from artifact or purposive movement in its pattern and amplitude of EMG recordings. Short phasic bursts in the 100–500 microvolt range characterize masseter contractions during shivering. A portable electromyogram designed specifically for facial muscle contractions (Myotronics, Inc., Seattle) will be used at the bedside. Data are collected via a Dolch portable microcomputer at the bedside. The software package captures EMG tracings over time, averages signals every 15 seconds, and graphs every 30 seconds. The event marker allows recording of other phenomenon occurring at any given point in time. Involvement of extremities in shivering will also be assessed by means of the *movement actigraph*, a motion sensitive wristband device attached to the Mini Logger II multichannel monitor.

<u>Temperature measurement</u>: *Core temperature* will be measured by infrared light reflectance tympanic membrane (TM) thermometer (Genius; Intelligent Medical Systems, Carlsbad, CA). This nonintrusive measurement is safe, rapid, and found accurate within .1°C and accurate up to 40.5°C in vitro in our preliminary work. During training for previous studies, in vivo inter-rater and intra-rater reliability was within .1°C after training to use the device with ear tug and "otoscope" approach. Continuous temperature monitoring with the Mini Logger II will record three sites of skin temperature and *aural canal temperature*, on separate channels for storage in computerized memory that can be later downloaded to the investigator's microcomputer. Disposable temperature probes (YSI 400, Yellow Springs, OH) with self-adhering contacts will be applied to the lateral thigh, approximately half the distance between knee and hip joints. *Heart rate* (HR) will also be obtained by cardiac monitor from another channel on the Mini Logger II. Self-adhering silver/silver chloride electrodes will be applied to the chest, and a flexible chest band applied to maintain contact. HR will be used with *blood pressure*, obtained from the automatic, battery-powered, oscillometric blood pressure cuff (Dynamap, Critikon, Tampa, FL) to calculate *rate pressure product* (RPP). RPP provides

an indirect estimate of myocardial oxygen consumption and cardiac effort. The *Mini Logger II* multichannel unit combines temperature, activity, and heart rate monitoring capability into a single compact unit. The unit is a refinement of the Mini Logger I, adding heart rate and an event marker. The basic unit has been a reliable, accurate, and rugged instrument for use in the field. The temperature units can be verified by water bath calibration to confirm accuracy (Appendix H). *Body water loss* will be measured by three criteria: (1) Physical assessment of skin moisture and turgor, (2) eyeball depression by gentle touch, and (3) dry tongue will be used to rate dehydration on an ordinal scale of 1 to 10, with 10 being extremely desiccated and 0 being well hydrated. *Sweating severity* will be rated on a 0–4 ordinal scale, with 0 = dry to touch, 1 = moist to touch, 2 = beads of sweat on brow and upper lip, 3 = sweat running down face and neck and spotting clothing, and 4 = clothes saturated with sweat. *Body weight* will be measured every day at the same time on a clinical balance scale. *Visual Analog Scales* (VAS): (Appendix H) will be administered by the investigator and include *thermal perception* (TP-VAS), meaning whether a person feels warm or cold, and *thermal comfort* (TC-VAS) meaning how comfortable a person is at that temperature. Subjects are asked to mark on a 100 mm line, bounded on each end by a descriptor. For thermal perception, the descriptors are "as cold as possible" and "as hot as possible" respectively. For thermal comfort the descriptors are "intense discomfort" on one end and "extreme comfort" on the other. The scale is scored by measuring the distance in millimeters from 0 at the cold end to the patient's mark, somewhere between 0 and 100 mm. VAS have been used in assessing a variety of subjective states. This scale was found to have construct validity and criterion validity with extant measures of thermal comfort used by environmental engineers *Fatigue* will be measured by the VAS for Fatigue (VAS-F) developed by Lee, Hicks, and Nino-Murcia. It is a VAS with 18 items (see Appendix H) with fatigue and energy subscales. It was found a valid and reliable VAS for normal and patient populations.

Justifying Alternate Instruments.   If alternate instruments are available or more traditionally used, the applicant will need to discuss the rationale for the selection of a particular instrument. A sample rationale for studying pain from an R15 application follows (Walden, 2001).

Pain research has produced several valid and reliable pain instruments, including the CRIES (Krechel and Bildner, 1995) and the Premature Infant Pain Profile (Stevens [et al., 1996).] While the CRIES has been validated for use in infants greater than 32 weeks gestational age, the PIPP can be used in preterm infants below 28 weeks gestational age. Furthermore, the PIPP is preferred over the CRIES in this study as it controls for two significant contextual factors (gestational age and behavioral state) known to modify pain expression in preterm neonates (Craig et al. 1993; Grunau and Craig 1987; Johnston et al. 1993; Stevens and Johnston 1994; Stevens, Johnston, and Horton 1994; Stevens et al. 1993; Johnston et al. 1999). The PIPP will be used to measure acute pain response in this study.

Describe any necessary training of research personnel in the use of each instrument. The researcher should report pilot data or if any is planned for new instruments. Finally, include copies of all instruments in an appendix.

Data Collection Procedures

The description of study procedures usually begins with a clear description of how potential subjects are identified and recruited as participants into the study. This is often followed by a clear description of how and when the intervention will be carried out. Provide the method of data collection and how often measurements are recorded. Include aspects of how, when, where, and who uses the instruments. If other study personnel are involved in data collection, a description of their training should be included. Describe the methods used to ensure inter-rater reliability. The researcher should address any potential problems that may be encountered during the study protocol and include the plan for how the problems will be addressed. If the study is complex, a step-by-step procedural checklist should be developed and used by data collectors to ensure that no procedural item is omitted during the course of the study (see Appendix D). If a checklist is used to simplify data collection procedures, include this checklist as an appendix for the reviewers to examine.

Finally, use diagrams of the data collection procedure to clarify the study design and timing of data collection for study instruments. For example, the diagram below (Figure 5-4) was used to illustrate the data collection procedures for the variables contained in the pain study (Walden, 2001).

Figure 5-4   Data Collection Protocol

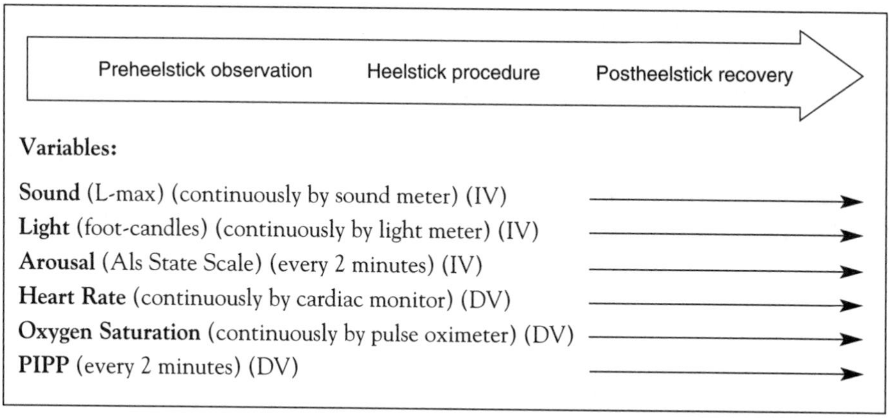

Notes: IV = independent variable; DV = dependent variable
    Sample: gestational age groups: 25–27 weeks (n = 51), 34–36 weeks (n = 51).

Data Analyses

This section should provide a clear description of plans for data management, refinement, and reduction. Proposals often adequately address the plans for statistical analyses but fail to provide sufficient detail on how large complex data sets will be reduced for analyses. The researcher should therefore take great care to describe how data will be collated, coded, keyed, and verified.

Base the selection of the statistical analyses on the level and type of data. Furthermore, the statistical analyses should match the specific aims and research questions or hypotheses. Organizing the presentation of data in this section by specific research question or hypothesis is often helpful for both the grant writer and reviewer. Constructing a table that shows each aim and its related hypothesis, the variables and instruments to measure them, the level of measurement for each variable, and the statistical test for each hypothesis, is an excellent way to organize this presentation. The principal investigator is wise to include a statistician on the research team. Involve the statistician early to assist with the development of the statistical plan of the study, including design, analyses, and plan for dissemination of project findings. Often, a biostatistician has the best knowledge and expertise to write the data analysis section of a proposal that involves biological assays, unusual statistics (such as those used in circadian rhythm measurements or genetics), or covariates of various variables (see the Sample Research Plan for examples of data analyses).

Study Timeline

The timeline is used to provide an anticipated time frame for project activities including start-up activities such as hiring and training of project personnel, identification of subjects, data collection, data preparation and analysis, and report writing. Be realistic in your time frame; projects always take longer than you expect. It is better to project a longer period of time for a certain aspect of the grant, say the hiring of personnel, so that you will have some extra time when other aspects of the grant take longer than expected. This information can be provided in narrative form, or the grant writer may choose to present this section in the form of a timeline table. Timelines can be simple with broad categories of activities listed (see Figure 5-5), or they can show phases and changes in personnel mandated by a more complicated study.

REFERENCES

The references, or Literature Cited section, is the final part of your research plan and contains references to journal articles, books, and other materials that you have cited in your grant proposal. Check for any inaccuracies and correct them. Reviewers

Figure 5-5   Timeline for a 3-Year Grant

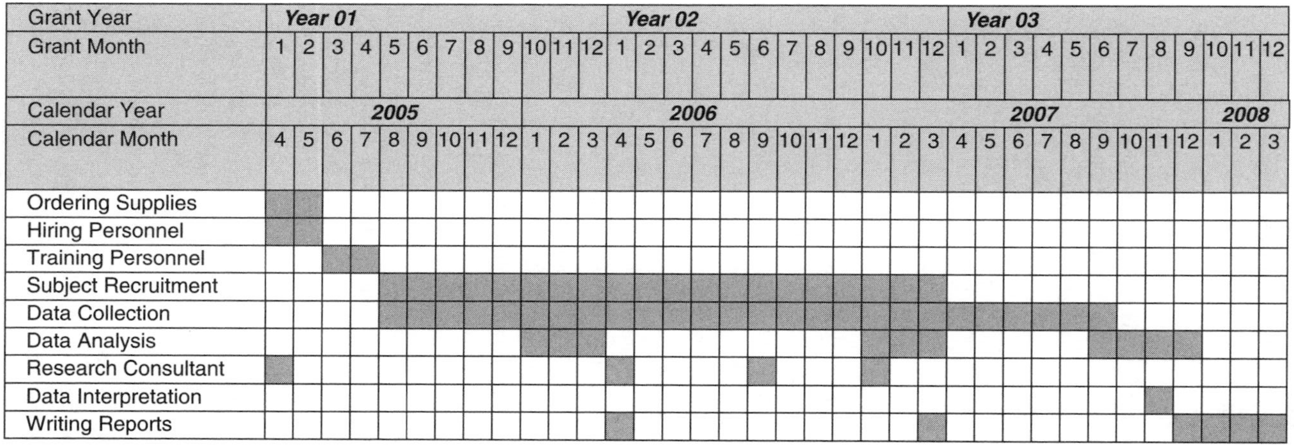

Grant Year	Year 01												Year 02												Year 03											
Grant Month	1	2	3	4	5	6	7	8	9	10	11	12	1	2	3	4	5	6	7	8	9	10	11	12	1	2	3	4	5	6	7	8	9	10	11	12
Calendar Year	2005												2006												2007									2008		
Calendar Month	4	5	6	7	8	9	10	11	12	1	2	3	4	5	6	7	8	9	10	11	12	1	2	3	4	5	6	7	8	9	10	11	12	1	2	3
Ordering Supplies																																				
Hiring Personnel																																				
Training Personnel																																				
Subject Recruitment																																				
Data Collection																																				
Data Analysis																																				
Research Consultant																																				
Data Interpretation																																				
Writing Reports																																				

83

may actually seek and retrieve literature you cite in order to verify your interpretation. Be sure to check the URL links on any references you have retrieved from the Internet. These sometimes change or become inactive between the time you accessed them and the time you prepare your proposal. Complete bibliographic information should be provided using a consistent referencing format, such as the American Psychological Association (APA) style. If you have used a superscript style reference format such as that required by the *Journal of the American Medical Association*, your reference list will be numbered in the exact order the references appeared in your proposal. This method saves you much-needed space in the proposal and is a favorite among NIH grant applicants.

BUDGET

The first important task in creating a budget for the proposal is to review the funding agency's budget criteria closely. The funding agency usually specifies what expenses are allowable and what is not fundable. For example, some grants will not allow for the salary of the principal investigator but will allow salary dollars allocated for consultants and research assistants. Some federal grants do not allow for travel costs related to dissemination, while others may. Foundation grants typically do not pay as high a rate of facilities and administrative (F&A) (also known as indirects) costs as federal grants. In fact, some pay none at all. If you are in an academic institution, part of your preparation for applying for a foundation grant will be to clarify F&A questions and possibly negotiate a waiver of the established institutional rate. If this is not possible, you will need to pay these administrative costs out of your grant budget. It is therefore extremely important to have a clear idea about the funding guidelines before you start to develop your budget for the proposal.

If you are in an academic center, there may be a research offices with personnel specifically trained to assist you in preparing the budget. The highly experienced staff in these offices can help you obtain salary information, benefit costs, cost of common budget items such as equipment, computers, pagers, mileage, and other costs. Salaries often are the largest budget item. For all persons listed on the grant, indicate the percentage of commitment to the grant and their salary and fringe benefits. The budget office will assist you in computing indirect costs and setting up subcontracts with other institutions.

Clearly match budget items to grant activities (research personnel, consultants, equipment, supplies, travel, computer costs, and other related expenses). The goal is to ask for what you need to conduct the study. Most funding agencies will require a budget justification for grant expenses. Budget justification is a specific description of each of the budget items requested and a rationale for why this expense is needed. Appropriate budget planning will help you to budget appropriately while avoiding the tendency to pad the budget. Although money often can shift within the same category of the budget, often the budget will not allow shifting of monies between categories such as salary dollars and equipment costs. Therefore, carefully consider where the monies are allocated within the budget.

Federal agencies often use a modular budget process for grant applications requesting up to $250,000 in direct costs per year. For these applications, total direct costs for the proposed study typically are divided into modules of $25,000. Although a standard modular grant application will request the same number of modules in each year of the grant, additional narrative budget justification provides a mechanism for researchers to request variation in the number of modules requested. For example, if the grant involves the purchase of expensive physiologic data acquisition equipment, the principal investigator may want to provide additional budget narrative to explain an increased number of modules for the first year of the grant.

The "cost of doing business" in carrying out a project of any kind often gets too little attention. As a result, there is sometimes a mismatch between what you need and what you've requested. It is never a good idea to skimp on the budget with the notion that it makes the grant more fundable. The contrary is true. Grant reviewers will likely see that you have no idea of how much support it takes to carry out the proposed work. On the other hand, reviewers are on guard for attempts to pad a budget. Salaries are likely to be the highest expenditure on extramural grant budgets, and principal investigators will often cut corners on their own salary in order to include colleagues as co-investigators or include travel to meetings to present their work. This is foolhardy and can jeopardize your review. If you are funded with such poor planning, you will find that your work is not compensated for in your budget. Map out the chores to be done on the grant, and figure as closely as possible how much time it will take you and your team to carry out the work. Request salary support for this amount and provide the rationale for each.

Budgeting salaries for smaller federal proposals, such as R03 and R15 grants, takes careful consideration. Salaries can take up much of a modular budget with a maximum allowable budget cap. Therefore, it is prudent to not allocate personnel when they are not needed. For example, if you are collecting samples that can be frozen for a laboratory assay, you could hire a lab tech near the end of the study. If you are using research assistants to collect data, you would not need their services during the last few months of the study when reports and analytic interpretation take place. These time-limited salaried positions can be shown clearly on your grant timeline and the rationale included in the budget justification.

Another misconception of novice researchers is that the indirect costs that are associated with the grant are taken out of the regular grant budget. The reality in many situations is that these are funds "on top" of the grant budget and are designed to cover operating or overhead costs. The amount or percentage of indirect costs is determined by the funding agency and the researcher's institution. There are some funding agencies that will not pay indirect costs, and this must be negotiated with the employing institution. Not all institutions will encourage researchers to apply for funds when no indirects are possible. For example at the University of Oklahoma the researcher must complete an "Exceptions" form that is signed by the College dean and then forwarded for signature of the vice president for research at the health sciences campus for any College of Nursing grants.

Finally, remember to update the budget as revisions are made throughout the grant-writing process to ensure the consistency of the proposal to funding requested. For example, if the sample size changes and thus the amount of time needed to pay a research assistant changes, adjust the budget to reflect these changes (see Appendix D).

HUMAN SUBJECTS CONSIDERATIONS

Human Welfare Protection

This grant section should provide a clear description of procedures for protecting subjects' rights and obtaining informed consent. Discuss measures to protect anonymity or confidentiality related to data collection, management, and storage. Identify potential risks and anticipated benefits of the study. Fully describe potential risks, measures to minimize those risks, and institutional resources available to treat clients who develop health-related complications that arise as a result of the study. Indicate whether the institutional review board (IRB) approval process is complete or pending.

Institutional Review Board Approvals

An IRB is a panel of health professionals across disciplines and at least one or two consumers. This panel is charged with reviewing any protocol that will be part of a research study involving humans. The IRB must ensure scientific merit and protection of human subjects. The IRB must question whether or not a study is ethical or not in relationship to protection of human subjects. For example, many years ago prisoners were used in studies to determine how infectious diseases progressed. These studies were later deemed unethical because a captive population was used. Prisoners were probably coerced into participating, and they were not informed of potential life-threatening dangers. Today an IRB would prevent this study from taking place. The IRB exists strictly to protect a person's rights and safety in any research study. IRB approval is an expectation for any grant award, and in most institutions studies are not allowed, even as staff projects, without IRB approval. The IRB reviews informed consent forms. The forms must be written at a low reading level (ideally third grade, but no higher than fifth or sixth grade), understandable to the population being tested, and in most instances translated into the population's native language. Protection of human subjects and disclosure of the intervention are important aspects of this process.

Timing of IRB Approvals

Beginning June 1, 2000, the NIH changed its requirement for IRB approval prior to submission of federal grant applications. Today, IRB approval is not required prior to NIH peer review of an application. Because fewer than half of all applications submitted to NIH are funded, the policy was modified to reduce the burden on applicants and submitting institutions. However, no grant award can be made without IRB approval. Applicants and research institutional offices have online access to their peer review scores and approval progress through the NIH electronic Research Administration Commons. Therefore, following NIH peer review and notification of priority score/percentile, institutions should proceed with IRB review for those applications that have not yet received IRB approval and that appear to be in a fundable range.

NIH Policies Affecting Human Subjects

Some of the significant changes affecting NIH grant applications have been in the area of human subjects. Legislation and policies that protect and allow more inclusiveness have created new section headings, review criteria, and oversight. It is therefore prudent to review these policies and grant application forms at the NIH Web site (http://www.nih.gov) to determine if you have the latest information. Your office of research administration will also be helpful in directing you to recently emerging new policies. Below are several changes that are already in effect.

Data Safety and Monitoring Plan

In 1998, NIH issued a policy stating that any research involving a clinical trial or intervention must have provision for data and safety monitoring to protect participants from physical and psychological injury or violations of privacy. Monitoring should be commensurate with size and complexity of the project. This means that a smaller project could be monitored by individuals or a committee, and a large multi-site project would engage a national committee. The complexity of a large phase III clinical trial requires an independent data and safety monitoring. If your study does not entail a clinical trial or test of an intervention, state so in this section of your grant application. However, it is also prudent to add that you are monitoring the progress of the study for adverse events and have a plan of action to address such possibilities. Describe the mechanism for reporting adverse events to the IRB, the Food and Drug Administration (FDA), and NIH program official responsible for the grant. Finally, include in your proposal your plans for ensuring data accuracy and study protocol compliance.

Inclusion of Women, Children, and Minorities

During the past two decades, it has become clear to the scientific community that most clinical research findings have been based on studies of adult white males. As more evidence emerged about genetic and gender-based differences in response to therapy, it became clear that treatment responses based upon research done on one population subgroup might lead to poor treatment choices in other groups. Today several groups—women, children, and minorities—are actively included in all NIH-funded studies, unless their exclusion is scientifically justified. The cost of including these groups is not considered an adequate reason for exclusion. If inclusion is expected to be difficult, a plan for recruitment is required.

In 1993, the NIH Revitalization Act wrote into law measures ensuring that women and members of minority groups are included as subjects in each project of clinical research. Amendments to this legislation were made in 2001 to clarify when and for what purpose modifications can be made. It remains the policy of the NIH that women and members of minority groups and their subpopulations must be included in all NIH-funded clinical research, unless a clear and compelling rationale and justification establishes to the satisfaction of the relevant NIH institute/center director that such inclusion is inappropriate with respect to the health of the subjects or the purpose of the research. Exceptions are frequently requested to study a disorder (e.g., prostate disease or ovarian cancer) that is specific to one gender, or to study problems that are specific to a subpopulation.

An NIH policy on inclusion of children in clinical research was developed in 1998 because medical treatments applied to children were too often based upon adult testing. The tendency to exclude children from research studies meant that their treatment was not scientifically evaluated for their age or development. The policy states that children (persons under the age of 21) must be included in all human subjects research, conducted or supported by the NIH, unless there are scientific and ethical reasons not to include them.

Targeted/Planned Enrollment Table. To facilitate your completing the section on inclusion of women and minorities, a "Targeted/Planned Enrollment Table" is required in a section of your NIH grant dealing with recruitment. Your planned enrollment should be based on some scientific approach, whether it is to try and duplicate the proportions of each minority category in a region or to ensure an equal number in a comparative study. There must first be a *plan* to include the targeted individuals (recruitment strategies, inclusion of additional sites if necessary, targeting minority agencies). Then your table should reflect that plan. All your planned participants are first divided into ethnic categories by gender. Ethnic categories in the table are (1) Hispanic and Latino, and (2) not Hispanic or Latino. Participants are then divided into racial categories by gender. Racial categories are (1) American Indian/Alaska Native, (2) Asian, (3) Native Hawaiian or other Pacific Islander, (4) Black or African-American, and (5) White. Done correctly, you will have the same totals in each category division.

ANIMAL WELFARE PROTECTION

Applications that involve research with animals go through a different ethical review process by an organization's institutional animal care and use committee (IACUC). This committee is as rigorous and concerned about animal welfare as the IRB is about the welfare of humans. Newer guidelines from the NIH ask applicants to check "Yes" to the question "Is the IACUC review pending?" even if the IACUC review/approval process has not yet begun at the time of submission. Even though an IACUC approval date is not required at the time of submission, this and other information may be requested later in the pre-award cycle. Because getting IACUC approval requires steps of training and review, it is prudent to submit the review request in a timely manner to avoid any delay in the grant review and award process. Just as the IRB approval must precede any research funding concerning humans, no grant award for animal research can take place unless IACUC approval is made.

APPENDICES

Appendices supplement key information contained within the research plan. Depending on the funding agency, not all accept appendices. In addition, all reviewers at the discussion table may not receive appendices. Ensure that both the abstract as well as the research plan include all pertinent information by which the scientific quality of the proposed study is to be evaluated. When they are allowed, the appropriate use of appendices may greatly enhance the research proposal submitted for review by allowing the applicant to provide examples of scholarly writings that show previous relevant work. Nearly all funding agencies will allow and expect inclusion of any data collection instruments to be used in the research. Schematics for an elaborate study apparatus or biomedical device that might interrupt the flow of the study description are often placed in the appendix. However, simple line drawings and conceptual maps that clarify your study belong in the body of the research plan. Other items commonly included in the appendices are letters of support from consultants and clinical agencies and subject consent forms.

CONCLUSION

There are several aspects that characterize a good grant proposal. First, a good grant proposal is based on a creative, well-articulated, research question and on a significant public health issue. For educational or special projects grant, the proposal must articulate the need and the potential pool of students or persons served. Second, the grant must be methodologically sound, well written, and carefully formatted. The presentation should convince reviewers that the research team is highly knowledgeable about the topic area and possesses the necessary skills in the research methods to expertly carry out the proposed work. Finally, the grant writer must check and recheck the proposal to ensure consistency from specific aims, research questions and hypotheses, background and significance, research design and methods, data analyses, and proposed budget. As a final parting word, do not assume that the reviewers will know what you mean. Putting on the hat of the reviewer versus that of the grant writer may help to clarify issues throughout the proposal that require further explanation.

"Do not write so that you can be understood; write so that you cannot be misunderstood."

—*Epictetus*

CHAPTER 6

Check Your Parachute! A Few More Hoops to Jump Through

GRANT JAIL: RECOGNIZING THE TIME COMMITMENT

Unless you have "been there and done that," you have no idea how time consuming grant writing is. Like childbirth, many who have experienced it once tend to forget the downside or discomfort with the passage of time. Granted, most of us write grants in between other professional and family responsibilities. But the reality is that at some point you must lock yourself up for a few hours or days to write and rewrite. It feels like grant jail! As the submission deadline gets nearer, numerous last-minute changes suggested or mandated by your institutional review board (IRB) or reviewers become necessary. This is a time when you cannot tolerate frequent interruptions if you plan to get the work done on schedule. Every change made in the grant may have ripple effects that make it necessary to make changes in the abstract, specific aims page, or methods. Failure to concentrate on the far-reaching effects of every revision will lead to flaws in the overall application. Plan on setting aside some concentrated work time to finalize your proposal for submission. It may be only 1 to 2 hours, but if possible plan 1 to 2 days to be strictly devoted to the grant; it will make a big difference in the outcome. Grant writing is not a quick process. Even short grants for foundations (10 pages) require a commitment of several days or weeks to actually write a tight, solid grant proposal.

WHAT TO INCLUDE (OR NOT)

As you near the submission of your grant, revisit what should and should not be included with your grant packet. All grants are not the same, and even grants submitted to the same funding agency may require different documents to be submitted with applications for different grant-funding mechanisms. The National Institutes of Health (NIH) is a good example of an agency that is progressively changing the items and configuration of pages required for a grant. A major change in NIH grant applications came when the itemized budget was eliminated from requested forms. Only a "consolidated" budget page is submitted to the NIH on large grants. Streamlining of the award process has brought about "modular budgets" for projects with budgets of $250,000 or less per year for direct costs. Even though you may have figured dollars and cents on individual items, personnel, and equipment, the budget

91

must conform to the modular amount allowed. Nursing pilot studies funded by the NIH most often fall into the modular budget group to fund studies awarded no more than $100,000 for the complete project. An example of how funds are allocated can be seen in the R03 award. Applicants may request a project period of up to 2 years and a budget for direct costs of up to two $25,000 modules or $50,000 per year.

CHECK YOUR NIH PASSPORT: REQUIRED eRA REGISTRATION

Today's gateway to the NIH grant submission process is the *electronic Research Administration (eRA) Commons* located at https://commons.era.nih.gov/commons/. Designed to be an interface between the newer electronic submission process, reviewers, and applicants, the Web site provides access to information, grant application status, and all things of importance to NIH applicants and awardees. With development of the eRA Commons, all grant applicants and applicant organizations must have a registration *username* and *password* in order to access the electronic submission process. Even those NIH grants still using paper submission formats are required to have an eRA Commons registration because, as of October 2007, grant review scores and feedback will be available only through the Web-based Commons. Most eligible institutions have already registered for a Commons registration, but if they have not, they must do so before you can submit your grant. In addition, you must register for your own unique username and password. This can be facilitated by your home institution's grant office.

PACKAGING YOUR GRANT FOR SUBMISSION: OTHER REQUIRED FORMS

Depending on the size and complexity of your home institution and the requirements of the grant-funding agency you apply to, the packaging and accompanying forms will vary. If you have followed our advice, you have already looked into the need for approval by your supervising administrator and department by the time you are ready to submit your grant proposal. Equally important are the approvals required by the overall university, hospital, or health science center that will house your research grant. The awardee's institution, *not* the principal investigator, in most cases becomes the *actual* grant recipient. As such, the institution must assure the grantor that it has met all the assurances and requirements of ethical and financial conduct in the management of awarded funds. When a grant is funded, the funding goes into institutional accounts and is allocated to the researcher only when requests match the specific budget details of the project. Recognizing the great responsibility of institutions in managing large awards of research funding for numerous applicants from different sources makes the need for careful accounting, rigorous attention to ethical practices, and internal revenue processes beyond reproach. Violations or failure to comply could result in institutional censure, charges of scientific misconduct, and loss of present and future federal funding.

ASSURANCES AND CLEARANCES

It should be absolutely understood that your own particular grant proposal requires IRB (human subject or animal protection) clearances before any research can take place. What new researchers may not know are the important assurances and clearances that your university, school, or healthcare institution must pass as well. A close look at the grant application form will clue you in to required specific assurance information and identification numbers that will necessitate a quick search. The best source of information about your particular institution's assurances, clearances, and internal requirements is your own Office of Research and Contracts or Research Administration Office. Many large institutions post these assurance documents and signoff procedures on their institutional Web site.

Assurances are required by institutions receiving any federal funds documenting that it has a formal human and animal protection committee that meets certain specifications for size and activities. Qualifying institutions are issued a human subjects assurance number and an animal welfare assurance number that must be included on the face page of federal grants. In addition, federal grants and most foundations require certification by the Internal Revenue Service of the institution's nonprofit status. This information is also required on the federal grant face page. There may be other assurances required by your institution, some of which may have already been filed, and for which there may exist a documented form.

Many institutions require an internal form to report disclosure of conflicts of interest in externally funded projects or external relationships and university activities. Another form may be required if the grant involves an employee jointly employed by two or more agencies (for example a person jointly employed by a university and a Veterans Administration agency). An internal memorandum of understanding must be filed prior to a grant submission to document that administration, clinical, research, and teaching activities add up to 100% of the person's total work activities. This serves to verify that no dual compensation for the same work is taking place and no actual or apparent conflict of commitment as well.

For federal grants from any of the agencies under the Department of Health and Human Services, an *entity number* is used to identify each institution eligible for funding. This number contains the employer identification number assigned by the Internal Revenue Service to be utilized for the submission of Social Security and income tax withholding payments. NIH grant applications require the entity identification number on the face page.

Since October 2003, federal grant applications or cooperative agreements have required institutions seeking grants to include a Dun and Bradstreet Data Universal Numbering System (DUNS) number in every application for a new or competing continuation grant or cooperative agreement. There is a spot to enter your institution's DUNS number on every NIH grant application face page. If you are not associated directly with an institution that has a DUNS number, you can apply for one through Dun and Bradstreet. For example, if you have a consulting business, you or your business can apply for this number. Go to http://www.dnb.com/US/duns_update/.

SHOWING RESEARCH PERSONNEL'S OTHER FUNDING

Listing of your key personnel's ongoing and completed grant funding is one way that your funding agency checks to see that there is not dual compensation for the same professional work or overlap of one grant's funding to another. This information formerly appeared in NIH grants in a section called "Other Support." Today's NIH streamlined grant process calls for this information to be included on the last page of each person's biographical sketch under the heading of "Research Support." In a prescribed format "Ongoing Research Support" is listed as well as "Completed Research Support." Grants are listed with their grant number and mechanism, the name of the principal investigator, the inclusive dates of the grant, funding agency, title, a brief 1–2 sentence description of the work, and role of the applicant on the grant.

SPECIALLY REQUESTED TABLES

Although we have discussed the need for targeted enrollment tables for ethnic minorities, women, and children in federal research grants, there may be other requirements in training or demonstration grants for minority, graduation, or faculty tables. Institutional training grants for doctoral study are enhanced by tables showing faculty/student assignments, publication collaboration, and previous institutions of enrolled students.

Tables for educational training grants present data on how many minority students are admitted to and have graduated from the institution submitting the grant. Graduation tables contain overall data on the number of students admitted and finally graduated from the various programs the school offers. Faculty tables are used by reviewers to see how many faculty are from ethnic minority groups, whether or not they are tenured, how many are full- versus part-time, the rank of each faculty member, and their areas of expertise. These data help reviewers know if there are enough internal resources and individuals with expertise specified in the grant to support the proposed program, special project, or research. These tables are usually not optional. Make sure they are included. Many grants are now reviewed by sections, such as the purpose and specific aims, the curriculum plan, and supporting data. Each section is given specific points so missing tables detract from the overall points in the grant. It also suggests to the reviewers that the grant writer is unable to follow directions or is not detail oriented. Because tables occupy space in your grant and present a graphic representation of your program, take pains to have them constructed neatly by an experienced staff member. Review them carefully for errors and missing information.

DATA TO SUPPORT CASE FOR GRANT

Data to support the rationale for the research, practice, or educational grant must be detailed enough to let the grant reviewer know that the writer is aware of the national, regional, and local needs and healthcare trends. For example, if a cancer rehabilitation center is proposed, the rates and types of cancer in Denver may greatly differ from Chicago. This should be reflected in the grant writing. Data need to be current, and if no current data are available at one of these levels, then make sure to state that and why. Even an informal needs assessment will strengthen the proposal. Include information on this assessment and how the data were collected. Giving only national data when the grant is administered locally is insufficient to provide a strong rationale for grant funding. Be as specific as you can in terms of each facet of the grant. Give the rationale to support your requests. Do not appear to the reviewers as if you are only trying to add to very adequate resources. Another important aspect is self-sufficiency. If the grant period is 3 years, how are you or your institution going to ensure that this program does not just die at the end of the funding cycle? The self-sufficiency statement, if requested, must be specific, with goals and acknowledgment of potential barriers. The potential barriers should have potential solutions built into the grant even though these are only projected. Not having a solid plan for sustainability can substantially reduce the funding chances.

PRE-SUBMISSION REVIEWERS

The need for good pre-submission review is so helpful to grant success that many nursing research centers build the process into their operation and hire experts to review grants before final submission. Schools of nursing conduct mock reviews or "modeling parties" where colleagues constructively critique grant applications to look for potential trouble spots. Hearing how discourse and discussion of a proposal can influence a group's scoring decision is helpful because this is exactly what a grant goes through at the funding agency. If getting a group together is not possible, or if you are fearful of your ability to tolerate honest feedback in a public forum, by all means get one or more individuals to review your proposal privately. Try to decide who might be very objective but will give you good, constructive criticism that can improve your grant. Have this person read the grant as if he or she were a peer reviewer. The person may be an expert in the area of the grant that can make sure that you are quoting the most recent researchers or educators in the area (grant reviewers want to make sure you know your grant area and the key names associated with the grant's content area). Another person might review the grant for flow and grammar and to make sure that you have built a credible case for why your grant should be funded. Even if this person has no knowledge of your grant area, he or she should be able to tell you if you have presented enough details to explain the rationale for the grant. An editor can also be extremely helpful in reviewing the grant by correcting grammar and cutting out excessive verbiage, formatting the application document, designing tables and figures, and checking references.

Pre-submission reviewers may include some of the internal people in your institution who must read and sign off on the grant prior to its submission. Their comments will also help in the peer review process. Of course, at some point you will have to decide how many of the suggestions from reviewers you will act on. The most important comments to warrant your attention are those that reflect confusion about what you have written. If your proposal has generated misunderstanding at any point, these are areas that must be corrected. If the person has been part of a previous grant review panel, please pay careful attention to comments. He or she knows what reviewers look for in grants and what constitutes a red flag.

AGENCY CONTACT PERSON FOR FINAL CHECKLIST OR TECHNICAL SUPPORT

As we have mentioned in earlier chapters, the contact person at your agency or technical support staff can be immensely helpful in the grant-writing process. Draw on this expertise. He or she will help you make sure your grant is complete. Use the checklist supplied with your grant application and, if included, the review criteria for the grant reviewers. Look at the criteria for selection and make sure your application addresses each of these points. Go over and over this checklist before you submit. Ideally, have someone else check the application with you; sometimes you cannot see your own omissions.

GRANT CHECKLIST

The grant checklist is the final step in the process. If one is not provided, create your own consisting of each required element and the materials required by the agency. Review the checklist for submission again, and make sure that each item required is included in the packet. The checklist is part of the application packet. The list does vary among funding agencies, but the basic elements are essentially the same. Look at the specific mailing instructions given in the packet. Grants mailed to the wrong person or the wrong addresses are often never reviewed. The NIH checklist for the PHS 398 form is used only for paper submissions. The checklist for the new SF242 electronic submission forms is checked off online by the person actually doing the electronic process. This may be your Office of Research Administration.

GUIDELINES: READ, REREAD, AND PRAY!

Just as with the checklist, go over the actual guidelines for the grant. Review the funding areas, and the key words or objectives that the application packet uses; in your grant use these terms as headers and descriptors. It shows the reviewers you read and paid attention to details. If you make a change in one section of the grant, make sure the table or other grant sections that also contain this information are changed as well. Depending on the type grant you are submitting or the type of institution in which you are working, determine whether there are optional tables or sections needed. These are small items that are often overlooked in the grant. If someone else is copying and compiling paper copies of your grant, make sure the final copies include all the pages in the order you want them. The copy machine can "eat" pages, making the grant incomplete and sometimes invalid for review. The need for photocopied pages with signatures to be inserted among pages of a document being produced by your printer makes it particularly easy for mistakes to occur in page numbering, inclusions, and order of pages in the packet. Once you have done your best to review these items, reviewed the guidelines, and checked the application checklist, put the package in the mail and sit back and pray.

CONCLUSION

A well-planned submission process makes grant writing much easier. The key is plan, plan, and plan. Be realistic in your timeline for completion. Dedicate time to the actual writing *and* editing of the project. Have it reviewed by others not involved in the grant, and be ready to revise your proposal if revision is warranted. If you are mailing a proposal, be sure to check the pages to be sure they have all been copied, printed, and numbered. Be sure to reexamine your grant proposal checklist just before the grant is mailed.

CHAPTER 7

The Electronic Flight Plan for Grant Submission

THE ELECTRONIC ENVIRONMENT OF GRANTSMANSHIP

Given the potential for saving costs in mailing, communication, and paper, it is not surprising that the federal government has been an early adopter for electronic submission of grants. The National Institutes of Health (NIH) expected that getting rid of paper copies would save approximately 200 million pieces of paper a year and reduce the costs of scanning, data entry, data validation, printing, and reproduction. The NIH rolled out its electronic submission process in October 2005 with the Small Business Innovative Research (SBIR) and Small Business Technology Transfer Program (STTR) grant proposals. Other federal agencies such as the Health Resources and Services Administration (HRSA) and the Agency for Healthcare Research and Quality (AHRQ) followed suit. The transition of all grant submissions at every level by electronic means is well on its way toward completion.

CYBER-SUBMISSION? IS THIS TRIP NECESSARY?

As with all new things, those involved with the process met the prospect of online submission with varying degrees of enthusiasm, delight, distress, and disgust. Potential grant applicants and their research administration offices shared anxieties about the process, access, and time needed for submission. Their primary fear was that the new process would be difficult and require excessive training. Grant reviewers accustomed to receiving paper copies fretted about whether they would be able to find an electronic copy legible. This fear was prompted in part by NIH's simultaneous move away from its old familiar PHS398 application form to a new one, called SF424 Research and Related (R&R) form, for all its electronic submissions. Instead of compiling a single document as in the past, the new electronic grant is built by filling out electronic forms and cutting and pasting grant proposals created with word-processing programs (such as Microsoft Word) into a template form. Do not try to fill out the forms without really reviewing your work. You need to really refine what is placed in the form. You want to put your best document and profile of your work forward. There were new requirements to download special software for creating the proposal, and all attachments such as letters and reprints had to be converted to portable document format (PDF) files for online submission. A cottage industry of consultants arose to offer assistance (and often at a hefty price!). At least one author has produced a book with NIH-specific directions for writing and submitting proposals electronically (Gerin, 2006). In most cases, the process has not been formidable, and help from the funding agency has been available. The NIH was proactive in making available free workshops and step-by-step procedures from its Web site to help alleviate fears and prepare institutional grant offices. Although there are still a few complaints from reviewers who dislike reviewing grants on a computer and object to printing out their own copies, the transition has not been as bad as expected. Other funding agencies, including the American Nurses Foundation, the Robert Wood Johnson Foundation (RWJF), Sigma Theta Tau International, and the regional research societies are joining the trend toward electronic proposals. Gone are the stacks of bulky proposals, the late-night trips to the FedEx office, and anxieties about ground mail delivery. But in their place are new mandates for planning ahead and timely submissions to institutional grant offices for sign-offs. Scenarios that involve staying up all night to complete a grant and hand carrying it by plane to Washington on its due date are outdated. If you wish to move along in this century, you must recognize that grants are now processed in an electronic environment. Be sure that you are on board and have electronic navigators to help you. These may be your research administration office, your technology staff, or a knowledgeable secretarial staff member. Get help early and plan ahead for your learning curve. Take advantage of institutional workshops and online training about electronic grant submission. Familiarity with the language, rules, and processes will make it less confusing. Remember, that many of the rules and information details are evolving. Look for the most recent versions of instructions, and be ready to encounter a few bumps in the journey. You can do this, and there is help available to you along the way.

CHECK OUT THE eRA COMMONS

In late October, 2007 the NIH completed its major update to its portal to electronic services, the electronic Research Administration Commons (eRA Commons). New access links and training features are in place, and others will undoubtedly appear as the electronic environment fully evolves. Accessed at http://commons.era.nih.gov/commons/, there are links to assist users that include the steps of the electronic application process, a demo of what the Commons offers, training events, and specific help buttons. Among the training features are videos that include guides to getting registered, using the new SF424 (R&R) forms, how to use the *status* feature to see where your grant is, and explanations of the many processes used by federal grant agencies (e.g., electronic Streamline Noncompeting Award Process (eSNAP), Status, and Just in Time).

Some Major Changes and Advantages Offered by NIH's Electronic Environment

A major advantage of having the review process enabled by electronic means is the ability for principal investigators (PIs) to view the status of their proposal. Your institution's research grant administrator also can access the status of your grant, see a summary view of grant applications, review the Notice of Grant Award, and access the Progress Report face page. This feature is helpful if you have questions about any of the postings and what they mean. Investigators can log on to the eRA Commons as their grant goes through committee review. The old familiar written notification of grant award (still called a "pink sheet" by some, even though it has not actually been pink for over a decade) is being replaced by electronic notification. Effective January 1, 2008, the NIH no longer provides paper notification of the Notice of Award letters. Instead, notices are sent solely via e-mail to grantee organizations and are accessible in the eRA Commons. This means that feedback is received when it is posted and does not have to wait for a form to be printed and mailed. Once a grant has been awarded, your institution can use the eSNAP to review noncompeting grant data and submit progress reports online.

Other benefits offered by the NIH electronic submission process are an easier compilation process. Page numbers and the table of contents are system generated and included in the final grant application. Because the system generates a customized table of contents based on each submission, any nonrelevant items that formerly appeared on the older standardized pages no longer appear.

NIH electronic submission also has advantages for grant reviewers who are able to access the grants and materials on the eRA Commons. The Internet Assisted Review process allows reviewers to submit critiques and preliminary scores for applications they are reviewing without having to worry about mail or e-mails arriving at their destination.

GENERAL RULES FOR ELECTRONIC SUBMISSION

- **Strive for error free originals:** Submitting any type of grant application online requires the development of error-free originals. Type your budget pages, biographical sketches, and research plan on paper forms first, print them out, and proofread carefully. Spell-check features in your word-processing program are helpful, but watch out for words that sound the same but have different meanings that are misused (the most common is using "principle investigator" when you mean "principal investigator"). Enlist at least one other person to follow behind you on your check for errors or missing items.
- **Software, format, and space issues:** Old rules about numbers of pages or words per page may not apply when document submissions move online. Be

sure to check the guidelines and regulations at the submission Web site and use the recommended format and headings if they are given. Double check to see what font is recommended and whether documents are single- or double-spaced. Check out the application Web site to be sure you are using the appropriate version of a word-processing program for online submissions. For NIH grants, the current software required for downloading and viewing the submission packet is *Pure Edge Viewer* and is available online from the Grants.gov Web site at http://www.grants.gov/resources/download_software.jsp. Testing of compatible versions of Adobe Reader in 2008 found them usable to download some application forms.

- **Use of a citation manager with your electronic proposal submission:** Take care to determine if your reference citations produced with a citation manager, such as EndNote (Carlsbad, CA: Thompson ResearchSoft) or ProCite (Carlsbad, CA: Thompson ResearchSoft) or Reference Manager (Carlsbad, CA: Thompson ResearchSoft), can be accepted by the online submission process. If not, you need not give up the citation manager. It means instead that once your proposal is complete, you must convert the document to plain text. Instructions for doing this are usually found in your citation manager "help" function under the topic "removing field codes." Removing these codes keeps all the citations and the reference list in place, but they are no longer interactive with your citation manager. Keep a copy with all the citation manager codes intact in case you have to return to the application and revise.
- **Check the source for updates and changes:** The NIH Web site and support facilities are rapidly changing; the guidelines for NIH grant applications have been revised three times as this book was in preparation. This makes it all the more important to *check the source* for new and evolving updates. The NIH electronic submission Web site at this time is http://era.nih.gov/ElectronicReceipt/. Other funding agencies may have moved from paper submission to partial online submission, with letters and signed documents mailed as paper files. More recently, it has become common for signed documents to be submitted as PDF files sent electronically.
- **Permission to apply:** Plan ahead if your grant application needs institutional or funder approval before you can apply. Some funding agencies require a letter of intent or a "mini-proposal" being approved before a full proposal will be accepted. TheRWJF and the National Palliative Care Research Center (NPCRC) streamline their selection and review process by asking for these abbreviated documents to help screen proposals. Full proposals "are accepted by invitation only." Some funding agencies allow only one application to be

submitted from a single institution or university. For example, the Nurse Education, Practice, and Retention (NEPR) program funded by the HRSA has nine purposes, but an applicant organization may only submit one application per NEPR purpose under this announcement.

- **Your NIH registration in eRA Commons:** The PI and key personnel should be registered in the eRA Commons and have usernames and passwords well in advance of an NIH grant submission. Registration can take several weeks to process, and you cannot submit an electronic federal grant without it. Your office of research administration is the best resource to help you obtain this registration. A PI's Commons account follows the PI throughout the PI's career, even if the PI moves to another institution. Also, if you become an NIH consultant or grant reviewer, you will keep the same Common account and username. Likewise, grant reviewers who acquire a Commons account and username during that activity will use the same registration, account, and username to submit a federal grant.

- **Your organization's eRA Commons registration:** All applicant organizations need to be registered in Grants.gov and the NIH Commons well in advance of the submission date and before you can submit an electronic federal grant. Any organization applying for registration must also supply taxpayer identification number, Dun and Bradstreet Data Universal Number System numbers, and Internal Revenue clearances, all which can take considerable time. Your office of research administration or grants office should be able to provide you with the institutional eRA Commons username. If you are not sure if the organization where you are a student, faculty member, or employee has a contracts office, contact your top administrative office early on. Other detailed information about registration appears at the eRA Commons Web site at http://commons.era.nih.gov/commons/.

- **Other points of reference for electronic searches:**
  - eRA Commons (http://commons.era.nih.gov/commons) provides information technology solutions and support for the full lifecycle of grants administration functions for the NIH, operating divisions of the Department of Health and Human Services, and other federal agencies.
  - Grants.gov (http://grants.gov) is the electronic source to find and apply for federal government grants.
  - HRSA (www.hrsa.gov) is an agency of the U.S. Department of Health and Human Services with a mission to improve access to healthcare services for people who are uninsured, isolated, or medically vulnerable. Their grant pages at http://www.hrsa.gov/grants/default.htm offer information on numerous funding opportunities in nurse training at several levels.

- The NIH (http://www.nih.gov) Web site offers access to NIH institutes and centers, training resources, research funding, initiatives, NIH employment, and publications. Web sites for specific institutes that fund pilot and major studies can be accessed from this site or from their own Web site addresses (e.g., National Institute of Nursing Research at http://www.ninr.nih.gov or National Institute on Aging at http://www.nia.nih.gov).

KEEPING A PAPER TRAIL IN A PAPERLESS ENVIRONMENT

Submitting grant proposals, or pieces of proposals, online tends to make researchers feel a bit fragmented. In fact, with NIH submissions, your proposal does not "come together" until the application data go through Grants.gov submission and the eRA system compiles the data fields and attachments into a single grant application. At that time, applicants are able to see the entire grant application for the first time in the eRA Commons. If your application had validation or missing identifiers and did not make it through the eRA Commons application checking process, you must correct any errors and submit a corrected application to Grants.gov before your application can proceed further. If something you omitted that was essential to your proposal, but not picked related to eRA checkers, is missing, check with your NIH science officer to determine if the missing element can be added or if it requires submission of an entire corrected application.

With small foundation or professional organization grant applications, you could find that you do not have a complete copy of your document unless you take precautions to print or electronically save each page you submit. It is in your best interest to have a complete copy to refer to during and after your grant has been reviewed. Print each screen before you submit the sections. Keeping a loose-leaf notebook with sections matching each grant section allows you to develop your paper copy as you submit pages. This notebook makes it easy to refer to sections if or when a funding agency calls you for specific information about your grant. Knowing what you submitted is key to keeping track of your commitments and obligations. It provides a framework for ongoing reports when a grant is finally funded.

If your grant administration office is submitting your online foundation or organizational grant, ask them to produce you a paper copy. Keep this copy in your loose-leaf notebook. NIH submissions produce a PDF copy of the compiled grant that your grant administration office will make available to you. This compiled copy will also be what is finally reviewed by your grant review committee. It is important that you examine it closely to be sure that you have included everything you intended. A trail of forgotten pages, letters, consent forms, and other missing items from grant submissions makes it clear that these errors are common. However, it is in your best interest to find such omissions early enough to correct them *before* they are found in review.

CONCLUSION

Electronic grant submissions are here to stay, with foundations and professional organizations following the lead of federal funding agencies in adopting them. These technological changes offer new advantages, including an online view of your grant status and final feedback. The new set of skills required to function in an electronic environment is not rocket science. Take them step by step, seek help when you need it, and enjoy the advantages.

CHAPTER 8

Gauging Progress and Reviewer Feedback

THE ENVELOPE PLEASE!

The results of your grant applications no longer are sent on "pink sheets"; however, they still hold the same weight. We still feel that they are either ego busters or ego boosters. Whether the notification of your grant status comes in an envelope, e-mail, or a Web site posting, the excitement and anxiety are palpable. In earlier days, some of us who received notification by mail at work would go into a restroom stall to read it. The results that followed were unpredictable. If the envelope held a grant score, the applicant often emerged puzzled and had to seek more information as to its meaning from a senior researcher. If the message was congratulatory, the bathroom trip was short, and we all soon shared in celebration. If the trip was prolonged, it likely meant that the message was disappointing, and we felt empathy amid tears and tissues. Disappointment should not be misinterpreted as failure. Even the experienced grant writer experiences disappointments as well as successes in proposal writing.

BEHOLD THE TURTLE!

A wise research mentor once shared an analogy that is true to the task of a successful grant applicant. "Behold the noble turtle. To get ahead he has to stick his neck out and carry a hard shell." The image of daring to enter the race, slow persistence, and the ability to take the critique process without feeling a personal affront are characteristics that keep a researcher on the path to success. Part of our difficulty comes from the love/hate relationship we have with reviews or evaluations of any kind. We can't wait to get feedback on our grant and are dying to know if we were funded, but we also have an awful dread of hearing any possibility that we weren't. This same dread of criticism tends to make us sidestep pre-submission reviews or avoid mock study sections of our grant in the first place. We quickly learn that it is crucial to develop a tough spine or some insensitivity to the process.

REVIEWERS ARE EXPERTS, BUT THEY ARE HUMAN

Bear in mind that the grant reviewers are enlisted to read and critique your proposal. They are often paid, or at least rewarded in some way for doing this, although seldom enough to truly pay for the time and effort they devote to the task. Because much is expected of the reviewers, they generally take great pains to do a thorough job and will find errors and inconsistencies you may have overlooked. National Institutes of Health (NIH) or Health Resources and Services Administration (HRSA) reviewers, for example, also write a narrative summary listing the strengths, weaknesses, and any changes they recommend. Because they are experts, they often go to great lengths to explain in detail where you have gone wrong. Contrary to what the applicant may feel, reviewers are not out to reject your proposal; they like nothing better than to find proposals that meet all the criteria for funding. On the other hand, they are not chosen to overlook shortcomings in a proposal, no matter how well intentioned it is. They also have low tolerance for sloppily written or submitted proposals. The fear is this is the way you would conduct the project as well. Another factor to remember is the likelihood that your grant was discussed in a group of several reviewers, so both positive and negative remarks in the critical review may influence the final review summary you receive. Often review of a proposal deemed highly acceptable by one reviewer will be dampened by that of another. This can happen in the other direction as well. One reviewer may have a hard time finding any redeeming features in a proposal but will change his or her mind when hearing the positive attributes found by another reviewer. All reviewers are reasonable human beings, and although they are experts with skills in reviewing, they hold subjective biases and opinions. They must come to an agreement to score or approve your proposal, so the final score is often a compromise among reviewers. If the review was positive and they thought your grant was innovative and wonderful, you're entitled to a huge ego boost. If it is clear that the comments are universally negative, allow yourself a brief pity party, then get back to work. The following tips are shared here to help you better understand and get the most out of reviewer feedback and use it to move forward. Begin by reading the review carefully, taking notes and highlighting the comments. Then begin translating what the review is really trying to tell you. Also remember if this is a resubmission review that you are receiving you may, in fact, receive a far different review. This difference may be the composition of the reviewers, or the landscape has changed in your area since your previous submission. For example, the first year that bioterrorism grants were requested, there was a "hunger" for these grants. But 2 to 3 years later, the science and educational strategies had advanced so just a simple resubmission of a rejected grant during the first year, 2 or 3 years later would have to be significantly more sophisticated.

TRANSLATING THE REVIEW

Grant reviews tend to fall into four categories. Reviews that say:

1. Yes, we love your proposal as it is.
2. Yes, this is acceptable with a few simple additions or revisions.

3. Possibly, in a resubmission with extensive revisions.
4. No, this isn't going to meet our needs, priorities, or standards.

The first category is fairly straightforward, and you may actually need to pinch yourself to be sure you fully understand that you've been funded! The second category may refer to some hoops you need to jump through, questions to be answered, or documents to be supplied before funding can be assured. Categories three and four are the hardest to decipher, especially if your results say that your study has been "approved, but not funded." Some foundations are likely to say that if it is a dissertation or thesis project, a student whose work has already been approved by a university committee should not be discouraged. However, sometimes a granting agency will approve a project on its merit, but not have sufficient funds to award all meritorious applications. If it is clear that is the case with regard to your grant, it should encourage you to seek another funder. Some applicants look for clues in their NIH or HRSA scoring to determine which category their review falls in, but this is not a reliable indicator. Excellent ideas are sometimes given less competitive scores if there is a clear omission of an important section, resource, or support. Look at the comments as indicators of whether it is your idea or the way it is implemented that has prompted your reviewers' response. On the other hand, a score that is near the top of the scoring range (1.0 for NIH reviews and 100 for HRSA), probably has fewer things that need to be revised for a resubmission.

WHAT YOU CAN LEARN

Try to interpret the meaning of the reviewers' message in light of your proposal. Did you have to submit the grant before you really had all the details worked out? Did the reviewers cast doubt on your abilities to carry out the project? Were you lacking a working team or resources to carry out the planned activities? These comments give you a fairly clear direction for a resubmission, and you know where you need to spend your efforts. Have the reviewers failed to understand what you had in mind? It may be that your writing skills need help and that you need technical assistance in the mechanics of grant writing. Making your idea more understandable is something a writing consultant can help you with. Most academic and hospital settings provide resources to assist with the grant-writing process. Commercial programs are also available that provide proposal master templates that help guide the grant writer through the process.

Do the reviewers express doubt that your idea will work? Pilot studies are the strongest evidence that an idea is workable or a phenomenon is measurable. Was there insufficient evidence that the problem, significance, or relevance was worthy of grant support? These comments require a more convincing argument that the problem is of concern and relevance to the funding agency. Less clear are comments that cast doubts on your ideas. Unfortunately, this is the area in which most grant applications are scored down in the review process. The idea itself may be something you are so close to and passionate about that you cannot be objective about its importance or significance. If your interpretation of the review is that the idea didn't measure up, engage an honest expert to level with you about its weaknesses and strengths. This needs to be a person you trust, but also someone knowledgeable about your scientific or scholarship area. Perhaps it is an idea whose time has not yet come. If that is the case, you can tuck it away in your treasure box and proceed to build some preliminary work that may show its relevance or replace it with a better idea.

Sometimes you are urged to submit an ill-prepared grant to meet needs of employing institutions. It may be that you had to submit the grant too quickly or too early in the process. For example, sometimes as educators we are forced, due to budget restraints, to submit a program grant well before the "idea" is really ready. Sometimes your institution includes barriers, such as courses that have little relevance to your proposed program but have been required by the system for decades. In such a case, harsh reviewers' comments may provide impetus for institutional change. So at your ego's expense you may have become a change agent!

Look to see if there is a hidden agenda in the review; perhaps the slant you took on the funding priority is not really congruent with what the foundation was looking for at this time. Perhaps the grant reviewers' comments were influenced by their own areas of expertise. You may determine you missed subtle cues in their application kit that you could address if given the opportunity to resubmit. If it is a foundation grant with a small overall budget, your rejection may simply be a case of many well-written grants being submitted but not enough money to fund them all. In this way, even a rejection may not mean that you wrote a bad grant, although it will certainly feel that way at first. If it is an NIH or other federal grant involving a two-tier review, the scoring is done on merit and grant criteria without regard to the funding budget. In this case, the reviewer comments are your best clue to the ultimate decision.

DEVELOPING A POSITIVE APPROACH TO CRITIQUE

You have led a sheltered life if you have not experienced disappointment or rejection of a prized idea. Remembering that grants are proposals, and that you are among many suitors, will help you develop a positive philosophy toward critique as a conditioning technique. Like any other learned pursuit, the more it is practiced, the better the performance. One must therefore decide how to respond to critical review, and practice it along the way. Here are some tips to guide you:

- **Expect to do alterations and revisions:** Do not fall into the trap of falling in love with your written words, but write and revise paragraphs often. See how many extraneous words you can remove but still be clear. This is called "crisping" your proposal.

- **Be prepared to submit a revised proposal:** It is a good idea to be prepared for the possible event of not being funded the first time around. Many grants have repeat submission cycles that allow you to revise and resubmit in a timely manner. Revisions of projects with good ideas generally have a better chance as resubmissions than simply turning to a different funding agency. The amended proposal allows you to show how responsive you have been to reviewer's comments. If you submit to a different agency, it is like starting over again, not like resubmitting to the same agency. The new review committee may have a whole new list of concerns about your proposal.
- **The more you write, the easier it gets:** It is hard for some people to believe that something hard gets easier when you keep doing it, but for the most part those who feel this way about writing are dealing with fear of failure. The beauty of computers is that you can write and write and never waste any paper. Set aside time to write, and then polish your writing. If you need some tools like a thesaurus, speller, or grammatical program, these are all available as computer aids. Taking a course in scientific writing can be helpful for those who tend to write copious prose or inverted sentences. Unlike a novel that holds the answer at the end, scientific writing needs to convey the idea up front and elaboration later.
- **Avoid getting wedded to your own words:** Unwillingness to give up a hard-earned paragraph is a symptom of those who struggle to write. Write it. Then use the Track Changes feature (in Microsoft Word) to record your efforts to make it better. If you think a phrase is "precious" and you are up against those suggesting it is inflated or pretentious, print it out on a piece of paper and put it in your jewelry box. You might use it later.
- **Invite review and critique of your work:** Finding someone who is willing to read and objectively critique your work is a gift worth millions. Oddly enough, most academic settings have mentors or experts who are willing to do that. If none are available to you, then push for your employing agency to hire consultants for this purpose. Often retired faculty are willing to do this type of consultation. On a much easier level, get together a group of colleagues who are in the same boat. Form a review group to go over one another's proposals or writing. Make a pact to give constructive criticism (it will be of no use to you if you only praise one another). Remember this is "conditioning" critique to better prepare you for the real show!
- **Build on reviewer comments:** Consider every comment as important. Reviewer comments are the only clues you have to evaluate the strength of your proposal. To build on positive comments, try to determine the difference

between enthusiastic comments and faint praise that the reviewer used to balance "strengths" with all of the weaknesses. Map out the "weakness" comments so that you fully understand what was missing, under supported, or a bad idea. Not all foundations give you a detailed review of your grant and nothing is less helpful than a rejected grant with little or no feedback. If your grant is rejected from a funding agency with little feedback, consult with a faculty member who is an experienced grant writer before you move to resubmit your proposal.

- **Dealing with rejected grant submissions:** If you are going to write grants, you will undoubtedly deal at some point with rejection. Submissions at the federal level often take three to four submissions of the same grant before it is actually funded. Out-and-out rejection is disappointing. But always remember, it was your *proposal*, not *you*, that was rejected. The proposal can be revised, even thrown out if you find it cannot be repaired, but you are now wiser and more experienced in grant writing than you were before. You have joined the ranks of experienced grant writers who know that this is an expected rough patch that you can move through. Regard the review process as a learning experience. If the review was extremely harsh, put it away for a while and then go back when you are ready to really read the comments instead of reacting to them. "Try, try again," must be your motto.

SUBMITTING AN AMENDED PROPOSAL

A revised grant application (now called an "amended" application by the NIH) is one that is resubmitted to the same funding agency. Federal grants, such as NIH, require an "introduction" to explain to the reviewers how you have addressed the previous critique. Carefully address specific comments and weaknesses pointed out in the earlier review and explain generally how you have corrected them. You will be expected to amend the earlier application by using a different font feature (italicizing, underlining, or bolding) any new additions or replacements. You will replace unwanted text with the amended text, so explain in your introduction which feature you are using to show changes. Your introduction should be respectful and not argumentative. If you decide that an aspect of your prior submission should stay in the proposal despite recommendations to remove it, respectfully provide new stronger rationale and support for its inclusion. Bear in mind, experts have told you to make a change, so be sure that your new argument is convincing. The funding agency will give instructions in its guide to revisions about how much space you are allowed for an introduction or explanation.

CONCLUSION

The dreaded grant review results and summary actually provide a great deal of good information. The comments, if specific enough, can help you to refine your grant even if it was funded. If the grant was not funded, use the comments to revise the grant for resubmission to the same funding agency or to another one that might be more appropriate. If you have received funding, your work has just begun! The next chapter will offer some tips for your journey.

CHAPTER 9

So Now You've Been Funded

THE GLOW OF SUCCESS!

Congratulations! What an accomplishment a funded research study is. You are finally out of grant jail! Take some time to bask in that reality when it happens. You earned it! Okay, take maybe one day, but then wake up and smell the coffee. This is when your work really begins. What will you do next? You will benefit by acknowledging some important facts to make your newly funded grant successful and enjoyable to all its participants. Probably the most important fact is that carrying out the research *takes time*. You need to carve out that time as if it were a job. If your grant includes some salary support, arranging time for the study is much easier to figure. If it does not, you must either negotiate the time to carry your project out from your regular employment or find time above and beyond your workday. We have dedicated this chapter to the importance of getting a grip on your time, organizing your work, and avoiding some common pitfalls in carrying out your work. The more you anticipate the real work of grantsmanship in your pre-submission plans, the easier the conduct of your project will be (Bergstrom & Baun, 1994).

DUST OFF THAT TIMELINE

Do you recall the timeline we discussed in Chapter 5? What might have been a skeleton plan for your proposal now becomes your map for action. This is the time to flesh it out with actual activities, dates, and assignments. Add dates for submitting annual reports, meeting with your team, and updating your institutional review board (IRB) reports. Enlarge and keep your timeline posted in a conspicuous place. Some items can be modified, while others are less flexible. Without a timeline, you are like a navigator without a map.

TIME TO GET ORGANIZED!

Many principal investigators (PIs) and project directors find a way to "bind" the project together. One simple way to do this is to begin putting documents in a 3-ring binder from the time you submit the grant to the end of the project. Use dividers with labels to separate sections of your proposal into those dealing with budget and those dealing with the project itself. This makes it easy to refer to the road map for the project and to keep the integrity of the plan intact. It is also useful if someone from the funding budget office or your own research administration office calls and needs some data from the original submission. Once the grant is funded, make a photocopy of the funding notice for your notebook and label that. It provides you with your grant number, the actual dollars funded, and other information you may need at a later date. The notebook can contain a section for correspondence about the grant between you, your funding agency, your consultants, and your clinical sites. Devote a section to personnel to keep names and contact information about key personnel, graduate assistants, data collectors, technicians, and consultants. Update this contact information regularly as people move and positions change. Annual reports can go in another section. If there have been changes for the IRB or the project must be reviewed, keep a section for just these reassurances. One section can be devoted to publications, abstracts, or news items about your study. For a multiyear grant, you may end up with a larger notebook, or even two or three. Binding your project together, both physically and virtually, in a retrievable form is essential to keeping track of your grant's history beyond the data you collect. It is more than a scrapbook of memorabilia; it is priceless when it comes time to write your final report to your grant funder.

ORDERING EQUIPMENT AND SUPPLIES

If you have planned well, you have figured into your timeline the time it takes to order essential equipment and supplies for your project (Bergstrom & Baun, 1994). This is particularly important when special instruments or devices must be made to order. Check with your institution's post-award accountant to see when you can actually start to spend funds. Some large institutions have mechanisms to order equipment when they receive a federal funding decision. Find out if you must make grant purchases through your institution's purchasing/receiving office. If so, clarify and supply information for sole-source items that cannot be replaced by less-expensive models for scientific reasons, and emphasize the urgency of expedient delivery to start your project. Also consider building on foundational equipment that is already in use at your institution. For example, if your research or educational project includes simulation equipment and there is already some equipment in place, buying from the same company often gains you discounts. Take advantage of loaner equipment to train your personnel and be innovative to avoid spinning your wheels.

WHEN CAN WE START?

Once your funds have been released to your institution, you will not be able to start your grant-funded project until several things are in place. If yours is a federal grant, your Office of Research Administration or Grants and Project Office will want to be sure that you have met all required special project assurances, such as Human Subjects Protection; Protections for Pregnant Women, Human Fetuses, and Neonates Involved in Research; Protections Pertaining to Biomedical and Behavioral Research Involving Prisoners as Subjects; and Additional Protections for Children Involved as Subjects in Research. If you are using animals, you must produce clearances of your project from your institution's institutional animal care and use committee. Any arrangements for ordering animals and housing them must also be cleared through your grants office. You will need to complete any Conflict of Interest forms and resolve any outstanding IRB issues before you can begin your study. Finally, expect to talk with your purchasing office to negotiate and resolve any issues about the items being purchased for your study.

RECRUITING AND TRAINING PERSONNEL

We discussed in Chapter 4 the need to make plans for personnel well in advance of your funding notice. Once the grant is funded, you can begin to formalize these appointments, set up payroll arrangements, and in cases of salaried faculty or agency employees, set up new and realigned positions within the institution. Keeping in close communication with your accounting office during the grant application process makes this transition much easier. Many institutions will require that you advertise positions for research staff with the Human Resources Office that were not named as key personnel in your grant in order to comply with equal opportunity guidelines. Graduate research assistants may fall under a different category at your institution, so clear how these team members can be recruited. Take time and effort in picking your team. Consider recruiting students for research assistants. Graduate students often are able to find spin-off projects from engaging in actual studies. We have had success with employing undergraduate students for clinical studies. With proper mentorship and supervision, they were reliable in collecting clinical data and enthusiastic about the work. Several of these students decided on graduate education, based on their experience with the study. Also, consider recruiting professional colleagues and nurses from clinical settings. Many would never consider embarking on a research study alone but are excellent data collectors or clinical experts. If you are posting an advertisement and interviewing persons you do not know, get professional references. Your project is a position of employment and requires reliable, ethical, and competent personnel.

Training personnel often takes considerable time. If possible, plan a get-acquainted meeting of all your personnel well in advance of your study's start. Give each team member an abbreviated version of your research plan and explain each team member's role. Get everyone's schedule of availability, exchange contact phone numbers, and set up a training schedule. For studies that require an elaborate protocol, specialized instruments, and unusual data collection schemes, have your team members practice the protocol on one another. Having someone serve as a surrogate subject may be helpful if you are training data collectors in dealing with a particular physical limitation or behavioral characteristic. Rehearsal of the protocol was most important in one study where various stages of shivering were to be detected. We conducted inter-rater reliability tests on patients who shivered while recovering from anesthesia.

Here are some things to remember in the care and feeding of a research team:

- **Build partnership/ownership among your team members.** Discuss study progress and acquaint them with the background and significance of the variables under study. Let them present parts of your orientation to the clinical sites.
- **Keep personnel happy and stimulated.** Grant teams are stimulated by learning more about the study. Celebrate holidays or special occasions with grant personnel with a cake or refreshments. Include them in seminar presentations when appropriate.
- **Give periodic orientation and updates.** You need not feel compelled to prematurely share study findings with your team, but focus instead on the variables, their improvement in measurement, and spin-off ideas arising from their observations.
- **Find right roles and replacements.** Don't be imprisoned by the chores. Try constantly to work smarter so that you let your team work for your study. If you are carrying out the work of others, stop and consider reassignments. You may find the person you have assigned to a project director role cannot direct others. If so, it is best to deal with this early; otherwise, you will be doing that person's job. If someone doesn't seem to fit in a research team role you first assigned him or her to, try something different. Let everyone experience success as much as possible, but do not neglect dealing with an absolute misfit in roles. Find the detail people on your team, and let them excel in record keeping and precision. Those that are better in social roles can be spokespersons or arrange meetings.
- **Clear understanding of data ownership.** Hard feelings arise after the fact if every team member thinks he or she can dip into the database and publish findings. Begin discussions early about who may do what with your study's data.
- **Clear authorship/presentation agreements.** As PI, you are responsible for the dissemination of research results, but you will likely generate findings that

provide interesting observations for secondary data analysis. Make it clear from the beginning that any use of the data must be cleared with you before dissemination. At the same time, share the load and the opportunity with those who are contributors to the project's scientific work. Include co-investigators in publication and presentations. If you have realistically included co-investigators who contribute to your work, they deserve to share in the fruits of dissemination. On the other hand, consultants, research assistants, and persons employed to do various tasks on the study should not expect to be included in publications.

REMEMBER TO CARE FOR YOUR RESEARCH SITES

Cooperation from your clinical or community research site can either make or break a research study. Finding helpers among employees in a hospital unit or clinical site can ease your access. Appointing clinical people as volunteer coordinators gives them a feeling of ownership and may be a necessity for navigating an institution's internal IRB. Always include an orientation about your study for each shift so they are aware what you are doing in the midst of their unit. If you have such valuable support from your research site, seek alternative rewards to show your gratitude. Sometimes this can be in the form of coffee and bagels or in contributions to their unit library. Always remember your research sites on holidays and special times. One way our project team chose to reward the clinical site over the December holidays was to bring a decorative bushel basket of apples (one for each shift). They loved the departure from candy and sweets over the holidays.

THINGS YOUR MOTHER MAY NEVER HAVE TOLD YOU

About Stewardship and Wise Spending

A grant is an endowment of trust. It is an investment in the future and sign of faith that you can carry out the project. You are expected to be a thoughtful steward of this funding. Treat it as if you are the trusted treasurer of a highly venerated order.

Who Keeps Books?

If you have a small grant with only a few items approved for purchase, keeping books is a snap. Your institution's accounting office will inform you how you may purchase the items and how you should keep records and receipts, because they will become part of your report as well. Things become less clear-cut when you employ research assistants, give cash as remuneration to subjects, or deal with purchasing hourly services from a transcriptionist. You should keep an accounting of your spending, but you should engage services from your institution's accounting office to keep a paper trail that is available for auditing. Each expenditure should be accounted for and clearly related to your budgeted award. There is some flexibility within categories for small changes in items, but always get clearance from your institution's post-award grant official for any changes you contemplate. Help dispel the myth that because you have a grant, that all manner of things can now be charged to it. Along with your own care and stewardship, there are several other mechanisms that routinely audit and follow up on grant expenditures. Be parsimonious in your spending and pristine in your accounting and record keeping ("purer than Caesar's wife" comes to mind!). Expect questions to arise that you haven't thought of. (How much does that lab rat cost? Who orders that lab rat? Where do we get pencils for those 100 people completing surveys today?). You can start your own collection of unanticipated questions. Try to keep a sense of humor. Some day they will make excellent anecdotes or the making of a book on lessons learned.

Whose Money Is It?

Although you may be the PI of a grant, the funds may actually not be awarded to *you* personally. Federal grants are typically awarded to the institution at which the PI is employed. Your own institution may require that all grants, no matter how small, be managed by its Office of Research Administration. Although this may offend your sensibilities somewhat (who wrote this grant anyway?), the benefits outweigh any drawbacks. You get the scholarly credit and recognition, but the institution takes care of much of the big accounting chores, maintains your funds in a safe place, and keeps you in line with institutional assurances to the funding agency. In return, your institution gets indirect costs from large grants above and beyond those funding your research. A well-run Office of Research Administration provides a repository for your funds and your information while making sure you maintain your fiscal agreements. If you change jobs and institutions during the period of the grant, be clear as to whether or not you can move the grant before you accept a new job and find out that the grant must remain behind.

A CAVEAT TO THE SUCCESSFUL

Once the fatigue of waiting for your grant results is extinguished by the exhilaration of a grant award, beware of the feeling you may have of being "on a roll." You may feel like turning around and writing still another grant while you have the spirit. The feeling is similar to that of a new mother of twins who looks at the angelic babes on her lap and says "Oh well, what's one more?" Unlike twins, you have a choice to put off taking on another grant until you have the first one well established. Your grant deserves undivided attention while you build your project team and nurture your project. Like twins, managing multiple studies takes more time. The more projects you are engaged in, the less time you have to write, think up new ideas, and relate to your project team. Stay focused. Delay dashing off to write another grant until your present project is functioning well. Use your grant team to help you flesh out ideas for your next grant application.

New investigators often fall into a similar situation when they apply for and receive several small grants. The grantee may be caught up in the thrill of getting small grants without thinking ahead to the work involved with each. This may not create a problem if the grants were awarded to carry out different parts of the same study. Where the rub comes is when a grantee is successfully awarded several small grants to carry out two or three different studies at the same time. In most cases, these are local grants from organizations or foundations with little knowledge of how overcommitted the grantee is. The grantee likewise has not thought ahead beyond the wonderful prospect of "being funded." Small grants offer no salary support for the investigator so, along with a regular work schedule, the PI soon realizes that "just one more" means double the time commitment.

PROGRESS REPORTS ONCE THE FUNDING BEGINS

The same care that you took to write the grant must go into the submission of the progress reports. Although the form of progress reports may vary with funding institutions, you must attend to details carefully to ensure continuation or successful completion of your grant.

The cycle of progress reports depends on the funding agency. For a grant that is awarded for several years, such as a National Institutes of Health (NIH) research grant or a Department of Health and Human Services (DHHS) Training grant, reports are annual *noncompeting* grant submissions. The acknowledgment of any changes that have occurred during the grant period and the progress made toward meeting the designated objectives/goals must be addressed in these reports. If a particular grant objective has not been met, then clearly state why. Ideally, you should be talking to your technical support person all along the grant's cycle, and the agency should already be aware of the problem. Even if the agency is aware, the problem and possible solution must be included in the report.

In the case of some grants, such as cooperative agreements from the Centers for Disease Control and Prevention, quarterly reports are required along with noncompeting grant renewals for each year of the grant. The guidelines for these reports must be followed to comply with the agency's regulations.

NONCOMPETING RENEWAL GRANTS

The funding cycle for a grant is 3 to 5 years for many federal grants. The second, third, and fourth years are referred to as *noncompeting grant renewal years*. This means that your project team or you, as the PI, are required to resubmit a streamlined *noncompeting continuation* grant application, including the grant's progress, budget usage or changes, and the proposed activities for the coming year. If federal funds to the NIH or DHHS are cut drastically by Congress, grants could theoretically be cut as well. Because it was previously approved, your grant will not compete with new grant applications for funding. However, if the funding agency is dissatisfied with the grant's progress, it has the option to either decrease the funds or not renew the grant. Funded grants are rarely terminated unless there is a very good reason.

During renewal may be the time to request changes in budget lines. You generally need to make these requests in writing before funds can actually be moved from one budget line to another. But such budgetary changes certainly can be made at the time of noncompeting renewal. It is advisable to discuss the budgetary changes with your contact person at the agency before submitting the request as a part of your noncompeting renewal grant. Be as careful with these applications as you were with the first submission; they will be reviewed and scrutinized in most instances. Today's competitive world dictates an eye for detail in the renewal process.

Timelines for submissions of these reports can be just as sticky as the original grant application. Annual reports are generally required well in advance of a year. Sometimes an institution has an internal process for how these reports are sent. They may need to be reviewed by the department head, senior administrator, comptroller, or budget officer. Know these key people, the process, and their time frame for reviewing these reports.

PLANNING THE CONTINUATION

A successful grant not only accomplishes the goals and specific aims of the project, but it generates meaningful questions that beg for answers. If your NIH research grant or training project has done that, you may wish to submit a *competing renewal* grant at the completion of your present grant if you have a compelling rationale to continue the same study with perhaps an enhanced population or approach. Not all levels of NIH funding allow competing renewals. Inquiries for all competing renewal applications should be directed to the NIH Program Officer for the current grant. What is more likely is that a new question or direction will cause you to write a new grant, perhaps moving from small grant funding (R03 or R15) to a large project (R01). Discuss your plans with your program office; write up a concept paper or abstract of what you are considering. Be sure to address information that your current funding has provided that moves you in this direction. Funding agencies look for their awards to generate new grant applications. Take advantage of the advice they offer.

LIFE AFTER GRANTS

There really is a life after grants! As a researcher/educator/practitioner, you must decide where you want your career to go after the grant is finished. It may be on to the next project or it may be to take a breather and really think about your next professional move. If you have not been successful at obtaining further funding, then perhaps this is a time to review other avenues for funding with a little different twist. For example, you might seek funds from Avon to examine the use of their skin care products in an adolescent population that has undergone chemotherapy with resultant dry skin. Or you might look at the use of complementary therapies in the treatment of women with endometriosis who are infertile. Although these two areas may not seem too out of line with current trends, they are not the usual mode of research for most nurses; the "twist" might give you a competitive edge. Another example is a nurse researcher with fibromyalgia who wants to compare time to diagnosis between health professionals and nonprofessionals. Again, this idea is not far from mainstream, but has a new twist and may produce cost-effective results if one group is determined to obtain a diagnosis of fibromyalgia sooner than the other.

The time after a grant also affords you space to get the manuscripts and presentations written that seemed so elusive during the day-to-day administration of the grant. Presentations can be a joy when they come from your passion. Tell your story. Get people excited about you and your work. These presentations can also bring you into contact with other researchers or persons responsible for funding in your area. Remember that these presentations are selling your expertise and your work. A well-articulated presentation will bring other opportunities for success. These opportunities may take your career in a slightly different direction than you had planned. Don't be afraid to go for the ride!

Don't underestimate the power of poster presentations. Many seasoned researchers or educators will not do posters. Personally, I find them very rewarding because novices will ask many questions when you are standing by a poster; few will ask these questions in a large audience listening to an oral presentation. For the seasoned researcher, this is a time to be a good role model and help shape the career of a junior researcher. You can provide mentorship to another person. If you are the novice researcher or educator, a poster presentation is less intimidating than standing before the masses to orally present.

Take this time to renew your life. Too many times, nurses in particular try to continue to do it all. Let's face it: a grant and the work associated with it takes its toll on our lives and those of our family and friends. The time after a grant lets you renew your ties with the outside world. Some of you may laugh at that statement, but others know this to be true of either yourself or some of your colleagues. So take the time. Take that vacation. Go to that play you have been putting off for months. Renew your soul so you are ready for the next project.

CONCLUSION

Your grant award is a remarkable hallmark of your scholarship and one you can be justly proud of. However, the award is just the beginning of the work. Pick your team well; nurture and care for them, and they will reward you with good service. Take equal care of your research sites, and show your appreciation in tangible ways. Maintain the confidence and goodwill of your funding agency by submitting meticulously written, timely reports. When the project director or PI does not follow the guidelines or is habitually late on reports, funding agencies tend to question the management of the project. They are concerned about the team's commitment to the project for which they have supported with funds. Do not put yourself in that position. Put your best foot forward, and keep on track of the endless paper trail.

Finally, take time. Take care and maintain balance in your life. Life does go on and really is not grant dependent. Keep your sense of humor and laugh often! You will rarely find one's grant history carved on his or her tombstone.

HELPFUL READING FOR THE FUNDED GRANT WRITER

Bergstrom, N., & Baun, M. M. (1994). The proposal-reality gap: The mechanics of implementing a funded research proposal. *Nursing Outlook, 42*(6), 272–278.

Brown, L. P., Meier, P., Spatz, D. L., Spitzer, A., Finkler, S. A., Jacobsen, B. S., & Zukowsky, K. (1997). Resubmission of a grant application: Breast-feeding services for LBW infants. *Nursing Research, 46*(2), 119–122.

Ingersoll, G. L., & Eberhard, D. (1999). Grants management skills keep funded projects on target. *Nursing Economics, 17*(3), 131–141.

Minnick, A., Kleinpell, R. M., Micek, W., & Dudley, D. (1996). The management of multisite study. *Journal of Professional Nursing, 12*(1), 7–15.

Ries, J. B., & Leukefeld, C. G. (1995). Funded. In *Applying for research funding: Getting started and getting funded* (pp. 225–236). Thousand Oaks, CA: Sage.

Selby-Harrington, M. L., Donat, P. L., & Hibbard, H. D. (1993). Guidance for managing a research grant. *Nursing Research, 42*(1), 54–58.

CHAPTER 10

Dissemination of Grant Findings

DISSEMINATION: HARVESTING THE PRODUCTS OF RESEARCH

Nursing scholarship cannot advance without dissemination of findings from scientific research. Although the funding agency usually asks for a written report to learn of your study outcomes, your dissemination of scientific findings to a wider audience is of an even greater contribution to universal knowledge. The evidence base of nursing science grows with each contribution of search and discovery to the literature. In today's world of translational science, professional silos are fast disappearing. Your published study in a nursing journal may pique the interest of a scientist in a different discipline and even in a different country.

ADVANCING YOUR CAREER THROUGH DISSEMINATION

It is imperative for any grant recipient to disseminate the outcomes of his or her funded research study. This final step in the grant process is a hallmark of an investigator's responsibility, capability, and contribution to scientific knowledge. Your scholarly career will be judged, not only by your ability to obtain grants but on your ability to follow through to completion by dissemination to others. Scientific publications are the gold standard for dissemination because they are widely distributed and easily retrieved through literature databases such as Medline or CINAHL. Publications of book chapters may give you entries in your curriculum vitae (CV) but are limited in distribution and nearly impossible for others to find from literature databases. One form of dissemination is an abstract/poster presentation. Podium or poster presentations can be ideal for dissemination of findings while awaiting journal publication if your selected scholarly journal allows it. However, podium or poster presentations should not take the place of a scientific publication. Sometimes numerous abstract and poster presentations limit your time for writing manuscripts so that you must be more selective about choosing speaking engagements in order to allow more time for writing. For some researchers, the poster or abstract presentations acts as the springboard for manuscript submissions. These presentations also bring you into contact with others who may be doing similar research and offer great opportunities for networking. Others may procrastinate by doing presentations and move on to the next study without a written publication. Written dissemination of your data has the potential to contribute more to the scholarship of practice, teaching, and research resulting from a broader and more permanent avenue of dissemination.

DEVELOP A PLAN

Develop a dissemination plan for all aspects of your scholarship. As you begin to develop a program of research, opportunities exist for dissemination at various levels including publication of literature reviews, theory development, pilot data, instrument development, primary and secondary research questions, serendipitous findings, and secondary analyses. A successful track record of dissemination can occur only if you make this aspect of your scholarship a priority. For most individuals, this means setting aside several hours a day or perhaps one day a week, depending on your schedule and writing style. Because writing often can take second place in a busy academic schedule, it is important to outline your publications and set timelines for submission to keep yourself on track.

As you begin your study, map out the articles and spin-off publications you wish to accomplish and set up a timeline. Engage your co-investigators and team members in presentations and publications appropriate to their contributions and interests. In our funded study on outcomes of fever in HIV, several spin-off projects emerged when doctoral students were involved. Some were able to participate in publishable literature reviews around variables under study. Others developed their own projects from secondary data. When writing for publication, target your journal carefully, based on the objectives you are trying to achieve. Know the audience of that journal. If the manuscript's goal is to reach clinicians in a timely manner, you may want to choose a clinical journal with a short publication schedule. If, however, the data are not as time sensitive and the goal is to reach a broader audience, you may choose to submit your manuscript to a well-recognized, scholarly journal that has a larger subscription base but where the timeline for publication following acceptance is longer. Clinical intervention research often lends itself to a scholarly publication in a research journal and a practice-oriented description of the intervention in a clinical practice journal. In this case, the research from the scholarly journal can be cited and can serve as a resource to the descriptive clinical article—but not a second research article. This approach makes it clear to a reader that you are not engaging in duplicate publication or "salami science" where an author slices a research study into the thinnest possible slices to maximize the number of publications (Feeg, 1992; Hoit, 2007). In choosing journals, consider nursing as well as nonnursing, discipline-specific journals if the topic is of interest to professionals outside of nursing. Please consider too that the reviewers may be researchers in your area or ones you have quoted, so make sure you are accurate. It is wise to see who is on the editorial board and review panel if possible to see who might have published in your area. There is nothing worse than to have a reviewer recognize that you have not acknowledged his or her work. Another word to the wise, following author guidelines is not optional. You must follow them. Once you have targeted a journal, see if there is a similar article on a different topic. Follow that format. If they published that article, then yours may have a greater chance of getting published. For example, Kenner's topic on "Transition from Hospital to Home for Mothers and Babies" might be similar to a hospital discharge and follow-up for an adult. If the latter article was published, then maybe mine would be too. In fact it was. So be savvy when it comes to selecting and targeting a journal for dissemination of your work.

PUBLISHING RESEARCH

Writing up research findings may involve a new learning curve for a beginning researcher. Even if you have published review or informative articles before, the process for publishing a research report is different. Unlike a dissertation, which may resemble a telephone book in size, the research article is usually no more than 16 pages and is crisp, concise, and free of extraneous verbiage. Your experience in writing a research grant is good preparation for writing research reports because it involves a stylized format and gets immediately to the point. Read examples of research reports from the journal in which you wish to publish. Their *Guide to the Author* page or Web site should tell you if they have a recommended style or format for your submission. Choose a journal that is likely to publish your methodology. Major nursing research journals, *Nursing Research, Research in Nursing and Health,* and *Western Journal of Nursing Research* now publish studies using both qualitative and quantitative approaches. Some have page limits that make it harder to include the rich narratives of qualitative studies. Others are highly supportive of this work, and there are a growing number of journals dedicated to or receptive of this methodology. A Web site sponsored by St. Louis University posts an extensive list of nursing and interdisciplinary journals accepting or focusing on qualitative research articles at http://www.slu.edu/organizations/qrc/QRjournals.html. Examine samples of articles from a variety of journals, and shop around before you choose a target to submit your article to.

EXPECT TO COMPETE

Getting published is not a shoo-in just because your grant was funded. Like grantsmanship, you must expect to compete. Get help if writing the manuscript seems an onerous task. Writing of any kind gets easier the more you practice it.

Engage help from your statistical consultant before writing quantitative findings. If someone on your grant team shines in writing, let that person help you organize the research report. Have plenty of review from colleagues and experts before submission. To increase your manuscript acceptance rate, you may want to consider setting up a process for scientific review of your manuscript prior to submission. Select the reviewers based on the type of feedback you are seeking for your manuscript (e.g., copyediting, design and methods, or clinical implications). Do not be discouraged or defeated by a rejected manuscript. Although rejection of a manuscript by a journal editor is difficult, remember it was the article, not *you*, being rejected. Articles can be reworked. Take the comments provided and use them to improve the manuscript. Ultimately you may choose to resubmit to the same journal or even a different journal after careful evaluation of the journal's target audience. Occasionally you may find that the same reviewer will receive your manuscript to review when you submit it to a different journal. This often happens when you write in a specialized area. For this reason, do take the time and effort to make any recommended changes and rethink areas that received negative comments. Ideally, when submitting a manuscript, have both a primary and secondary journal in mind. This method will facilitate the resubmission process.

Finally, you need to evaluate your dissemination plan periodically and adjust it as necessary. This evaluation should include your publication submission-to-acceptance ratio. You might find that you need to reorganize your scholarship priorities to increase your publication output. Perhaps you need to develop more realistic goals and timelines for publications.

CONCLUSION

Dissemination of your findings is exciting. Few ego boosts equal seeing your name in print on a widely disseminated article. Publication allows you to share your information and build a niche for yourself as you build a professional career. The writing and dissemination through presentations becomes your legacy to the profession and to your family. Like any scholarly endeavor, the more you practice, the greater the ease and elegance of your product. Look for opportunities and contribute your work to the world around you!

References

Abraham, I. L., & Wasserbauer, L. I. (2006). Quasi-experimental research. In J. Fitzpatrick & M. Wallace (Eds.), Encyclopedia of Nursing Research (2nd ed., pp. 506–507). New York: Springer.

American Association for the Advancement of Science. (2007). New congress wraps up 2007 budget with increases for key R&D programs; overall research funding flat (AAAS R&D Funding Update). Retrieved June 6, 2007, from http://www.aaas.org/spp/rd/upd107.htm.

American Psychological Association. (2001). Publication manual of the American Psychological Association (5th ed., p. 6). Washington, DC: Author.

Benefield, L.E. (2005). Distance caregiving of CI elders living alone at home. NIH/ National Institute for Nursing Research Grant 7R03NR009512-02.

Bergstrom, N., & Baun, M. M. (1994). The proposal-reality gap: The mechanics of implementing a funded research proposal. Nursing Outlook, 42(6), 272–278.

Birkett, M. A., & Day, S. J. (1994). Internal pilot studies for estimating sample size. Statistics in Medicine, 13(23–24), 2455–2463.

Bravo, N. R., & Olsen, K. L. (2007). NIH-NSF Definition of Postdoctoral Scholar, NIH-NSF Definition of Postdoctoral Scholar (January 29, 2007 Letter to National Postdoctoral Association) (02/22/2007) – (PDF - 76 KB) Bethesda MD: NIH. Retrieved 4/1/08 from http://grants.nih.gov/training/Reed_Letter.pdf

Burns, N., & Burns, S. K. (2005). The practice of nursing research: Conduct, critique and utilization (5th ed., p. 71). St. Louis: Elsevier Saunders.

Cohen, J. (1988). Statistical power analysis for the behavioral sciences (2nd ed.). Hillsdale, NJ: Erlbaum.

Cohen, J. (1990). Things I have learned (so far). American Psychologist, 45(12), 1304–1312.

Department of Health and Human Services. (2004). FY 2004 budget in brief. Retrieved February 9, 2008, from HYPERLINK "http://www.hhs.gov/budget/04budget/fy2004bib.pdf" http://www.hhs.gov/budget/04budget/fy2004bib.pdf.

Feeg, V. D. (1992). Duplicate publication or salami science? Pediatric Nursing, 18(6), 550.

Gerin, W. (2006). Writing the NIH grant proposal: A step-by-step guide. Thousand Oaks, CA: Sage.

Grunau, R. V., Whitfield, M. F., Petrie, J. H., & Fryer, E. L. (1994). Early pain experience, child and family factors, as precursors of somatization: A prospective study of extremely premature and full-term children. Pain, 56(3), 353–359.

Health Resources and Services Administration (1998). Nursing: Title VIII Program Legislation / Retrieved February 9, 2008, from HYPERLINK "http://bhpr.hrsa.gov/nursing/legislation.htm" http://bhpr.hrsa.gov/nursing/legislation.htm.

Hoit, J. D. (2007). Salami science. American Journal of Speech-Language Pathology, 16(2), 94.

Holtzclaw, B. J. (1994). Febrile symptom management for persons living with AIDS. R01, NIH/ National Institute for Nursing Research (R01 NR03988).

Holtzclaw, B. J. (2006). In good company: Celebrating 50 years of American Nurses Foundation research scholars. Nursing Outlook, 54(1), 17–22.

Holtzclaw, B. J. (2007, April). Characteristics of a fundable research grant. Paper presented at the Second Research Conference of the Association of Nurses in AIDS Care (ANAC), San Antonio, TX.

International Committee of Medical Journal Editors. (2006). Uniform requirements for manuscripts submitted to biomedical journals: Writing and editing for biomedical publication. Retrieved September 28, 2007, from HYPERLINK "http://www.icmje.org/#author" http://www.icmje.org/#author.

Jones, C. B., Tulman, L., & Clancy, C. M. (1999). Research funding opportunities at the Agency for Health Care Policy and Research. Nursing Outlook, 47 (4), 156-161.

Kron, R. E., & Litt, M. (1971). Fluid mechanics of nutritive sucking behaviour: the suckling infant's oral apparatus analysed as a hydraulic pump. Medical & Biological Engineering, 9(1), 45-60.

Levine, E. (2006). Quantitative research. In J. Fitzpatrick & M. Wallace (Eds.), Encyclopedia of Nursing Research (2nd ed., pp. 503–504). New York: Springer.

Medoff-Cooper, B., McGrath, J. M., & Bilker, W. (2000). Nutritive sucking and neurobehavioral development in preterm infants from 34 weeks PCA to term. MCN, American Journal of Maternal Child Nursing, 25(2), 64-70.

Mitchell, P. H. (2006). Research and development in nursing revisited: Nursing science as the basis for evidence-based practice. Journal of Advanced Nursing, 54(5), 528–529.

National Institutes of Health (NIH). (2005). Multiple-PI versus single-PI NIH applications. In Frequently asked questions. Bethesda, MD: Author. Retrieved September 28, 2007, from http://grants2.nih.gov/grants/multi_pi/Mult_PI_FAQ_6_Feb_2006.doc.

NIH Office of Portfolio Analysis and Strategic Initiatives. (2007). NIH Roadmap Initiatives. , Bethesda, MD: Author. Retrieved September 28, 2007, from HYPERLINK "http://nihroadmap.nih.gov/initiatives.asp" http://nihroadmap.nih.gov/initiatives.asp.

NIH Office of Portfolio Analysis and Strategic Initiatives. (2006). Overview of the NIH Roadmap. Retrieved June 18, 2007, from http://nihroadmap.nih.gov/overview.asp.

Parker, B., & Steeves, R. (2005). The National Research Service Award: Strategies for developing a successful proposal. Journal of Professional Nursing, 21(1), 23–31.

Sackett, D. L., Rosenberg, W. M., Gray, J. A., Haynes, R. B., & Richardson, W. S. (1996). Evidence-based medicine: What it is and what it isn't. British Journal of Medicine, 312, 71–72.

Sandelowski, M. (1995). Sample size in qualitative research. Research in Nursing & Health, 18(2), 179–183.

Speziale, H. J. S., & Carpenter, D. R. (2007). Qualitative research in nursing: Advancing the humanistic imperative (4th ed., p. 20). Philadelphia: Lippincott Williams & Wilkins.

Tripp-Reimer, T., & Kelley, L. S. (2006). Qualitative research. In J. Fitzpatrick & M. Wallace (Eds.), Encyclopedia of Nursing Research (2nd ed., pp. 497–499). New York: Springer

Walden, M. (2001). Environment and sleep on preterm infants pain response. 1R15NR007731-01 NIH/ National Institute for Nursing Research.

Glossary

Academic Research Enhancement Award (R15)—NIH mechanism used to support small-scale research projects conducted by faculty in educational institutions that have not been major participants in NIH programs.

Application identification numbers—A unique number assigned to a submitted NIH application that identifies (in this order): Type of application (e.g., 1 = new, 2 = competing continuation, etc.); activity code (e.g., R01); serial number assigned by the Center for Scientific Review (e.g., 143723), suffix showing the support year for the grant (e.g., the first year of a grant would be -01), and other information identifying a supplement (e.g., S1), amendment (e.g., A1), or other modifying data. A sample application identification number would be 1 R01 AI 143723 -01 A1 S1.

Career Development Awards (K awards)—NIH series of grant awards to support PhDs and clinicians wishing to develop careers in biomedical research. The level of award (K1 through K99) depends on the type and level of training, research, or mentorship.

Contract—An award that establishes a binding legal procurement relationship between NIH and an award recipient obligating the latter to provide a product or service defined in detail by NIH and binding the institute to pay for it.

Cooperative agreement—This form of grant usually requires the grantee and grantor work together after the funding begins to formulate research protocols.

CRISP—CRISP (Computer Retrieval of Information on Scientific Projects) is a biomedical database system containing information on research projects and programs supported by the Department of Health and Human Services. Searchable by name, institution, funding institute, date, and topic, the CRISP Web site is a good place to search for scientific concepts, emerging trends and techniques, or to identify specific projects and/or investigators.

Direct costs—Expenses, such as salaries, equipment specifically designated for the project, and other monies that go to support the actual project.

Evidence-based practice—The use of scientific data or a large collection of practical knowledge that supports clinical interventions.

Facilities and administrative costs (F&A)—Costs that are budgeted on grants for several common or joint objectives and cannot be specifically identified with a particular project or program. These costs are commonly known as *indirect costs*.

Funding mechanism—The type of funded application or transaction used at the NIH and which falls into one of three types: grants, contracts, and cooperative agreements.

GANTT chart—A visual use of bar graphs to depict timelines for various aspects of a project.

Indirect costs—The expenses or overhead that it takes to run a grant: the benefits packages, cost of utilities, phone cost, and other hidden costs that are part of the bricks and mortar of conducting daily business in any institution. Also known as facilities and administrative costs (F&A).

Institutional review board (IRB)—A review panel made up of health professionals and at least one or two laypersons that examines the grant for research safety and scientific merit only in relationship to participant rights and safety. This panel resides either in the hospital where the research, educational, or special project is conducted; in the academic center; or both.

Noncompeting continuation—Continued support for an NIH-funded grant. Progress reports for continued support do not undergo peer review but are administratively reviewed by the institute/center and receive an award based on prior award commitments. Also known as a Type 5.

Noncompeting grant—An ongoing grant whose award is contingent on the completion of a progress report as the condition for the release of money for the following year. Award is predicated on solid evidence that the grant is doing what it set out to do.

Pink sheets—Term formerly used to describe NIH summary statements (which were at one time printed on pink paper).

Power analysis—A method by which a sample size is calculated to achieve significance. This analysis considers the level of significance of the variable of interest, the effect size desired, and finally what number of subjects it will take to achieve significance results.

Qualitative research—A method of research that looks at the subjective worldview. The concern is to describe "what is" rather than be able to predict why an event occurred.

Quantitative research—A research method interested in quantifying or counting responses. This type of research answers questions of relationships, probability, causality, and predictability. Objective, verifiable data are of interest.

Request for applications (RFA)—A call for grantees to apply for research or educational funds. These calls designate the objectives for the grant monies, the type of grant that will be accepted for review, and the cycle for the grant from application to the funding announcement.

Request for proposals (RFP)—This is another name for the call for grant applications. It is basically the same as an RFA, but applications are accepted on a broad range of research priorities versus solicitation of proposals for a specific designated priority area.

Scientific review administrator (SRA)—An NIH scientist-administrator who presides over a scientific review group, coordinates the meeting, and reports the review of each application assigned to it. The SRA serves as an intermediary between the applicant and reviewers and prepares summary statements for all applications reviewed.

Small Business Innovation Research (SBIR) and Small Business Technology Transfer (STTR) grants—NIH-sponsored programs that support projects to establish the technical merit and feasibility of research and development ideas leading to commercial products or services.

Special Projects of Regional and National Significance (SPRANS)—Grant funds to support projects that support a regional or national healthcare need.

Summary statements—Combined reviewers' written comments and the SRA's summary of the review panel's discussion during the study section meeting. It includes the recommendations of the study section, a recommended budget, and administrative notes of special considerations.

Systematic or integrated reviews—Reviews of literature, usually of randomized clinical control trials, that represent the state of the science on a specific topic. Databases on the Internet house these reviews that provide evidence to support a grant area or an intervention.

Resources: Printed or Web Based

An abundance of grant resources is available through the print media or the Internet. This list is not meant to be all-inclusive, but to give a start to early search efforts. Listing of a resource does not imply an endorsement of the institution or product. Because Web sites or addresses of businesses and foundations can change periodically, use names and titles on the list as Internet browser search terms for finding new addresses and emerging resources.

GRANTFUNDING SOURCES FOR HEALTHCARE SUBJECTS

The following list represents foundations and other funding agencies that support research, education, scholarships, or special projects. The funding areas listed will help you to determine exactly what type of project each agency supports.

American Nurses Foundation
8515 Georgia Avenue
Suite 400 West
Silver Spring, MD 20910
E-mail: anf@ana.org
Phone: (301) 628-5227
Fax: (301) 628-5354
Web site: http://www.anfonline.org

Funding Areas
Beginning and advanced nurse researchers who are developing a research career. There are several cosponsored grants that have a specific area of nursing research that is specified; otherwise, funds are available for general nursing research.

Archstone Foundation
401 E. Ocean Boulevard, Suite 1000
Long Beach, CA 90802
E-mail: archstone@archstone.org
Phone: (562) 590-8655
Fax: (562) 495-0317
Web site: http://www.archstone.org/

Funding Areas

Health and well-being of seniors and supporting their choices in health care throughout the aging process. The majority of grants support senior programs in Southern California. Demonstration projects and programs that have a regional or national impact on senior issues are considered from any part of the country.

Association of Women's Health, Obstetric and Neonatal Nurses (AWHONN)

AWHONN Research Grants
2000 L Street, NW, Suite 740
Washington, DC 20036
Phone: (800) 673-8499 x2431 (U.S.)
Phone: (800) 245-0231 (Canada)
Fax: (202) 728-0575
Web site: http://www.awhonn.org/awhonn/

Funding Areas

The AWHONN small research grants program is designed for researchers who are working on first-time efforts at beginning development of a program of research. The purpose of the funding is to provide seed money, pilot funding, or total funding for small projects with promising contributions to nursing knowledge in clinical practice. The focus of the research is women's health, obstetric, or neonatal nursing phenomena. All AWHONN grants are awarded to members only. Membership must be current at the time of application, selection, and funding. An application for membership may accompany the proposal. If there are multiple investigators, the individual named as principal investigator must be a member. Researchers who are currently principal investigators on a federally funded grant or who have already received an AWHONN-funded research grant in the past five years are not eligible.

Centers for Disease Control and Prevention (CDC)

1600 Clifton Road
Atlanta, GA 30333
Phone: (404) 639-3311 or (404) 639-3534 or (800) 311-3435
Web site: http://www.cdc.gov/ or www.cdc.gov/od/pgo/funding/funding.htm or http://www.cdc.gov/od/pgo/forminfo.htm

Funding Areas

Multiple program and research grant opportunities exist with the CDC:

1. Agency for Toxic Substances and Disease Registry Public Health Conference Support Grant Program
2. *HIV Prevention Projects*: HIV/AIDS Surveillance and HIV Incidence and Prevalence Surveys; Leadership and Investment in Fighting an Epidemic (LIFE)—Global AIDS Activity; National Partnerships for Human Immuno-deficiency Virus (HIV) Prevention with a Focus on Business and Labor, Youth at High Risk, and Migrant Workers; Public Health Conference Support Cooperative Agreement Program for Human Immunodeficiency Virus (HIV) Prevention
3. *Chronic Disease Prevention/Health Promotion*: Postinfective Fatigue: A Model for Chronic Fatigue Syndrome; Health Promotion and Disease Prevention Initiatives Related to Chronic Disease Prevention and Health Promotion; Initiative to Educate State Legislatures About Priority Public Health Issues
4. *Emerging Infections*: Epidemiology and Laboratory Capacity for Infectious Diseases
5. *Environmental Health*: Childhood Lead Poisoning Prevention Programs
6. *Injury and Violence Prevention and Control*: Grants for Acute Care; Rehabilitation and Disability Prevention Research; Grants for Traumatic Injury Biomechanics Research; Grants for Violence-Related Injury Prevention Research
7. *Minority Health/Health Promotion*
8. *Occupational Safety and Health*: Beryllium-Induced Diseases; Occupational Safety and Health R01s; Research Methods for Occupational Cancer; State Fatality Surveillance and Field Investigations of Occupational Injuries: Fatality Assessment and Control Evaluation; Career Development Grants in Occupational Safety and Health Research (K01s); Small Grants in Occupational Safety and Health Research (R03s); Community-Based Interventions to Prevent Childhood Agricultural Injury and Disease; Worldwide Occupational Safety and Health Program; Centers for Agricultural Disease and Injury Research, Education, and Prevention; Traumatic Occupational Injury Research—Science for Prevention; Extended Work Schedules in the New Economy—Health and Safety Risks to Workers; Occupational Exposure to Putative Reproductive/Developmental Toxicants in Humans
9. *Public Health Laws and Practices*: Association of State and Territorial Directors of Health Promotion and Public Health Education (ASTDHPPHE)
10. *Sexually Transmitted Diseases*: Competitive Supplemental Funds for Comprehensive STD Prevention Systems—Monitoring STD Prevalence and Reproductive Health Services for Adolescent Women in Special Settings
11. *Tuberculosis*

CDC Foundation
50 Hurt Plaza
Suite 765
Atlanta, GA 30303
Phone: (404) 653-0709 or (888) 880-4CDC or (888) 880-4232
Fax: (404) 653-0330
Web site: http://www.cdcfoundation.org/index1.shtml

Funding Areas
Price Fellowships for HIV Prevention are awarded to build relationships between governmental and nongovernmental agencies to provide HIV prevention programs. Grants are given to support information programs that build partnerships to promote health.

China Foundation
9216 Falls Chapel Way
Potomac, MD 20854
E-mail: info@chinafoundation1.org or education@chinafoundation1.org, or health@chinafoundation1.org
Phone: (301) 340-2065
Fax: (301) 340-3814
Web site: http://www.chinafoundation1.org/

Funding Areas
Think tank to support health care, education, and social security reform in China. Projects that provide basic medical services to remote China villages; renovation or building of China elementary schools; or working with other nonprofit organizations, foundations, and think tanks to develop and improve healthcare systems, health insurance, education, and environmental protection for China.

The Commonwealth Fund
One East 75th Street
New York, NY 10021-2692
E-mail: nb@cmwf.org
Phone: (212) 606-3800
Fax: (212) 606-3500
Web site: http://www.commonwealthfund.org/fellowships/index.asp

Funding Areas
Research on health and social policy issues
Fellowship Programs
The Commonwealth Fund/Harvard University Fellowship in Minority Health Policy; Harkeness Fellowships in Health Care Policy; and Ian Axford Fellowships in Public Policy

Program Grants
Research on health and social issues with emphasis on practice and policy. The fund is most concerned about vulnerable populations. Specific programs areas are improving access to care, improving quality of healthcare services, international healthcare policy and practice, and improving public spaces and services.

Charles E. Culpeper Foundation and the Rockefeller Brothers Fund
These funds have merged.
437 Madison Avenue, 37th Floor
New York, NY 10022-7001
E-mail: info@rbf.org
Phone: (212) 812-4200
Fax: (212) 812-4299
Web site: http://www.rbf.org/

Funding Areas
Health, education, arts and culture, and administration of justice

Nathan Cummings Foundation
1926 Broadway
Suite 600
New York, NY 10023-6915
E-mail: grants@cummings.ncf.org
Phone: (212) 787-7300
Fax: (212) 787-7377
Web site: http://www.ncf.org/

Funding Areas
Environment, health, Jewish life, spirituality, and democratic values

Department of Health and Human Services (DHHS)
Grants Management Branch
Bureau of Health Professions
Health Resources and Services Administration
8C-26 Parklawn Building
5600 Fishers Lane
Rockville, MD 20857
Web site: http://www.hrsa.dhhs.gov/bhpr/

Funding Areas
Academic administrative units in primary care, predoctoral training in primary care, physician assistant training in primary care, advanced education nursing

grants, advanced education nursing traineeship grants, advanced education nursing-nurse anesthetist traineeship grant program, residency training in primary care, faculty development in primary care, residencies in the practice of pediatric dentistry, residencies and advanced education in the practice of general dentistry, basic nurse education and practice grants, and public health nursing experiences in state and local health departments for baccalaureate nursing.

Foundation for Neonatal Research and Education
c/o Anthony J. Jannetti, Inc.
Box 56
Pitman, NJ 08071-0056
Phone: (856) 256-2300
Fax: (856) 589-7463
Web site: http://www.ajj.com

Funding Areas
Neonatal healthcare issues and application of research to neonatal practice

Friends Research Institute, Inc.
505 Baltimore Avenue
PO Box 10676
Baltimore, MD 21285
Phone: (410) 823-5116
Fax: (410) 823-5131
Web site: http://www.friendsresearch.org/

Funding Areas
Research for medical, drug, mental treatments, and pharmaceutical studies

Fulbright Scholar Program
Institute of International Education
809 United Nations Plaza
New York, NY 10017-3580
E-mail: info@iie.org
Web site: http://www.iie.org/fulbright/

Funding Areas
Fellowships and programs aimed at university coursework, independent library or field research, classes in a music conservatory or art school, special projects in the social or life sciences, or a combination. The scholarships can be for U.S. international students and scholars or part of faculty/student exchanges.

Bill and Melinda Gates Foundation
William H. Gates Foundation
PO Box 23350
Seattle, WA 98102
Web site: http://www.gatesfoundation.org

Funding Areas
Innovations in education, technology, and world health. Special emphasis on use of technology in developing countries. Health care, health promotion, and other health-related issues involving technology for education or care delivery are acceptable areas.

John Simon Guggenheim Memorial Foundation
90 Park Avenue
New York, NY 10016
E-mail: fellowships@gf.org
Phone: (212) 697-4470
Fax: (212) 697-3248
Web site: http://www.gf.org

Funding Areas
Fellowships for advanced professionals in all fields except performing arts

Walter and Elise Haas Fund
One Lombard Street
Suite 305
San Francisco, CA 94111-1130
E-mail: Brenda@haassr.org
Phone: (415) 398-4474
Fax: (415) 986-4779
Web site: http://www.haassr.org/

Funding Areas
Leadership development

Health Resources and Services Administration (HRSA)
5600 Fishers Lane, Rockville, MD 20857
Phone: (877) HRSA-123
Grants Application Center
E-mail: hrsagac@hrsa.gov
Web site: http://www.hrsa.dhhs.gov/grants.htm

Funding Areas

This is the Bureau of Primary Health Care, the Bureau of Health Professions, Bureau of Maternal and Child Health, and HIV/AIDS Bureau. Funding areas are education and training of health professionals. See DHHS for more information.

Howard Hughes Medical Institute
4000 Jones Bridge Road
Chevy Chase, MD 20815-6789
E-mail: webmaster@hhmi.org/
Phone: (301) 215-8500
Web site: http://www.hhmi.org/

Funding Areas

Strengthening science education from kindergarten through graduate school; graduate program awards for graduate education and medical student research training fellowships. Biomedical research is also supported.

Institute of Medicine Office of Health Policy Educational Programs and Fellowships
Marion Ein Lewin
Office of Health Policy
Programs and Fellowships
2101 Constitution Avenue, NW
Washington, DC 20418
E-mail: iomwww@nas.edu
Phone: (202) 334-1506
Web site: http://www.nas.edu/iom/hppf/hppfhome.nsf

Funding Areas
Advancement of scientific knowledge to improve health

International Research & Exchanges Board
1616 H Street, NW
6th Floor
Washington, DC 20006
E-mail: irex@irex.org
Phone: (202) 628-8188
Fax: (202) 628-8189
Web site: http://www.irex.org/

Funding Areas

Exchange of U.S. scholars to conduct research in Central and Eastern Europe (CEE), the New Independent States (NIS), Mongolia, and China.

Ittleson Foundation
Anthony C. Wood, Executive Director
15 East 67th Street
New York, NY 10021
Phone: (212) 794-2008
Web site: http://www.IttlesonFoundation.org/

Funding Areas
Resources for organizations that serve the environment, those with AIDS, and those with mental health problems

W. M. Keck Foundation
555 South Flower Street
Suite 3230
Los Angeles, CA 90071
E-mail: info@wmkeck.org
Phone: (213) 680-3833
Web site: http://www.wmkeck.org/

Funding Areas
Grants in the areas of outstanding science, engineering and medical research, undergraduate science and engineering and liberal arts education.

W. K. Kellogg Foundation
One Michigan Avenue East
Battle Creek, MI 49017-4058
Phone: (616) 968-1611
Fax: (616) 968-0413
Web site: http://www.wkkf.org/

Funding Areas
Building the capacity of individuals, communities, and institutions to solve their own problems

Lymphoma Research Foundation of America, Inc.
8800 Venice Boulevard, #207
Los Angeles, CA 90034
E-mail: LRFA@aol.com
Phone: (310) 204-7040
Fax: (310) 204-7043
Web site: http://www.lymphoma.org/

Funding Areas
Research and providing patient resources, including support groups, educational materials, clinical trials, information, and a periodic newsletter

A. L. Mailman Family Foundation
707 Westchester Avenue
White Plains, NY 10604
E-mail: betty@mailman.org
Phone: (914) 681-4448
Fax: (914) 686-5519
Web site: http://www.mailman.org/

Funding Areas
Children and families, with a special emphasis on early childhood
Priorities
Infant/toddler care, professional development and compensation, quality, advocacy, strengthening diverse leadership

Magic Johnson Foundation, Inc.
600 Corporate Pointe
Suite 1080
Culver City, CA 90230
Phone: (888) MAGIC-05 or (888) 624-4205
Web site: http://www.magicjohnson.org/

Funding Areas
Community-based organizations serving the health, educational, and social needs of children residing in inner-city communities. This is a for-profit group that provides grant consultants and proposal writers. Their mission is to provide the finest grants consulting service available.

March of Dimes
1275 Mamaroneck Avenue
White Plains, NY 10605
Phone: (888) 663-4637
Web site: http://www.marchofdimes.com

Funding Areas
Educational programs related to maternal-child health; innovative programs and research projects that concern prevention of birth defects

McGovern Family Foundation
The Terry McGovern Foundation
Janine L. Clarke, Executive Director
PO Box 33393
Washington, DC 20033
E-mail: jeffjay@terrymcgovern.org
Phone: (202) 463-8750
Web site: http://www.mcgovernfamily.org/

Funding Areas

Research into alcoholism, to assist in fund-raising for treatment and recovery, and to increase public understanding of addiction.

Merrill Lynch Forum: The Innovation Grants Competition
c/o Katia Mujica Communications & Public Affairs
2 World Financial Center, Floor #6
New York, NY 10281-6106
E-mail: InnovationGrants@ml.com
Phone: (888) 33-FORUM
Web site: http://www.merlyn.com/woml/forum/innovation/

Funding Areas

Doctoral students whose topic could be converted into a commercial product or service

National Hospice Foundation
1700 Diagonal Road
Suite 300
Alexandria, VA 22314
E-mail:info@nhpco.org
Phone: (703) 516-4928
Fax: (703) 525-5762
Web site: http://www.nho.org/foundation.htm

Funding Areas

Increasing awareness of and access to hospice care education and research

National Institutes of Health
Center for Scientific Review
6701 Rockledge Drive, Room 1040-MSC 7710
Bethesda, MD 30892-7710 or Bethesda, MD 20917 (for express/courier service)
Grants Information
National Institutes of Health
E-mail: grantsinfo@nih.gov
Phone: (301) 435-0714
Fax: (301) 480-0525
Web site: http://www.grants.nih.gov/grants/oer.htm

Funding Areas

These are all found in the *NIH Guide for Grants and Contracts* available weekly online at http://grants.nih.gov/grants/guide/index.html. All types of research regarding health-related issues are funded. Each institute lists funding priorities, RFAs, and PAs.

National Science Foundation
4201 Wilson Boulevard
Arlington, VA 22230
E-mail: info@nsf.gov
Phone: (703) 306-1234 or (800) 877-8339
Web site: http://www.nsf.gov/home/grants.htm

Funding Areas
Broad areas that include education, research, and small businesses. Areas include biology, computer and information sciences, crosscutting programs, education, engineering, geosciences, international, math, physical sciences, polar research, science statistics, and social and behavioral sciences.

New England Biolabs Foundation
Martine Kellett, Executive Director
32 Tozer Road
Beverly, MA 01915
E-mail: cataldo@nebf.org
Phone: (978) 927-2404
Fax: (978) 921-1350
Fax e-mail: kellett@nebf.org
Web site: http://www.nebf.org/

Funding Areas
Supports grassroots organizations working with the environment, social change, the arts, elementary education, and scientific research.

Onassis Public Benefit Foundation
Alexander S. Onassis Public Benefit Foundation
Athens 7 Eschinou Str.
GR 105 58, Athens, Greece
Phone: (+301) 37 13 000
Fax: (+301) 37 13
Web site: http://www.onassis.gr/

Funding Areas
Scholarships and research grants, international competitions

David and Lucille Packard Foundation
300 Second Street
Suite 200
Los Altos, CA 94022
Phone: (650) 948-7658
Web site: http://www.packfound.org/

Funding Areas
Supports universities, community groups, national institutions, and community agencies. They publish *The Future of Children*.

Pew Charitable Trusts
2005 Market Street
Suite 1700
Philadelphia, PA 19103-7077
E-mail: info@pewtrusts.com
Web site: http://www.pewtrusts.com/

Funding Areas
A portion of the annual grantmaking budget is dedicated to serving the needs of the Philadelphia community in the areas of culture, education, environment, health and human services, public policy, and religion.

RGK Foundation
Gregory A. Kozmetsky, President
1301 West 25th Street
Suite 300
Austin, TX 78705-4236
Phone: (512) 474-9298
Fax: (512) 474-7281
Web site: http://www.rgkfoundation.org

Funding Areas
Medical, educational, and community programs and research

Sarnoff Endowment for Cardiovascular Science, Inc.
731 G-2 Walker Road
Great Falls, VA 22066
Phone: (888) 4-SARNOFF
Fax: (703) 759-7838
Web site: http://www.sarnoffendowment.org/

Funding Areas
Medical students must perform one year of research in the cardiovascular sciences at an institution other than their own.

Sigma Theta Tau International
550 West North Street
Indianapolis, IN 46202
E-mail: stti@stti.iupui.edu
Phone: (317) 634-8171 or (317) 634-8171 or (888) 634-7575
Fax: (317) 634-8188
Web site: http://www.nursingsociety.org/

Funding Areas
- Virginia Henderson Clinical Research Grant: Clinical issues
- Rosemary Berkel Crisp Research Award: Women's health, oncology, and infant/child care
- Mead Johnson Nutritionals Research Grant: Nutrition and health
- Small Grants: No specific target area

Society of Pediatric Nurses
7794 Grow Drive
Pensacola, FL 32514-7072
Phone: (800) 723-2902
Fax: (850) 484-8762
Web site: http://www.pedsnurses.org/

Funding Areas
Grants for research and education that focus on children's health

Paul and Daisy Soros Fellowships for New Americans
Warren F. Ilchman, Director
400 West 59th Street
New York, NY 10019
E-mail: pdsoros_fellows@sorosny.org
Phone: (212) 547-6926
Fax: (212) 548-4623
Web site: http://www.pdsoros.org

Funding Areas
Graduate study for new Americans

Spencer Foundation
875 North Michigan Avenue
Suite 3930
Chicago, IL 60611-1803
Phone: (312) 337-7000
Fax: (312) 337-0282
Web site: http://www.spencer.org/

Funding Areas
Faculty research and fellowships that contribute to the understanding and improvement of education

Stuart Foundation
50 California Street
Suite 3350
San Francisco, CA 94111-4735
Phone: (415) 393-1551
Fax: (415) 393-1552
Web site: http://www.stuartfoundation.org/

Funding Areas
Help children and youth of California and Washington states become responsible citizens. The three programs of support are Strengthening the Public School System, Strengthening the Child Welfare System, and Strengthening Communities to Support Families.

Priorities
Policy analysis and development; stronger connections among policy makers, practitioners, and researchers; collaboration across agencies and disciplines; building public understanding of key issues in community well-being; improving practice, innovations/demonstrations; and dissemination.

Texas A & M Research Foundation
Box 3578 TAMUS
College Station, Texas 77843
E-mail webmaster@rf-mail.tamu.edu
Phone: (979) 845-8600
Fax: (979) 845-7143
Web site: http://www.rf-web.tamu.edu/

Funding Areas
Provides network on developments in funding sources, sponsor requirements, and regulations

Verizon Foundation (formerly Bell Atlantic Foundation)
1095 Avenue of the Americas
New York, NY 10036
E-mail: Verizon.Foundation@Verizon.com
Phone: (800) 360-7955
Fax: (908) 630-2660
Web site: http://foundation.verizon.com/

Funding Areas

Best-in-Class Model Technology Grants in Delaware, Maine, Maryland, Massachusetts, New Hampshire, New Jersey, New York, Pennsylvania, Rhode Island, Vermont, Virginia, Washington, DC, and West Virginia.

Technology integration is priority. Main areas of interest are literacy, the digital divide, workforce development, employee volunteerism, and community technology development. These funds are disseminated for program and research efforts.

Weingart Foundation
1055 West Seventh Street
Los Angeles, CA 90017-2305
E-mail: info@weingartfnd.org
Phone: (213) 688-7799
Fax: (213) 688-1515
Web site: http://www.weingartfnd.org/

Funding Areas

Grants to human service organizations, educational and health institutions, and cultural centers throughout Southern California

White House Fellowships
President's Commission on White House Fellowships
712 Jackson Place, NW
Washington, DC 20503
E-mail: info@whitehousefellows.gov
Phone: (202) 395-4522
Fax: (202) 395-6179
Web site: http://www.whitehousefellows.gov

Funding Areas

Provides gifted and highly motivated young Americans experience in the process of governing the nation. Nurses are included in this group. This fellowship is an excellent opportunity for gaining firsthand knowledge of policy making.

U.S. DEPARTMENT OF HEALTH AND HUMAN SERVICES RESOURCES AND OTHER GOVERNMENTAL AGENCIES

These agencies of the federal government often support research, education, some educational scholarships, and special projects themselves or have links to agencies that do. They are a good resource for gaining information for a grant's background and significance section.

U.S. Department of Health and Human Services Resources

- Adolescent pregnancy program: www.hhs.gov/opa/titlexx/oapp
- Adoption: www.acf.dhhs.gov/programs/cb
- Adoption/abductions: www.travel.state.gov
- Aging-eldercare information and research: www.aoa.dhhs.gov
- AIDS/HIV prevention, testing, treatment, and prevention information: www.cdc.gov/dstd/dstdp.html
- Alcohol: www.niaaa.nih.gov
- Alcohol/drug: www.nida.nih.gov
- Arthritis/bone diseases: www.nih.gov/niams
- Autism: www.ninds.nih.gov
- Birth defects: www.nih.gov/nichd
- Blindness/eye information: www.nei.nih.gov
- Brain tumors: www.nci.nih.gov
- Breast cancer information and support: www.nci.nih.gov
- Breast implants: www.fda.gov/opacom/morechoices/breastim.html
- Breast-feeding: www.hhs.gov/hrsa/mchb
- Cancer information service: www.cancernet.nci.nih.gov
- Cerebral palsy: www.ninds.nih.gov
- Child abuse and neglect: www.acf.dhhs.gov/programs/cb
- Child care bureau: www.acf.dhhs.gov/programs/ccb
- Child health and development: www.nih.gov/nichd
- Child support enforcement: www.acf.dhhs.gov/programs/CSE
- Childhood immunization information: www.cdc.gov/nip
- Chronic diseases: www.cdc.gov/nccdphp
- Civil rights offices: www.hrsa.gov/oa.html
- Clinical practice guidelines: www.ahrq.gov/clinic/cpgsix.htm or www.ihs.gov/csp/customer.html
- Consumer affairs inquiries: www.ihs.gov/csp/customer.html

- Consumer complaint/fraud/referral help: www.hhs.gov/progorg/oig
- Consumer product safety hotline: www.cpsc.gov
- Cosmetics: www.vm.cfsan.fda.gov/~dms/cos-toc.html
- Deafness, speech, communication disorders: www.nih.gov/nidcd
- Dental/tooth decay: www.nidr.nih.gov
- Depression helpline: www.nimh.nih.gov
- Developmental disabilities: www.acf.dhhs.gov/programs/ADD
- Diabetes: www.niddk.nih.gov
- Digestive diseases: www.niddk.nih.gov
- Disabled infants: www.acf.dhhs.gov
- Disease prevention and health promotion: www.cdc.gov/nccdphp
- Drug/alcohol treatment referral: www.nida.nih.gov
- Drugs, adverse reactions: www.fda.gov/medwatch
- Drugs, prescription and OTC: www.fda.gov
- Drug use, adolescents: www.health.org or www.nida.hih.gov.html
- Eldercare: www.aoa.dhhs.gov/naic/ or www.aoa.dhhs.gov/elderpage.html
- Epilepsy: www.ninds.nih.gov
- Family planning: www.hhs.gov/progorg/opa
- Foster care: www.acf.dhhs.gov/programs/cb
- Fraud and abuse/Medicaid: www.hhs.gov/progorg/oig
- Food and Drug Administration: www.fda.gov/foi/foia2.htm
- Genome (human) research: www.nhgri.nih.gov
- Hazardous substances/Superfund sites: www.cdc.gov/niosh/homepage.html
- Headache: www.ninds.nih.gov
- Head injury: www.ninds.nih.gov
- Head Start: www.acf.dhhs.gov/programs/hsb
- Healthcare technology: www.ahrq.gov
- Health information: www.hhs.gov
- Health maintenance organizations: www.hcfa.gov/medicare/mgdcar.htm
- Health professionals education: www.hrsa.dhhs.gov
- Herpes: www.niaid.nih.gov
- High blood pressure/cholesterol: www.nhlbi.nih.gov
- HIV/AIDS: www.hab.hrsa.gov
- Hospice: www.medicare.gov/publications.html
- Indian Health Service: www.ihs.gov
- HIS publications: www.ihs.gov/PublicInfo/index.asp
- Infectious diseases: www.cdc.gov/ncidod.htm
- International and refugee health: www.cdc.gov
- Juvenile justice/delinquency information: www.ncjrs.org/ojjdp/juvoff/ojjdp.html or www.fedstats.gov
- Kidney/urologic diseases: www.niddk.nih.gov

- Lead poisoning: www.hiehs.nih.gov
- Learning disabilities: www.ninds.nih.gov
- Leprosy (Hansen's disease): www.niaid.nih.gov
- Liver diseases: www.niddk.nih.gov
- Lung diseases: www.nhlbi.nih.gov
- Mammography: www.nci.nih.gov
- Medicaid/Medicare: www.hcfa.gov or www.hcfa.gov/medicaid/medicaid.htm
- Medicaid/Medicare fraud: www.hcfa.gov
- Medical devices: www.fda.gov/cdrh
- Medical school grants: www.hrsa.dhhs.gov
- Medicare (including Medigap): www.hcfa.gov
- Medicine, National Library of: www.nlm.nih.gov
- Mental health: www.samhsa.gov
- Mental retardation: www.acf.dhhs.gov/programs/pcmr
- Migrant worker health care: www.bphc.hrsa.dhhs.gov
- Missing children/runaways: www.missingkids.com
- National Cancer Institute: www.cancernet.nci.nih.gov
- National Health Service Corps: www.hrsa.dhhs.gov
- National Practitioner Data Bank: www.npdb-hipdb.com
- Nutrition: www.fns.usda.gov/fncs
- Occupational safety: www.osha.gov/index.html
- Organ and other transplantation: www.hrsa.dhhs.gov/osp
- Outcomes research: www.ahrq.gov
- Pain disorder/trauma helpline: www.ninds.nih.gov
- Paralysis, spinal cord injury: www.ninds.nih.gov
- Pregnancy, prenatal care, childbirth: www.hhs.gov/hrsa/mchb
- Pregnancy and substance abuse: www.cdc.gov/nccdphp/osh
- Radiological health: www.fda.gov/cdrh
- Radon safety helpline: www.ebtpages/airairporadon.html
- Rape Crisis Hotline: www.members.aol.com/NCMDR/index.html or www.bphc.hrsa.dhhs.gov/omwh/omwh_8.htm
- Refugee resettlement, immigration: www.acf.dhhs.gov/programs/orr
- Runaway youth and homelessness: www.nrscrisisline.org
- Rural health services: www.ruralhealth.hrsa.gov
- School health education: www.cdc.gov/nccdphp/dash/cshedef.htm
- Sexually transmitted disease helpline: www.cdc.gov/nchstp/dstd/dstdp.html
- SIDS (sudden infant death syndrome): www.nichd.nih.gov
- Statistics—Health care and vital: www.ahrq.gov/data
- Stroke and neurological disorders: www.ninds.nih.gov
- Teen pregnancy: www.teenpregnancy.org or www.hrsa.dhhs.gov
- Toxic substances: www.niehs.nih.gov

- Travelers health information: www.cdc.gov/travel/index.htm
- Treatment and referral assistance: www.cdc.gov/travel/index.htm or www.ahrq.gov
- Uninsured assistance: www.hrsa.gov/cap/default.htm
- Urban Indian Health Programs: www.ihs.gov/Healthcare/general/programs.asp
- Vaccine—to report adverse event: www.fda.gov/medwatch/ or www.fda.gov/cber
- Vaccine injury compensation: www.hrsa.dhhs.gov
- Veterinary medicine: www.fda.gov/cvm/default.htm
- Weight control and obesity information: www.niddk.nih.gov/health/nutrit.htm
- Welfare and AFDC jobs programs: www.acf.dhhs.gov/programs/cb
- Women's health: www.fda.gov/womens
- Women's health research: www.fda.gov/womens{/UL}

Other Agencies

- Allergies and asthma: www.AAFA.org
- Alzheimer's disease: www.alzheimers.com
- Disabled children and youth: www.dredf.org
- Domestic violence: www.igc.org/fund/healthcare/res_center.htm
- Drug and alcohol information: www.health.org
- Environmental health: www.neha.org
- Helene Fuld: www.fuld.org/welcome.htm
- Homelessness: www.prainc.com/nrc/info.htm
- Marrow donor program: www.marrow.org
- Osteoporosis: www.osteo.org
- Sickle cell disease: www.SickleCelldisease.org
- Smoking and tobacco: www.health.org
- Welfare information: www.welfareinfor.org
- Youth crisis hotline: www.nrscrisisline.org

SUGGESTED READINGS ON RELATED ISSUES

The suggested readings are some resources for grant writing or ideas for future grants.

Anonymous. (1999). Apolipoprotein E epsilon 4 allele (APOE epsilon 4) and Alzheimer's disease: role of genetic testing for diagnosis and risk assessment. *Tecnologica MAP Supplement*, 4-7. Blue Cross and Blue Shield Association. Medical Advisory Panel.

Brakely, M. R. (1997). Tips for the novice grant-seeker: Implications for staff development specialists. *Journal of Staff Development, 13*(3), 160–163.

Gaberson, K. B. (1997). What's the answer? What's the question? *Association of Operating Room Nurses Journal, 66*(1), 148–151.

Kahn, C. R. (1994). Picking a research problem: The critical decision. *New England Journal of Medicine, 330*(21), 1530–1533.

Lorentzon, M. 1995. Multidisciplinary collaboration: Life line or drowning pool for nurse researchers? *Journal of Advanced Nursing, 22*(5), 825–826.

Malone, R. E. (1996). Getting your study funded: Tips for new researchers. *Journal of Emergency Nursing, 22*(5), 457–459.

Marshall, M. N., Shekelle, P. G., Leatherman, S., and Brook, R. H. (2000). Public disclosure of performance data: Learning from the U.S. experience. *Quality Health Care, 9*(1), 53–57.

Patterson, E. R., & Bakewell-Sachs, S. (1998). Toward evidence based-practice. *Maternal Child Nursing, 23*, 278–280.

Ries, J. B., & Leukefeld, C. G. (1995). *Applying for research funding: Getting started and getting funded.* London: Sage.

Sage, W. M. (1999). Regulating through information: Disclosure laws and American health care. *Columbia Law Reviews, 99*(7), 1701–1829.

Triendl, R. (2000). World's academies seek a sustainable future [news]. *Nature, 405*(6786), 501.

Van Dyke Hayes, K. (1999). Research grants and you: Perfect together. *SCI Nursing, 17*(3), 104–107.

Woolley, M. (1996). What are you waiting for? *Circulation, 94*(8), 1802–1803.

OTHER INTERNET RESOURCES

These resources are on the Internet. They represent tools for grant writing, statistical analyses, systematic reviews, or potential sources for project ideas. Included are literature search engines such as ERIC and Medline.

Systematic Reviews: For Evidence-Based Practice and Integrated Literature Reviews

- Cochrane Collaborative: www.hiru.mcmaster.ca/cochrane/centres/canadian/
- The Joanna Briggs Institute for Evidence-Based Nursing and Midwifery: Systematic Reviews: www.joannabriggs.edu.au/sysmenu.html

- Systematic Reviews on Childhood Injury, Prevention, and Interventions: www.depts.washington.edu/hiprc/childinjury/
- Thomas C. Chalmers Centre for Systematic Reviews: www.cheori.org/tcc/index.htm
- Vermont Oxford Network: www.vtoxford.org/

Grant Resources

- COS funding opportunities, funded research: www.fundedresearch.cos.com
- Department of Education Technology Innovation Challenge Grants: www.ed.gov/Technology/challenge
- Federal government grants, loans and financial aid: www.americanfinance-center.com
- Financial Aid Resource Center—Scholarships, Grants, Loans for College: www.theoldschool.org
- The Foundation Center: www.fdncenter.org
- Food: www.fda.gov
- Grants and related resources: www.lib.msu.edu/harris23/grants/federal.htm
- Grants Resources on the Internet: A Detailed Guide: www.library.wisc.edu/libraries/Memor
- Grants Web: www.infoserv.rttonet.psu.edu/gweb.htm
- HRSA grants and contracts: www.hrsa.dhhs.gov/grants.htm
- Internet Grateful Med V2.6: www.igm.nlm.nih.gov
- Justice Information Center (NCJRS)—Justice grants: www.ncjrs.org/fed-grant.htm
- Medline—Entrez-Pubmed: www.ncbi.nlm.nih.gov/PubMed
- NIH Center for Scientific Review: www.drg.nih.gov
- NIH Guide index: www.med.nyu.edu/hih-guide.html
- NIH Office of Extramural Research—Grants: www.nih.gov/grants/oer.htm
- Office of Educational Technology: www.ed.gov/Technology
- Office of Science Grants and Contracts: www.er.doe.gov/production/grants/grants
- Pell Grant Program: www.ed.gov/prog_info/SFA/StudentGuide/1998-9/pell.html
- The Grants Information Center: www.library.wisc.edu/libraries/Memor
- TRAM—Texas Research Administrators Group hosted by Arizona State University East: www.tram.east.asu.edu
- U.S. Department of Education—Grants and Contracts: www.gcs.ed.gov
- Welcome to GrantsNet: www.grantsnet.org

Grant Writers/Reviewers

The Grant Doctors
PO Box 417212
Sacramento, CA 95841
Phone: (888) 208-2441
Fax: (800) 783-0238
E-mail: dave@thegrantdoctors.com
Web site: http://www.thegrantdoctors.com/

This is a for-profit group that provides grants consultants and proposal writers. Their mission is to provide the finest grants consulting service available.

Literature Searches

- Scientific Information: www.biolinks.com
- CINAHL Database—Cumulative Index to Nursing and Allied Health Literature: www.cihahl.com
- ERIC (Educational Research Information Collection) database: http://www.eric.ed.gov/
- Google: www.google.com
- Governmental information: www.google.com/unclesam
- Legal data: www.findlaw.com
- Medline database—Search using either PubMed or Internet Grateful Med: www.nlm.nih.gov/databases/freemedl.html
- Ingenta—The Global Research Gateway: www.ingenta.com/home/

Statistical Resources

Interactive Statistical Calculation Pages: This resource provides over 550 links to assist with statistical analyses: www.members.aol.com/johnp71/javastat.html

Power Analysis—Step by Step: An easy-to-follow format to estimate a power for the correct sample size: www.mp1-pwrc.usgs.gov/powcase/steps.html

Power Analysis Monitoring Programs—A Power Primer: This resource is just what it says—a primer on the how to do a power calculation: http://www.mbr-pwrc.usgs.gov/software/monitor.html

Power Calculator: With this resource, you choose a model and plug in information and out comes the power for a given sample: www.ebook.stat.ucla.edu/calculators/powercalc

Power Analysis of ANOVA Designs: This Web site explains power calculations—what they are and how to do a power analysis: www.math.yorku.ca/SCS/Demos/power

SAS e-Intelligence: SAS software for power calculations and other statistical analyses: www.sas.com

This site is a portal to online information around the world. The center is in the United Kingdom, but it has merged with the Carl Organization that runs the Uncover and Reveal service from Denver, Colorado. These services assist researchers and educators to set up delivery of literature reviews on a weekly basis or tables of contents for a designated number of journals for an annual subscription rate. The Carl Organization Web site is www.carl.org.

Healthy People 2010
Goals and Objectives

Healthy People 2010 is a national health promotion and disease prevention initiative. Its goals are to increase the quality and years of healthy life and eliminate health disparities. Grants that focus on healthcare practice, education, or research often require a clear tie to at least one goal and objective of this initiative.

This list is a brief synopsis of the *Healthy People 2010* Goals and Objectives. One specific example is given for each category.

Goals
1. Increase Quality and Years of Healthy Life
2. Eliminate Health Disparities

Objectives:
Promote Healthy Behaviors
Physical Activity and Fitness

Goal: Improve the health, fitness, and quality of life of all Americans through the adoption and maintenance of regular, daily physical activity.

Objectives:
1. Leisure Time Physical Activity
   Example: Increase to 85 percent the proportion of people aged 18 and older who engage in any leisure time physical activity.
2. Sustained Physical Activity
3. Vigorous Physical Activity
4. Muscular Strength and Endurance
5. Flexibility
6. Vigorous Physical Activity, grades 9–12
7. Moderate Physical Activity, grades 9–12
8. Daily School Physical Education
9. Physical Education Requirement in Schools
10. School Physical Education Quality
11. Inclusion of Physical Activity in Health Education

Source: Office of Disease Prevention and Health Promotion. (2001). *Healthy People 2010* Goals and Objectives. Retrieved from http://web.health.gov/healthypeople.

12. Access to School Physical Activity Facilities
13. Worksite Physical Activity and Fitness
14. Clinician Counseling about Physical Activity

Nutrition

Goal: Promote health and reduce chronic disease risk, disease progression, debilitation, and premature death associated with dietary factors and nutritional status among all people of the United States.

Objectives:
1. Healthy Weight
   Example: Increase to at least 60 percent the prevalence of healthy weight (defined as a BMI [Body Mass Index] equal to or greater than 19.0 and less than 25.0) among all people aged 20 and older.
2. Obesity in Adults
3. Overweight and Obesity in Children/Adolescents
4. Growth Retardation
5. Fat Intake
6. Saturated Fat Intake
7. Vegetable and Fruit Intake
8. Grain Product Intake
9. Calcium Intake
10. Sodium Intake
11. Iron Deficiency
12. Anemia in Pregnant Women
13. Meals and Snacks at School
14. Nutrition Education, Elementary Schools
15. Nutrition Education, Middle/Junior High Schools
16. Nutrition Education, Senior High Schools
17. Nutrition Assessment and Planning
18. Nutrition Counseling
19. Food Security

Tobacco Use

Goal: Reduce disease, disability, and death related to tobacco use and exposure to secondhand smoke by (1) preventing initiation of tobacco use, (2) promoting cessation of tobacco use, (3) reducing exposure to secondhand smoke, and (4) changing social norms and environments that support tobacco use.

Objectives:
1. Adult Tobacco Use
   Example: Reduce to 13 percent the proportion of adults (18 and older) who use tobacco products.
2. Cigarette Smoking During Pregnancy

3. Adolescent Tobacco Use
4. Age at First Use of Tobacco
5. Adolescent Never Smokers
6. Smoking Cessation
7. Smoking Cessation During Pregnancy
8. Smoking Cessation by New Mothers
9. Smoking Cessation Attempts among Adolescents
10. Advice to Quit Smoking
11. Treatment of Nicotine Addiction
12. Providers Advising Smoking Cessation
13. Physician Inquires about Secondhand Smoke
14. Tobacco-Free Schools
15. Worksite Smoking Policies
16. Smoke-Free Air Laws
17. Enforcement of Minors' Access Laws
18. Retail License Suspension for Sales to Minors
19. Adolescent Disapproval of Smoking
20. Adolescent Perception of Harm of Tobacco Use
21. Tobacco Use Prevention Education
22. Cigarette Price Increase
23. Tobacco Product Price Increase
24. State Tobacco Control Programs
25. Preemptive Tobacco Control Laws

Promote Health and Safe Communities
Educational and Community-Based Programs

Goal: Increase the quality, availability, and effectiveness of educational and community-based programs designed to prevent disease and improve the health and quality of life of the American people.

Objectives:
1. High School Completion
   Example: Increase the high school completion rate to at least 90 percent.
2. School Health Education
3. Undergraduate Health Risk Behavior Information
4. School Nurse-to-Student Ratio
5. Worksite Health Promotion Programs
6. Participation in Employer-Sponsored Health Promotion Activities
7. Patient Satisfaction with Health Care Provider Communication
8. Patient and Family Education
9. Community Disease Prevention and Health Promotion Activities
10. Community Health Promotion Initiatives
11. Culturally Appropriate Community Health Promotion Programs
12. Elderly Participation in Community Health Promotion

Environmental Health

Goal: Health for all through a healthy environment.

Objectives:
1. Air Quality
   Example: The air will be safer to breathe for 100 percent of the people living in areas that exceed all National Ambient Air Quality Standards (NAAQS).
2. Emission Reduction
3. Cleaner Alternative Fuels
4. Waterborne Disease
5. Water-Related Adverse Health Effects
6. Surface Water Health Risks
7. Beach Closings
8. Discharge from Livestock Production Operations
9. Watersheds with Contaminant Problems
10. Poisonings from Contaminated Fish
11. Blood Lead Levels
12. Risks to Human Health and Environment by Hazardous Waste Sites
13. Pesticide Poisonings
14. Energy Recovery
15. Municipal Solid Waste
16. Exposure to Tobacco Smoke
17. Testing for Lead-Based Paint
18. Exposure to Household Hazardous Chemicals
19. Household Levels of Lead Dust and Allergens
20. Carbon Monoxide Poisonings
21. Radon Testing
22. Exposure to Household Chemicals
23. Exposure to Persistent Chemicals
24. Monitoring of Exposure to Selected Chemicals
25. Environmental and Environmental Health Information Systems
26. Monitoring Diseases Caused by Environmental Hazards
27. Global Burden of Disease
28. Infectious and Parasitic Diseases
29. Consultation on Environmental Issues
30. Tracking Mechanism of Exported Pesticides
31. Diseases Among U.S. Travelers Overseas
32. Total Pesticide Exposure
33. Uniform International Guidelines for Environmental Quality

Food Safety

Goal: Reduce the number of foodborne illnesses.

Objectives:
1. Foodborne Infections
   Example: Reduce, by 50% for bacteria and 10% for parasites, the proportion of infections caused by key foodborne pathogens.
2. Salmonella and *Escherichia coli*
3. *Listeria monocytogenes* and *Vibrio vulnificus*
4. Antimicrobial-Resistant Bacterial Pathogens
5. Food-Induced Anaphylaxis
6. Food Handling by Consumers
7. Food Handling in Retail Establishments
8. Pesticide Residue Tolerances
9. Limits for Mycotoxins

Injury/Violence Prevention

Goal: Reduce the incidence and severity of injuries from unintentional causes, as well as violence and abuse.

Objectives:
Injuries That Cut Across Intent
1. Nonfatal Head Injuries
   Example: Reduce nonfatal head injuries so that hospitalizations for this condition are no more than 74 per 100,000 people.
2. Nonfatal Spinal Cord Injuries
3. Firearm-Related Deaths
4. Homes with Firearms
5. Laws Requiring Proper Firearm Storage
6. Child Death Review Systems
7. Injury Prevention and Safety Education

Unintentional Injuries
8. Deaths from Unintentional Injuries
9. Emergency Department Visits
10. Nonfatal Unintentional Injuries
11. Motor Vehicle Crashes
12. Pedestrian Deaths
13. Nonfatal Motor Vehicle Injuries
14. Pedestrian Injuries
15. Safety Belts and Child Restraints

16. Primary Enforcement Laws for Safety Belt Use
17. Use of Motorcycle Helmets
18. Motorcycle Helmet Laws
19. Graduated Driver Licensing
20. Residential Fire Deaths
21. Smoke Alarms
22. Deaths from Falls
23. Hip Fractures
24. Drowning Deaths
25. Bicycle Helmet Laws
26. Bicycle Helmet Use, High School Students
27. Bicycle Helmet Use
28. Nonfatal Poisoning
29. Deaths from Unintentional Poisoning
30. Nonfatal Dog Bite Injuries
31. Head, Face, Eye, and Mouth Protection in School Sports
32. Injury Prevention Counseling

Violence and Abusive
33. Homicides
34. Maltreatment of Children
35. Physical Abuse by Intimate Partners
36. Forced Sexual Intercourse
37. Emergency Housing for Battered Women
38. Sexual Assault Other Than Rape
39. Physical Assaults
40. Physical Fighting among Adolescents
41. Weapon Carrying by Adolescents

Occupational Safety and Health

Goal: Promote worker health and safety through prevention.

Objectives:
1. Deaths from Work-Related Injuries
   Example: Reduce deaths from work-related injuries to no more than 3.6 per 100,000 workers.
2. Work-Related Injuries
3. Workplace Injury and Illness Surveillance
4. Overexertion or Repetitive Motion
5. Pneumoconiosis Deaths
6. Work-Related Homicides
7. Workplace Assaults

8. Noise-Induced Permanent Threshold Shift
9. Blood Lead Levels Greater than 25 g/dL
10. Blood Lead Levels Greater than 10 g/dL
11. Occupational Skin Diseases/Disorders
12. Latex Allergy
13. Tractor Rollover Protection Systems
14. Worksite Stress Reduction Programs
15. Hepatitis B Infections
16. Hepatitis B Vaccinations

Oral Health

Goal: Improve the health and quality of life for individuals and communities by preventing and controlling oral, dental, and craniofacial diseases, conditions, and injuries and improving access to oral health care for all.

Objectives:
1. Caries Experience
   Example: Reduce dental caries (cavities) in primary and permanent teeth (mixed dentition) so that the proportion of children who have had one or more cavities (filled or unfilled) is no more than 15% among children aged 2–4, 40% among children aged 6–8, and 55% among adolescents aged 15.
2. Untreated Dental Decay
3. Root Caries
4. No Tooth Loss
5. Complete Tooth Loss
6. Gingivitis
7. Periodontal Disease
8. Stage I Oropharyngeal Cancer Lesions
9. Dental Sealants
10. Water Fluoridation
11. Topical Fluorides
12. Screening/Counseling for 2-year-olds
13. Screening, Referral, Treatment for First-Time School Program Children
14. Adult Use of Oral Health Care System
15. School-Based Health Centers with Oral Health Component
16. Community Health Centers with Direct Oral Health Service Component
17. Exams and Services for Those in Long-Term Care Facilities
18. Referral for Cleft Lip/Palate
19. State-Based Surveillance System
20. State and Local Dental Programs
21. Screening for Oropharyngeal Cancer

Improve Systems for Personal and Public Health
Access to Quality Health Services

Goal: Improve access to comprehensive, high-quality health care across a continuum of care.

Clinical Prevention Services

Objectives:
A 1 Uninsured Children and Adults
   Example: Reduce to 0% the proportion of children and adults under 65 without healthcare coverage.
A 2 Insurance Coverage
A 3 Routine Screening about Lifestyle Risk Factors
A 4 Reporting on Service Delivery
A 5 Training to Address Health Disparities

Primary Care
B 1 Source of Ongoing Primary Care
B 2 Failure to Obtain All Needed Health Care
B 3 Lack of Primary Care Visits
B 4 Access to Primary Care Providers in Underserved Areas
B 5 Racial/Ethnic Minority Representation in the Health Professions
B 6 Preventable Hospitalization Rates for Chronic Illness

Emergency Services
C 1 Access to Emergency Medical Services
C 2 Insurance Coverage
C 3 Toll-Free Poison Control Center Number
C 4 Time-Dependent Care for Cardiac Symptoms
C 5 Special Needs of Children
C 6 Follow-up Mental Health Services

Long-Term Care and Rehabilitative Services
D 1 Functional Assessments
D 2 Primary Care Evaluation
D 3 Access to the Continuum of Services
D 4 Pressure Ulcers

Family Planning

Goal: Every pregnancy in the United States should be intended.

Objectives:
1. Planned Pregnancy.
   Example: Increase to at least 70% the proportion of all pregnancies among women aged 15–44 that are planned (i.e., intended).

2. Repeat Unintended Births
3. Contraceptive Use, Females
4. Contraceptive Failure
5. Postcoital Hormonal Contraception
6. Male Involvement in Family Planning
7. Adolescent Pregnancy
8. Sexual Intercourse Before Age 15
9. Adolescent Sexual Intercourse
10. Pregnancy and STD Preventive Methods
11. Pregnancy Prevention Education
12. School Requirement for Classes on Human Sexuality, Pregnancy Prevention, etc.
13. Impaired Fecundity

Maternal, Infant, and Child Health

Goal: Improve maternal health and pregnancy outcomes and reduce rates of disability in infants, thereby improving the health and well-being of women, infants, children, and families in the United States. The health of a population is reflected in the health of its most vulnerable members. A major focus of many public health efforts, therefore, is improving the health of pregnant women and their infants, including reductions in rates of birth defects, risk factors for infant death, and deaths of infants and their mothers.

Objectives:
1. Infant Mortality
   Example: Reduce the infant mortality rate to no more than 5 per 1,000 live births.
2. Infant Mortality from Birth Defects
3. SIDS Mortality
4. Child Mortality
5. Fetal Death
6. Perinatal Mortality
7. Maternal Mortality
8. Maternal Morbidity
9. Preconception Counseling
10. Prenatal Care
11. Quality of Prenatal Care
12. Serious Developmental Disabilities
13. Childbirth Classes
14. Postpartum Visits
15. Very Low Birthweight Babies Born at Level III Hospitals
16. Cesarean Delivery

17. Low Birthweight
18. Preterm Birth
19. Weight Gain During Pregnancy
20. Infant Sleep Position
21. Alcohol Use During Pregnancy
22. Tobacco Use During Pregnancy
23. Drug Use During Pregnancy
24. Fetal Alcohol Syndrome
25. Prenatal Exposure to Teratogenic Prescription Medication
26. Neural Tube Defects
27. Folic Acid Intake
28. Folate Level
29. Breast-feeding
30. Exclusive Breast-feeding
31. Newborn Screening
32. Sepsis Among Infants with Sickling Hemoglobinopathies
33. Newborn Hearing Screening
34. Training in Genetic Testing
35. Understanding of Inherited Sensitivities to Disease
36. Genetic Testing
37. Primary Care Services for Babies 18 Months and Younger
38. Screening for Vision, Hearing, Speech, and Language Impairments
39. Service Systems for Children with Chronic and Disabling Conditions

Medical Product Safety

Goal: Ensure the safest and most effective possible use of medical products.

Objectives:
1. Monitoring of Adverse Drug Reactions
   Example: By the year 2010, compatible with a requirement to protect the privacy of each individual, there will be a population base of 20,000,000 individuals under close electronically monitored safety surveillance for indicators of adverse events associated with medical therapies.
2. Approval of Medical Products
3. Response from Managed Care Organizations Regarding Adverse Drug Reactions
4. Linked Automated Information Systems
5. Drug Alert Systems
6. Provider Review of Medications Taken by Patients
7. Complementary and Alternative Health Care
8. Safety-Related Labeling Changes
9. Updates to Drug Alert Systems
10. Patient Information about Prescriptions

Public Health Infrastructure

Goal: Ensure that the public health infrastructure at the federal, state, and local levels has the capacity to provide essential public health services.

Objectives:
1. Competencies for Public Health Workers
   Example: Increase the number of states and local jurisdictions that incorporate specific competencies for public health workers into their public health personnel system.
2. Training in Essential Public Health Services
3. Continuing Education and Training by Public Health Agencies
4. Use of Standard Occupational Classification System
5. Onsite Access to Data
6. Access to Public Health Information and Surveillance Data
7. Tracking *Healthy People 2010* Objectives for Select Populations
8. Data Collection for *Healthy People 2010* Objectives
9. Use of Geocoding in Health Data Systems
10. Performance Standards for Essential Public Health Services
11. Health Improvement Plans
12. Access to Laboratory Services
13. Access to Comprehensive Epidemiology Services
14. Model Statutes Related to Essential Public Health Services
15. Data on Public Health Expenditures
16. Collaboration and Cooperation in Prevention Research Efforts
17. Summary Measures of Population Health and the Public Health Infrastructure

Health Communication

Goal: Improve the quality of health-related decisions through effective communication.

Objectives:
1. Public Access to Health Information
   Example: Increase the proportion of cities and counties that have a publicly or privately funded program or activity to promote and enhance public access to health information for underserved populations.
2. Centers for Excellence
3. Evaluation of Communication Programs
4. Satisfaction with Health Information
5. Health Literacy Programs
6. Quality of Health Information
7. Health Communication/Media Technology Curricula

Prevent and Reduce Diseases and Disorders
Arthritis, Osteoporosis, and Chronic Back Conditions

Goal: Reduce the impact of several major musculoskeletal conditions by reducing the occurrence, impairment, functional limitation, and limitation in social participation (i.e., disability) due to arthritis and other rheumatic conditions; reducing the prevalence of osteoporosis and resulting fractures by increasing reducing activity limitation due to chronic back conditions.

Objectives:
Arthritis
1. Mean Days Without Severe Pain
   Example: Increase mean days without severe pain for U.S. adults with arthritis to more than 20 of the past 30 days.
2. Activity Limitations
3. Personal Care Limitations
4. Help in Coping
5. Labor Force Participation
6. Racial Differences in Total Knee Replacement Rate
7. Failure to See a Doctor for Arthritis
8. Early Diagnosis and Treatment of Systemic Rheumatic Diseases
9. Arthritis Education among Patients
10. Provision of Arthritis Education
11. Dietary Practices and Physical Activity

Osteoporosis
12. Prevalence
13. Counseling about Prevention, 13 and over
14. Counseling about Prevention, Women 50 and Over

Chronic Back Conditions
15. Activity Limitations

Cancer

Goal: Reduce the burden of cancer on the U.S. population by decreasing cancer incidence, morbidity, and mortality rates.

Objectives:
1. Cancer Deaths
   Example: Reduce cancer deaths to a rate of no more than 103 per 100,000 people.
2. Lung Cancer Deaths
3. Breast Cancer Deaths
4. Cervical Cancer Deaths
5. Colorectal Cancer Deaths

6. Oropharyngeal Cancer Deaths
7. Prostate Cancer Deaths
8. Sun Exposure
9. Provider Counseling about Preventive Measures
10. Pap Tests
11. Colorectal Screening Examination
12. Oral, Skin, and Digital Rectal Examinations
13. Breast Examination and Mammogram
14. Physician Counseling of High-Risk Patients
15. Statewide Cancer Registries
16. Cancer Survival Rates

Diabetes

Goal: Reduce needless disease and economic burden for all persons with, or at risk for, diabetes mellitus.

Objectives:
1. Type 2 Diabetes
   Example: Decrease the incidence of type 2 diabetes to 2.5 per 1,000 persons per year.
2. Diabetes Prevalence
3. Diagnosis of Diabetes
4. Diabetes-Related Deaths
5. Diabetes-Related Deaths among Known Persons with Diabetes
6. Cardiovascular Deaths
7. Perinatal Mortality in Infants of Mothers with Diabetes
8. Congenital Malformations in Infants or Mothers with Diabetes
9. Foot Ulcers
10. Lower Extremity Amputations
11. Visual Impairment
12. Blindness
13. Proteinuria
14. End-Stage Renal Disease
15. Lipid Assessment
16. Glycosylated Hemoglobin Measurement
17. Urinary Measurement of Microalbumin
18. Controlled Blood Pressure
19. Dilated Eye Examinations
20. Foot Examinations
21. Aspirin Therapy
22. Self-Blood Glucose Monitoring
23. Diabetes Education

Disability and Secondary Conditions

Goal: Promote health and prevent secondary conditions among persons with disabilities, including eliminating disparities between person with disabilities and the U.S. population.

Objectives:
1. Core Data Sets
   Example: Include a comparable core set of items to identify "people with disabilities" in all data sets used for *Healthy People 2010*.
2. Depression
3. Days of Anxiety
4. Healthy Days Among Adults with Activity Limitations Who Need Assistance
5. Personal and Emotional Support
6. Satisfaction with Life
7. Print Size on Medicine, Patient Instructional Materials, and Syringe Markings
8. Employment Rates
9. Inclusion of Children with Disabilities in Regular Education Programs
10. Compliance with Americans with Disabilities Act
11. Environmental Barriers
12. Disability Surveillance and Health Promotion Programs

Heart Disease and Stroke

Goal: Enhance the cardiovascular health and quality of life of all Americans through improvement of medical management, prevention and control of risk factors, and promotion of healthy lifestyle behaviors.

Objectives:
1. Coronary Heart Disease Deaths
   Example: Reduce coronary heart disease deaths to no more than 51 per 100,000 population.
2. Female Deaths after Heart Attack
3. Knowledge of Early Warning Symptoms of Heart Attack
4. Provider Counseling About Early Warning Symptoms of Heart Attack
5. Females Aware of Heart Disease as the Leading Cause of Death
6. High Blood Pressure
7. Controlled High Blood Pressure
8. Action to Help Control Blood Pressure
9. Blood Pressure Monitoring
10. Serum Cholesterol Levels
11. Blood Cholesterol Levels
12. Blood Cholesterol Screening
13. Treatment of LDL Cholesterol

14. Stroke Deaths
15. Knowledge of Early Warning Symptoms of Stroke
16. Provider Counseling about Early Warning Symptoms of Stroke

HIV

Goals: Prevent HIV transmission and associated morbidity and mortality by (1) ensuring that all persons at risk for HIV infection know their serostatus, (2) ensuring that those person not infected with HIV remain uninfected, (3) ensuring that those person infected with HIV do not transmit HIV to others, and (4) ensuring that those infected with HIV are accessing the most effective therapies possible.

Objectives:
1. AIDS Incidence
   Example: Confine annual incidence of diagnosed AIDS cases among adolescents and adults to no more than 12 per 100,000 population.
2. HIV Incidence
3. Condom Use
4. Screening for STDs and Immunization for Hepatitis B
5. HIV Counseling and Testing for Injecting Drug Users
6. HIV Counseling and Testing for Prison Inmates
7. Knowledge of HIV Serostatus among People with Tuberculosis
8. Classroom Education on HIV and STDs
9. Compliance with Public Health Service Treatment Guidelines
10. Mortality Due to HIV Infection
11. Years of Healthy Life Following HIV Diagnosis
12. Perinatally Acquired HIV Infection
13. Treatment for Injecting Drug Use

Immunization and Infectious Diseases

Goal: Prevent disease, disability, and death from infectious disease, including vaccine-preventable diseases.

Objectives:
1. Vaccine-Preventable Diseases
   Example: Reduce indigenous cases of vaccine-preventable disease.
2. Impact of Influenza Vaccinations
3. Hepatitis A
4. Hepatitis B in Infants
5. Hepatitis B, under 25
6. Hepatitis B in Adults
7. Deaths from Hepatitis B-Related Cirrhosis and Liver Cancer

8. Hepatitis C
9. Identification of Persons with Chronic Hepatitis C
10. Deaths from Hepatitis C-Related Cirrhosis and Liver Cancer
11. Tuberculosis
12. Hospital-Acquired Infections
13. Hospital-Acquired Infections from Antimicrobial-Resistant Microorganisms
14. Antimicrobial Use in Intensive Care
15. Occupational Needle-Stick Exposure
16. Bacterial Meningitis
17. Invasive Pneumococcal Infections
18. Invasive Early-Onset Group B Streptococcal Disease
19. Lyme Disease
20. Peptic Ulcer Hospitalizations
21. Immunization of Children 19–35 Months
22. States with 90% Immunization Coverage
23. Immunization Coverage for Children in Day Care, Kindergarten, and First Grade
24. Immunizations among Adults
25. Curative Therapy for Tuberculosis
26. Preventive Therapy among High-Risk Persons with Tuberculosis
27. Antibiotics for Ear Infections
28. Antibiotics Prescribed for Colds
29. Inappropriate Rabies Post-Exposure Prophylaxis
30. Two-year-olds Receiving Vaccinations as Part of Primary Care
31. Provider Measurement of Immunization Coverage Levels
32. Immunization Registries
33. Vaccine-Associated Adverse Reactions
34. Febrile Seizures Caused by Pertussis Vaccines
35. Preventions Services for International Travelers
36. Laboratory Confirmation of Tuberculosis Cases

Mental Health and Mental Disorders

Goal: Improve the mental health of all Americans by ensuring appropriate, high-quality services informed by scientific research.

Objectives:
1. Suicide
   Example: Reduce suicides to no more than 9.6 per 100,000 people.
2. Injurious Suicide Attempts
3. Unipolar Major Depression
4. Mental Disorders among Children and Adolescents
5. Serious Mental Illness among Homeless People

6. Employment of Persons with Serious Mental Disorders
7. Disabilities Associated with Mental Disorders
8. Mental Health Services for People with Mental and Emotional Problems
9. Culturally Competent Mental Health Services
10. Provider Training in Screening for Mental Health Problems in Children
11. Provider Training in Addressing Mental Health Problems in Children
12. Provider Review of Patients' Cognitive, Emotional, and Behavioral Functioning
13. Primary Care Provider Assessment of Mental Health of Children
14. Mental Health Benefits
15. Access to Mental Health Benefits
16. Children's Access to Mental Health Services
17. Comparability of Mental Health Insurance
18. Children with Mental Health Insurance
19. Jail Diversion for Seriously Mentally Ill Adults
20. Mental Health Screening by Juvenile Justice Facilities
21. Crisis and Ongoing Mental Health Services for the Elderly
22. State Plans to Address Co-Occurring Disorders
23. Consumer Satisfaction with Services
24. Offices of Consumer Affairs of Mental Health Services

Respiratory Diseases

Goal: Raise the public's awareness of the signs and symptoms of lung diseases and what to do when they experience them—specifically symptoms of asthma, chronic obstructive pulmonary disease (COPD), and obstructive sleep apnea, and promote lung health through better detection, treatment, and education.

Objectives:
Asthma
1. Deaths
   Example: Reduce asthma death rate to no more than 14 per million population.
2. Hospitalizations
3. Emergency Department Visits
4. Activity Limitations
5. School or Work Days Lost
6. Patient Education
7. Continuing Medical Education
8. Written Asthma Management Plans
9. Counseling on Early Signs of Worsening Asthma
10. Instruction on Peak Expiratory Flow Monitoring
11. Short-Acting Inhaled Beta Agonists
12. Long-Term Management
13. Surveillance System

Chronic Obstructive Pulmonary Disease

14. Prevalence
15. Deaths
16. Culturally Competent Care
17. Training in Early Signs of COPD

Obstructive Sleep Apnea

18. Medical Evaluation
19. Follow-up Medical Care
20. Vehicular Accidents
21. Training in Sleep Medicine

Sexually Transmitted Diseases

Goal: A society where healthy sexual relationships, free of infection as well as coercion and unintended pregnancy, are the norms.

Objectives:

1. Chlamydia
   Example: Reduce the prevalence of *Chlamydia tracheomatis* infections among young person (15 to 24 years old) to no more than 3%.
2. Gonorrhea
3. Primary and Secondary Syphilis
4. Herpes Simplex Virus Type 2 Infection
5. Human Papilloma Virus Infection
6. Pelvic Inflammatory Disease
7. Fertility Problems
8. Congenital Syphilis
9. Neonatal STDs
10. Heterosexually Transmitted HIV
11. STD Clinics
12. School-Based Services
13. Medicaid Contracts
14. Reimbursement for Treatment of Partners of STD Patients
15. Training in STD-Related Services
16. Television Messages
17. Screening for Genital Chlamydia
18. Screening of Pregnant Women
19. Screening in Youth Detention Facilities and Jails
20. Compliance with CDC Guidelines for Treatment of STDs
21. Provider Referral Services for Sexual Partners
22. Reimbursement for Counseling on Reproductive Health Issues
23. Provider Counseling During Initial Visits

Substance Abuse

Goal: Reduce substance abuse and thereby protect the health, safety, and quality of life of all Americans, especially the Nation's children.

Objectives:
1. Motor Vehicle Crashes
   Example: Reduce deaths and injuries caused by alcohol and drug-related motor vehicle crashes.
2. Cirrhosis Deaths
3. Drug-Related Deaths
4. Drug Abuse-Related Emergency Department Visits
5. Drug-Free Youth
6. Adolescent Use of Illicit Substances
7. Binge Drinking
8. Riding with a Driver Who Has Been Drinking
9. Alcohol Consumption
10. Steroid Use
11. Inhalant Use
12. Alcohol and Drug-Related Violence
13. Alcohol-Related Drowning
14. Peer Disapproval of Substance Abuse
15. Perception of Risk Associated with Substance Abuse
16. Treatment Gap for Illicit Drugs
17. Treatment Gap for Problem Alcohol Use
18. Services for School-Aged Children
19. Screening and Treatment of Patients 60 and Older
20. Lost Productivity
21. Community Partnerships and Coalitions
22. Administrative License Revocation Laws
23. Blood Alcohol Concentration Levels

Standard Forms, Grant Examples, and Other Documents

INTRODUCTION

Standard Forms

Grants require several fairly standard forms. This appendix gives examples of these forms:

- Letter of intent: A letter of intent should be sent to indicate to a funding agency that you plan on submitting a grant.
- Concept paper: A concept paper should briefly describe the project to a funding agency.
- Abstract (dissertation proposal): An abstract gives a very brief sketch of the project.
- Abstract (NIH proposal): This is a concise paragraph conforming to space limitations that briefly introduces the research problem, and then summarizes the specific aims, background and significance, and research design and methods sections.
- Research plan: The research plan is the brief outline of the step-by-step project blueprint found in each example of the NIH grant application.
- Example of an R03 NIH grant application: Qualitative methods
- Example of an R15 NIH grant application: Quantitative methods
- Protocol worksheet: The protocol worksheet found in the NIH application is an example of a form that a researcher can follow to make sure that the intervention steps are carried out appropriately.
- Example of a final report for an NIH Grant

NIH Forms

Samples are shown from Form SF 424 used by NIH and other PHS agencies:

- Cover sheet
- Senior/Key Person Profile

- Research & Related Budget—Section A & B, Budget Period 1
- Research & Related Budget—Cumulative Budget
- R&R Subaward Budget Attachment(s) Form
- Biographical Sketch Form

Pink Sheet and GAPPT

The final sections of this appendix offer an example of the NIH Grant Summary Statement (formerly known as the Pink Sheet), followed by the Grant Application Process Planning Tool (GAPPT).

SAMPLE FORMS

Letter of Intent

January 23, 2001
Applications Officer
March of Dimes Birth Defects Foundation
Greater Cincinnati Chapter
Cincinnati, Ohio

RE: Call for Educational Grants

Dear Grant Applications Officer:

As a practicing nurse and educator I am seeing an increasing number of infants born alcohol exposed. Yet, in our prenatal clinics the report rates average about 2 percent. We have found that some perinatal health professionals still advocate use of alcohol to women during the last trimester if the fetus is too active. Having completed substance abuse training through NIAAA, I know the dangers of this practice.

I am submitting a grant to the CDC for Fetal Alcohol Syndrome Prevention. As a corollary part to this project, I want to provide education to the health professionals in eight perinatal clinics in Cincinnati. My research team and I believe that with education we can heighten the awareness and increase the number of women identified during pregnancy that use alcohol. It is our hope that such education will result in a decreased incidence of Fetal Alcohol Syndrome. This proposed project fits well with your mission to decrease birth defects and increase awareness of potential perinatal problems that result in birth defects. I would like to submit this proposal for your next funding cycle.

Thank you in advance for your consideration of this proposed project. We look forward to hearing from you.

Sincerely,

Carole Kenner, DNS, RNC, FAAN
Professor of Clinical Nursing, University of Illinois at Chicago

Concept Paper

January 23, 2001

Agency for Healthcare Research and Quality
2101 E. Jefferson Street, Suite 501
Rockville, MD 20852

RE: Call for Health Care Policy Research

Dear Applications Officer:

As a neonatal nurse and an educator, I have become increasingly aware of the need for health policy research in the area of Last Precepts and End-of-Life Care in the newborn/infant population. Below you will find the concept paper outlining this issue.

Background/Significance

Low-birthweight infants (under 5.5 pounds) remain a problem in the U.S. despite educational efforts to promote good prenatal care. Since 1984 the incidence of low-birthweight births has increased to the present level of 7.5 per 1,000 live births. This steady rise contributes to the increase in mortality rate during the first month of life. Notably, two thirds of all infant deaths are neonatal (first 28 days of life) death (http://www.childstats.gov). Morbidity and mortality are only part of the issue. Questions are being raised about what healthcare professionals are doing to assist the child who is dying and his/her family. The answer is little in terms of palliative or hospice care for the newborn and infant populations. Most of the emphasis of end-of-life care and last precepts centers on the child with cancer or adult health care issues. Little health policy reflects the younger population.

Palliative care is a "philosophy of care that provides a combination of active and compassionate therapies intended to comfort and support patients and families who are living with life-threatening illness, while being sensitive and respectful of their religious, cultural, and personal beliefs, values, and traditions" (Canadian Palliative Care Association, 1995). End-of-Life (EOL) Care encompasses palliative care. EOL refers to care for the terminally ill who are not likely to survive.

In December 1997, the Task Force on Palliative Care developed the *Last Acts, Care and Caring for the End of Life Precepts of Palliative Care*. To date more than 30 professional associations have endorsed these precepts; few are child oriented. The precepts are broad and need to be translated to fit the child and family model of care. To this end professional organizations were brought together by Johns Hopkins to work on this national problem, EOL across the lifespan. Leaders from 22 national nursing organizations representing 463,000 nurses met in September 2000 in Baltimore to attend the Nursing Leadership Academy in End-of-Life Care. This Academy was funded by a grant from the Open Society Institute's Project on Death in America. Following this meeting the charge was given to participants to work with like associations to gain strength in numbers to adapt the Last Precepts to their population. The National Association of Neonatal Nurses (NANN), Society of Pediatric Nurses (SPN), and Association of Pediatric Oncology Nurses (APON) joined to work toward this goal.

Conceptual Model

Dame Cicely Saunders developed a Model of Whole Person Suffering (Krammer, Muri, Gooding-Kellar, Williams, & von Gunten, 1999). The model considers four aspects: physical, psychological, spiritual, and social. The emphasis is on maximizing quality of life and function and not the medical model of cure. This model requires a collaborative approach to care with all healthcare professions represented. One difficulty in implementing this model is the push for cost containment in healthcare delivery. Ethical challenges arise from the desire to provide EOL care and the need for cost containment measures. When working with newborns and infants, the family is the unit of care just as Saunders' model suggests (Krammer, Ring, Martinex, Jacobs, and Williams, 2001).

Health Policy Implications and Projected Research

To date there is little support by Medicaid for EOL care. Healthcare policies need to be changed to include EOL benefits. The nurse coordinates care as a family prepares for discharge. For the newborn or infant who is dying, there are few options if the family cannot pay. This situation must be changed. The magnitude of this problem is not well defined so the first step is to conduct a pilot study to determine the number of children and their families who require hospice or palliative care and who are Medicaid eligible but who cannot receive support for these services. This pilot will be conducted as a prospective study of families discharged from the Children's Hospital since 1999 to present and whose child is still alive but would benefit from hospice or palliative care. Concurrently the researchers will conduct a national survey of legislators to determine if they support inclusion of such care under Medicaid benefits—why or why not. This research is to determine the barriers to changing health policy. The final step in the research is to formulate policy based on the preliminary findings that will then be tested in the full research study. The project's timeline is one year.

REFERENCES

Canadian Palliative Care Association. (1995). *Canadian palliative care association: Palliative care: Towards a consensus in standardized principles of practice.* Ontario, Canada.

Krammer, L.M., Muir, J.C., Gooding-Kellar, N., Williams, M.B., and von Gunten, C. F. 1999. Palliative care and oncology: Opportunities for oncology nursing. *Oncology Nursing Updates* 6: 1–12.

Krammer, L.M., Ring, A.A., Martinex, J., Jacobs, M.J., & Williams, M.B. (2001). The nurse's role in interdisciplinary and palliative care. In M.L. Matzo and D.W. Sherman (Eds.), *Palliative care nursing: Quality care to the end of life.* New York: Springer, pp. 118–139.

Note: This concept paper is fabricated. It would need many more details in terms of statistics and more details about the project than space will allow. If the legislators were truly to be polled, a representation of some current policies that either support or refute Medicaid benefits should be included. A very defined target for the study would include hospital data, statistics of the surrounding area, and state statistics.

Abstract Example from Dissertation

Purpose:	To identify physiologic and behavioral responses of extremely preterm infants to a routinely administered painful stimulus (heelstick for necessary blood sampling) and to determine how postconceptional age (PCA) may influence pain responses.
Subjects:	Nonprobability convenience sample of 11 preterm infants born at 24–26 weeks PCA
Design:	Quasi-experimental, repeated measures design
Methods:	The Neonatal Individualized Developmental Care Assessment Program (NIDCAP) method was used to assess infant responses prior to, during, and following a heelstick procedure performed at weekly intervals between ages 27–32 weeks PCA.
Main Outcome Measures:	Univariate indicators of pain including physiologic (heart rate, oxygen saturation, and respiratory rate) and behavioral (brow bulge, eye squeeze, and 45 NIDCAP variables) responses were examined. Additionally, the Premature Infant Pain Profile (PIPP) was used as a composite measure to assess pain.
Principal Results:	Heart rate increased while oxygen saturation and respiratory rate decreased during the most invasive phase (stick/squeeze) of the procedure for infants between 27–32 weeks PCA. Increased PIPP scores and increased percent of occurrence of brow bulge and eye squeeze were also noted during the stick/squeeze phase. Although trends were noted towards increased behavioral stress between baseline and stick/squeeze values, these behaviors were not statistically significant across phases of the heelstick procedure. Finger splay increased significantly in magnitude of occurrence between 27 and 32 weeks PCA, while other NIDCAP variables, physiologic measures, facial variables, and PIPP scores were not sensitive to differences in PCA.

Conclusions: Former 24–26 week preterm infants who are between 27 and 32 weeks PCA are capable of expressing pain through physiological measures and facial actions in a manner similar to more mature preterm and healthy term infants. While NIDCAP behaviors failed to reach statistical significance, this method may be helpful in providing information about the physiologic and behavioral cost of the heelstick event on preterm infants. The PIPP is a valid instrument for assessing pain in infants as young as 27–32 weeks PCA.

Keywords: pain; postconceptional age; premature newborn; heelstick procedure; neonatal intensive care

Source: Walden, M. (1997). *Changes over Six Weeks in Multivariate Responses of Premature Neonates to a Painful Stimulus.* Unpublished doctoral dissertation, University of Texas at Austin, School of Nursing, Austin.

Abstract from NIH R03 Application*

*This is a single-spaced abstract as it appears on a completed NIH grant form.

Informal caregivers, often family members, care for 22 million older adults in the US, including 3 million with cognitive impairment. Nearly one-third of these families provide care coordination, independence maintenance, and socialization for elders from a distance greater than a 60 minute drive from the caregiver. Caregiving for cognitively impaired (CI) elders on-site imposes a heavy emotional, physical, and financial toll on caregivers. Caring at a distance further complicates caregiving roles. The exact nature of distance caregiving needs for families caring for CI elders living alone at home is unexplored, yet essential for planning clinically significant interventions to address the needs. At issue are problems of less physical contact with elders and greater coordination of services from afar. Modern computer / video technology with telecommunication innovations suggest a means for dialogue, remote wellness checking, information seeking and decision-support that could potentially bridge significant socialization and communication gaps by distance. However, these modalities remain relatively untapped. There is a need to provide evidence to inform the selection/customization of technology interventions to support distance family caregivers in a way that fosters independence and quality of life for CI elders. This study is a first step in a program of research to accomplish this goal. Aims of this preliminary, descriptive study are to describe and prioritize caregiving concerns of distance caregivers, identify caregiving facilitators, identify technology-based interventions to address priority concerns, and explore caregivers views of feasibility of the selected interventions. Focus group interviews of a purposive sample of culturally diverse distance family caregivers (n=48) of CI elders will be qualitatively analyzed to identify caregiving concerns and facilitators. A panel of experts in technology, elder care and cognitive impairment, and caregiving, and a long distance caregiver, will identify technology-based interventions to address priority concerns. Caregivers who composed the focus groups will then assess feasibility and usability of the recommended technologies. Understanding caregiving needs of distance caregivers should enable development and testing of user-friendly interventions for caregivers and promote cost-effective care delivery and beneficial outcomes for CI elders.

Source: Benefield, L.E. (2005). *Distance Caregiving of CI Elders Living Alone at Home.* NIH/NINR Grant 7R03NR009512-02.

Research Plan

Example of an R03 NIH Grant Application: Qualitative Methods

RESEARCH PLAN

A. SPECIFIC AIMS

Informal caregivers, often family members, are responsible for home care of about 22 million older adults in the US,[1] including 3 million with cognitive impairment.[2] This number is increasing, and the costs associated with care are significant.[2-4] Estimates of costs of family caregiving for community care of elders with mild to moderate dementia total $7.1 billion annually with $36.5 billion to businesses in lost caregiver productivity and absenteeism.[2, 5] Nearly one-third of informal caregiving occurs at a distance with family members coordinating provision of care, maintenance of independence, and socialization for elders living alone at home.[6, 7] Caregivers live, on average, 450 miles from care recipients and spend about 7 hours traveling to their homes to reach the care recipient.[7] Distance caregivers report an average of 35-41 hours per month providing care and lose 15 million days of work each year to perform care.[8] Distance caregiving, as compared to on-site caregiving, includes additional responsibilities, and roles become more complex when cognitively impaired (CI) elders require distance care.[7, 9-11] In order to plan interventions to support distance caregivers of CI elders, the scope and complexity of their role must be better understood.[10, 12] Interventions to lower healthcare costs, promote quality of life, and foster functional independence for the elder are more effective if they reflect perceived concerns of distance caregivers.[13] Therefore, it is essential to identify the nature and characteristics of these concerns. Caring for a CI elder is likely to include the processes of monitoring, interpreting, making decisions, taking action, making adjustments, assessing resources, providing hands-on care, working together with the care recipient, and negotiating the healthcare system.[14] Distance caregivers must develop and coordinate these same processes from a distance by enlisting assistance from family, friends, social networks, and formal agencies.[6, 9] Unfamiliarity with local and state assistance and regulations that affect the elder make the task more difficult. Distance caregivers may find it difficult to locate assistance to navigate the healthcare system, or knowing which local providers to consult about care issues.[15] While it may be assumed that some needs of distance caregivers are similar to those living near the elder, the extent to which geographical distance between family members and CI elders affects caregiving remains largely unknown. Once needs are identified, technology-based interventions that include

Source: Grant example with permission from Benefield, L.E. (2005). *Distance Caregiving of CI Elders Living Alone at Home.* NIH/NINR Grant 7R03NR009512-02.

computer and communication technology may offer potentially strong support for distance caregiving,[16-19] yet little is known about how such technology might address specific distance caregiving needs. A crucial first step is to have caregivers identify, in their own words, the concerns and perspectives of providing care. A second step is to identify and develop interventions aimed at making meaningful differences to the caregiver and promoting the ability of CI elders to remain at home.[1, 12, 20, 21] By better understanding the needs of distance caregiving for CI elders who live alone, more meaningful,[22] user-friendly, technology-based interventions for caregivers can be developed and tested. Use of effective and efficient interventions, tailored to the needs of the consumer, should lead to more productive and cost-effective healthcare delivery[12] and beneficial outcomes for both caregivers and elders.[23] The integration of consumer and technology expertise represents an innovation in pushing exploration and knowledge transfer from needs to feasible solutions. Therefore, the purposes of this exploratory study are: (1) to identify the caregiving needs of distance caregivers who care for CI elders living alone at home and (2) explore possible technologies to address the expressed concerns. Specific aims of the study are to:

1. Describe perceived caregiving concerns of distance caregivers of CI elders living alone at home.
2. Prioritize the caregiver-identified concerns most difficult to resolve from a distance.
3. Identify perceived facilitators to distance caregiving of CI elders.
4. Identify current and emerging technology-based interventions to address priority caregiving concerns.
5. Explore caregivers' views of the feasibility of the selected technology-based interventions.

B. BACKGROUND AND SIGNIFICANCE

Family caregiving from a distance and the numbers of CI elders remaining at home who require care are increasing.[3, 7, 24] A MetLife study reported the percentage of distance caregivers helping a CI person increased from 20% in 1997 to 33% of respondents in 2004.[7] However, consumers often lack the caregiver education, training, skills and support services to provide distance caregiving for CI elders. Research findings suggest that quality caregiving is possible, provided ample resources for caregivers are present.[25] Although capabilities of everyday and emerging technology offer potentially strong resource support for distance caregiving, it is noteworthy that neither specific caregiving needs nor tailoring technology-based interventions for caregiver-identified needs have been studied. Eighty percent of elders, totaling 22 million adults in the US, live at home or in independent care settings,[26] including 3 million with cognitive impairment.[2] Most older people prefer to remain at home, and 95% receive some level of caregiving from family and friends.[1, 20, 26] The presence of family caregiving for elders promotes good quality of life, functional independence, delays functional decline and institutionalization,[27, 28] and saves healthcare dollars. However, caregiving becomes increasingly heavy over time, making caregiver burden, stress, strain, and depression common.[29-31] The caregiving experience is influenced by caregiver and care recipient profiles and by caregivers' perceived level of burden.[32] *Family caregiving* is a multidimensional construct including cognitive, psychomotor, and affective dimensions that involve complex reasoning and behavioral processes.[14] The caregiving process involves physiological, social, contextual, and physical location dimensions for which the caregiver may not be prepared.[33] Even when families embrace caregiving, it can impose a heavy emotional, physical, and financial toll on the caregiver.[8, 14, 22, 26, 32, 34-43] *Caregiving for an elder with cognitive decline* differs from caring for an elder without impairment.[2, 44-50] Despite the growing body of literature addressing caregiving, the conceptual underpinnings of the actual process of doing the caregiving have historically received limited attention.[51] *Distance caregiving:* In nearly one-third of caregiving families, caregiving must occur at a distance.[7] The preference of frail elders to remain at home in declining years is made more difficult when primary caregivers live at a distance from the elder. Approximately five to seven million Americans are long-distance caregivers for elders, and this number is expected to escalate, doubling in the next 15 years.[6, 7] Distance caregiving is different than on-site caregiving, and caregivers report that distance caregiving impacts personal, social, and family needs, and that family, friends, and formal social and health services are enlisted to assist.[7, 10, 11, 52] Distance caregivers may monitor, if not actively participate in, activities similar to those ascribed to family caregivers of nursing home residents including the interpersonal quality of assistance, promotion of function, access to assistive devices, providing and decision making regarding ongoing activities of care planning and determination of health status and changes.[53] Additionally, distance caregivers often coordinate caregiving activities including the provision of care, maintenance of independence, and socialization of the elder from a distance. Thus, distance caregivers may experience emotional stress or burden and an increase in isolation related to these special activities and responsibilities.[54] *Distance caregiving of elders with CI:* Whereas there is considerable research evidence on family caregiving of elders and CI elders, little is known about distance caregiving of CI elders. Little is known about what is needed, from the family's perspective, to provide distance care to CI elders. The problems of caring for CI elders living alone at home can be expected to reflect those of family caregiving in general. However, when elders require distance care, the caregiving role becomes more complex and difficult.[6, 7, 9, 10, 55] When elders have mild to moderate cognitive impairment, they are dependent in one or more activities of daily living (ADLs) and may lack ability to make appropriate decisions about safe and dangerous situations.[28, 56, 57] When the environment of care for the CI elder is distant from the family caregiver, issues of safety, socialization, assistance with ADLs, and finding and using formal and informal resources become even more difficult to manage. Distance caregivers of CI elders must enlist assistance from family, friends, social networks, and formal agencies.[7, 9] While some caregiving needs of distance caregivers of CI elders living alone at home may be similar to those living with or nearby the elder, the extent to which the distance between caregiver and the CI elder affects caregiving needs and their ability to provide care remains largely unknown. In order to sustain elders in their home, we must plan interventions to support the role of distance caregivers. *Interventions for family caregivers*: Interventions have been developed to modify burden and role strain of caregivers of CI elders.[38, 58] Research suggests that interventions for caregivers of Alzheimer's patients may achieve small to moderate success due, in some measure, to limited information from the caregiver about the clinical significance and relevance of the interventions being tested.[59] Research suggests a conceptualization is needed of actually performing the in-home family caregiving that includes monitoring, interpreting, making decisions, taking action, making adjustments, assessing resources, working together with the care recipient, and negotiating the healthcare system.[14] Distance care for a CI elder living alone at home may include these processes, yet little attention has been paid to the family's perspective and the needs of family members providing distance care to CI elders. In 2001, the NINR identified a need for research to address caregiving issues including chronic illness, aging, technology-dependence, cognitive impairment, and caregiver support systems. The workgroup recommended research efforts to better understand generic caregiver knowledge, skills, and support, including "caregiver needs related to sorting through their options and then making decisions on behalf of their family members and themselves."[60] Although caregivers in special categories such as those caregiving CI elders may face unique challenges when geographically distant from the care recipient, their perceived needs have not been addressed when designing interventions. Certainly, developing skill in the caregiver role is an important issue and more resources are needed to address special assistance to long-distance caregivers. *Technology-based interventions*: Numerous high technology-based interventions, defined as devices that use microprocessors/computer chips,[61] are being developed and tested to assist with aging in the home environment.[62-65] Through high-technology transfer, space-age and amplified intelligence, new innovations are possible. Historically, most technology-based assistive devices and home modifications have addressed problems of caring for elders including wandering and rummaging; more recent technologies addressed enhancing or maintaining functional status.[62, 64, 66] Intelligent assistive technology such as activity cueing, autominders, televideo monitoring, or a ComputerLinks network could assist in remote wellness checking, providing information and decision support, and provide telecommunication innovation to address distance caregiving needs.[16, 64, 67-69] Technology-based interventions could virtually connect the caregiver and elder and provide strong support for distance caregiving that addresses the elder's physical, social, cognitive, and/or sensory impairments.[19, 64] Computer-based two-way video dialogue and remote wellness checking, computer networks to provide information and decision support, and telecommunication innovations could potentially bridge some of the socialization and communication gaps imposed by distance and assist the caregiver in assessing and enhancing the elder's functional status. Using technology to communicate and interact with CI elders offers avenues for novel approaches to care and opens new areas to be explored. The challenge to using advanced technology-based interventions is to match technological capabilities to actual caregiving needs, understand how people prefer to interact with technology, and learn how it fits into caregivers' lives without introducing new burdens associated with technology use.[17, 69] *Conceptual basis of the study*: A conceptual model of caregiving "skill," including the processes and properties of caregiving, informs this study and is proposed as the basis for measurement of family caregiving ability.[33] Skill indicators of caregiving include monitoring, interpreting, making decisions, taking action, making adjustments, accessing resources, providing hands-on care, working together with the ill person, and negotiating the healthcare system.[70] This model provides a powerful visualization of the complex, multidimensional, cognitive, and psychomotor nature of "doing the caregiving." Except for "providing hands-on care," the remaining processes seem intuitively valid for caregiving from any location. This model of caregiving processes may inform distant as well as direct family caregiving, since there is overlap in activities and responsibilities. Therefore, this model will serve as the sensitizing framework for this study. The model supports the assumption that caregiving processes and needs can be identified and quantified by asking the caregivers currently immersed in this process to identify caregiving concerns and facilitators. *Importance of the proposed study*: The exact nature of caregiving at a distance for a CI elder remains illusive, yet the need for caregiver relief is apparent. This innovative study provides an opportunity to identify needs and perspectives of the family caregiver in their own words and is a critical first step in selecting and testing interventions that might make a meaningful difference to the caregiver.[12, 21, 71] This study is the first step of a multistage plan to select, tailor, and test technology-based interventions to address the needs of distance caregivers and the CI elders living alone at home. If distance caregivers can receive technology support to address their expressed needs in distance caregiving for the CI elder, improvements in healthcare quality and outcomes are more achievable. In many cases, assistance can be provided that can prevent premature decline.[16] Use of effective and efficient interventions, tailored to the needs of the consumer, should lead to more productive and cost-effective healthcare delivery[12] and beneficial outcomes for both caregivers and elders.

C. PRELIMINARY STUDIES

The principal investigator's program of research centers on family caregiving of elders with cognitive impairment. The proposed study is a logical extension of the PI's earlier program of research and professional roles. The PI has been actively involved in home care services since 1981 including: (1) two years as administrator of a Medicare-certified home healthcare agency serving elders and their caregivers; (2) site-visitor with the national Community Health Accreditation Program of the NLN; and (3) author, consultant, researcher, and educator in home care and caregiving. The PI is currently a Postdoctoral Fellow at the University of ——. During the fellowship with Dr. ——, Dr. Benefield is gaining methodological skill in gerontological health services research, conducting preliminary studies related to distance caregiving for frail elders, and gaining skill in the design and implementation of gerontological intervention research. In addition, she is gaining knowledge of advanced technologies and technology transfer to home and clinical settings. She is meeting and forming collaborations with researchers in academic and business settings who are using technology-based interventions to assist elders and caregivers. *Study # 1*: Dr. Benefield, as Senior Chiron Fellow with Sigma Theta Tau 2001–02, conducted a study Home Healthcare Nursing: A Domain Analysis to identify the state of the science in home healthcare nursing as reflected in the periodic literature for the timeframe 1990–2000. Of 157 qualified studies, 25 addressed intervention research, five of these related to caregiving. Gaps were identified in the science, particularly the lack of family caregiver-identified role and functions and interventions to assist caregivers.[72, 73] Under contract with editors of *Online Journal of Clinical Innovation,* Dr. Benefield is conducting a follow-up integrative review specific to distance caregiving (completion date December, 2004). *Study # 2*: Dr. Benefield conducted a program evaluation of caregiver education programming through the Area Agency on Aging, part of the National Family Caregiver Support Program, to identify factors associated with program success among six local agencies. Using case study methodology, Dr. Benefield conducted individual and group interviews with key agency informants to determine structural and procedural factors within and across programs that influenced caregiver education program outcomes. Characteristics of more successful programs included targeting specific groups of caregivers by geographic or work location, specific care recipient profiles and diseases (e.g., elders with Alzheimer's disease), and/or carer-to-care-recipient relationship, e.g., female spouses, adult-children caregivers. Items from the caregiver demographic data sheet developed during this study have been adapted for use in the current study.[74-76] *Study # 3*: The purpose of this case study was to explore caregiving concerns of an adult daughter caregiver who provided distance care for her elder parent with Alzheimer's disease who was living alone at home, then made the transition to a specialized Alzheimer's Disease Care Unit. Data collection consisted of an interview using open-ended questions related to caregiving concerns, role of the primary and secondary family caregivers, changes in caregiving after the parent was placed in the specialized unit, and supports and difficulties in caregiving. Content analysis of interview responses suggested caregiving needs including coordination of care, direct physical care, and creating opportunities to provide "tender loving care." The major theme illustrated in the caregiver's dialogue was the need to maintain virtual and physical connectedness with the parent across locations as the elder progressed from moderate to severe dementia. During this case study (1) the wording and sequencing of questions for this proposed study were tested and modified, (2) methods proposed for this study were reviewed to determine whether this caregiver would find the methods acceptable, and (3) the acceptability of the purposive sample recruitment process was validated by this caregiver.

D. RESEARCH DESIGN AND METHODS

Designs for this *three*-phase descriptive study follow. **Phase 1** uses focus group methodology[71] employing in-depth interviewing to elicit distance caregivers' of CI elders views of caregiving concerns (Aim 1), prioritized caregiving needs related to the concerns (Aim 2), and caregiving facilitators (Aim 3). **Phase II** uses a consensus development process modeled after the National Institutes of Health (NIH) Consensus Development Panel process[77] with a panel of a caregiver and experts in aging-in-place technology, engineering technology transfer, Alzheimer's disease, and caregiving. The panel will review prioritized caregiving concerns and the list of facilitators of Phase I and a listing of technologies, then, for concerns amenable to technology interventions, recommend advanced technology-based interventions that can be deployed in new ways to address the concerns (Aim 4). **Phase III** reconvenes all members of the focus groups into two larger groups to evaluate feasibility and usability of technology interventions recommended by the expert panel (Aim 5). Although the ideal design would include eliciting the views of the distance caregiver, the care recipient, and the larger community, due to budget limitations this study will address only the perceptions of distance caregivers. A strength of this innovative design is the combined use of caregiver perspective and experts well-informed on clinical issues and technology transfer to explore the human interface in technology and distance caregiving. Each phase of the study is described separately below and will be shared with participants. See Table 1 for the project timeline.

Phase I: Describe Distance Caregiving Needs (Focus Group Sessions)

Sample: A purposive nonprobability sample of 48 self-identified adult distance caregivers of elders with mild to moderate cognitive impairment will be selected from among 494 faculty and 1013 staff of _____ University and 400+ caregivers accessing the Alzheimer's Association XXXX Chapter. Criteria for selection include (1) self-reported adult child, [78, 79] distance caregiver of a mild to moderately CI elder ≥ 60 years old living alone at home, primary or secondary caregiver to the elder and assisting or providing for activities of daily living (ADLs) and/or instrumental activities like transportation, shopping, and managing finances;[7] (2) has provided distance care for at least three months and is currently providing caregiving; (3) ability to speak, read, and write in English; (4) access to a telephone; and (5) the elder living beyond the 60-minute driving [6] radius of the local area and residing in the United

Table 1 Timeline

Activity	Study Phase indicated in columns below; X = Not phase specific																	
Study Year	**Year 01**												**Year 02**					
Calendar months	9	10	11	12	1	2	3	4	5	6	7	8	9	10	11	12	1	2
Study months	1	2	3	4	5	6	7	8	9	10	11	12	13	14	15	16	17	18
Hire and train staff; procure equipment	1	1											3					
Develop recruitment, screening scripts	1	1	1															
Recruit focus group participants			1	1														
Refine interview guides and procedures			1	1									3					
Secure meeting dates and times			1	1							3	3						
Conduct focus group sessions 1 & 2					1	1	1											
Interpret and analyze findings					1	1	1	1	1									

Table 1 Timeline *(continued)*

Complete final report from Phase I									1									
Set up expert panel conference						2	2	2										
Complete list of technologies for panel												2	2					
Convene expert panel													2					
Develop the report of expert panel													2	2				
Approval of report by panel members														2				
Caregiver feasibility of technologies																3		
Analyze caregivers' feasibility assessment																3	3	3
Preparation of manuscripts		X	X						X	X	X	X	X	X	X	X	X	X
Prepare study report																		X

Source: Grant example with permission from Benefield, L.E. (2005). *Distance Caregiving of CI Elders Living Alone at Home.* NIH/NINR Grant 7R03NR009512-02.

States. Limiting the study to those caring for elders with mild to moderate cognitive decline offers the greatest potential for technology to extend the elder's independent living and quality of life.[16] Although limiting the sample to caregivers of CI elders with a *medically documented* diagnosis of cognitive impairment was considered, this would exclude distance caregivers whose parent exhibits impairment without a formal diagnosis. In order to include the widest range of caregivers, medical diagnosis of the elder's cognitive impairment is not a criterion for participation in the study. After considering a sample from the larger _____ area, we chose the university community because it is representative of the _____ area in cultural, socioeconomic, and educational diversity, and provides ease in accessing participants due to the established relationship between the PI and the Human Resource Department. The use of the Alzheimer's Association is specifically included to (1) solicit distance caregivers who have connected with formal support systems and (2) solidify our commitment during this and future studies to partnering with provider constituents. Purposive sampling principles[71] will be used to select from a range of caregivers including family relationship (daughter, son), and occupation and cross-cultural diversity (an African-American and Hispanic sample representative of the region) with the goal of achieving heterogeneity across groups and homogeneity and compatibility within each focus group.[71, 80] The university sample (53% female, 47% male) is culturally and economically diverse and includes 77% non-Hispanic white, 14% Hispanic, 6% African-American, 2% Asian, and 1% American Indian. Fifteen percent of university staff earn $\leq$ \$20,000, and 15% of faculty earn $\geq$ \$70,000 in annual salary. The Alzheimer's Association audience is similarly diverse and includes caregivers who have used the resources of the Association at least once and the service area includes urban, suburban, and rural locales. Based on previous sampling in these settings, we anticipate no difficulty recruiting 48 participants: approximately 30 from faculty/staff participants and 18 from the Alzheimer's Association. The standard focus group consists of 6–10 participants[71] and sampling will provide for six separate focus groups of eight persons each that will meet twice. Based on established focus group size and composition protocols,[81] since caregivers will be emotionally involved in the topic and the topic itself is complex, each group is limited to eight participants to allow adequate time for all participants to respond to questions within the 90-minute focus group session. The six groups provide opportunity for separation of supervisor-employee dyads, and male versus female caregivers.[82-84] Although we considered not segmenting participants into specific groups, we feel it necessary to separate supervisor-employee dyads and to provide opportunity for male and female caregivers, who may relate different caregiving experiences, to respond within homogeneous groups.[7, 10, 85, 86]

Recruitment: The PI will recruit potential participants from the university and the Alzheimer's Association, obtain consent from the participants, and gather preliminary demographic data including documenting caregiver status and perception of their parent's level of cognitive impairment (Appendices). The PI, a member of the university, will not participate in selecting participants into groups or moderating the focus group interviews to avoid biasing selection or influencing open dialogue. (An experienced focus group moderator will conduct all focus groups.) Recruitment procedures differ for the university and Alzheimer's Association sites. Recruitment from the university community includes sending an e-mail announcement of the study and contact information to all faculty and staff at their university e-mail address. This has been approved by administrators at the university. Nonprofessional staff (e.g., housekeepers, groundskeepers, maintenance personnel) who do not have ready computer access at work but may have home access will receive both e-mails to their university e-address and hardcopy letter to their university box. One follow-up reminder will be posted in the general university announcement page, distributed electronically and as a hardcopy. Additional postings in staff meeting areas will be used to recruit participants. Potential participants will be asked to seek out other potential participants with distance caregiver experience. Announcements to the local Alzheimer's Association staff and volunteers, newsletter, support groups, website, and educational programs will be used to access caregivers. Because distance caregivers may not self-identify as a caregiver, announcements and advertisements include prompts describing caregiving, e.g., make telephone calls on behalf of another, check on the person on a regular basis, assist with coordinating health care, and/or help manage bills and finances. To promote retention, each participant will receive a $10 local department store gift card and $10 gasoline voucher at the conclusion of each of the 2 focus group sessions. Other strategies include refreshments during the sessions, meeting locations close to the university or at local library sites used successfully for previous Alzheimer's Association programming, free convenient parking, meeting times convenient to participants' work schedule, and an opportunity to be involved in future studies that may evaluate interventions. **Instruments and Tools:** Data will be generated from demographic data sheets and guided interviews using focus groups consisting of distance caregivers (Appendices). Each of the six focus groups will meet twice as part of Phase I, first to respond to semistructured interview questions about caregiving concerns and a second time to review, validate, and prioritize[87] concerns identified from the first session and identify facilitators to caregiving. Interview questions for session 1 will address "doing" the caregiving and the concerns and needs that impact the process. For the first interview session, global questions[71] include "What kind of support are you providing for your parent?" (We expect to see comments related to emotional connectivity and physical, social, financial, and/or spiritual support.) and "Where do you need support?" In addition, questions from the Family Caregiver Skill Profile Interview Schedule have been adapted for use as interview probes with the focus groups. This schedule is being used in a current NIH-funded study of in-home caregiving skill[70] and the originator, Dr. _____, is a consultant to this study. The question "I heard you say that (insert concern) also was an issue in (CI elder's) care; this is something that is important and yet can be difficult to manage at home, so I would like to talk in a little more detail about how that is going for you" will be used in focus group session #1 (Aim 1). The purpose of session 2 is for participants to prioritize their concerns identified in session 1; we will use the question from Schumacher's guide "We have talked about a number of things that you are involved in as a caregiver. Which of these have been of greatest concern to you?" (Aim 2). In addition, participants will be queried about facilitators to distance caregiving using a final probe "What has helped or would help you provide better care from a distance?" (Aim 3) The PI currently is conducting pilot work to evaluate the global questions and probes with focus groups of a purposive sample of distance caregivers. She will revise the questions and interview guide based on results of this work and review by study consultants. The focus group moderator will use these questions and additional probes to elicit caregivers' views of concerns important to caregiving. To establish consistency, the same and only moderator and RA will be involved in the group interviews. **Procedures:** After the PI has telephoned the participants for consent, the completed demographic sheets on participants will be forwarded to the research assistant (RA) to place caregivers into focus groups. Each of the six focus groups will meet twice as part of Phase I, first to respond to semistructured interview questions about caregiving and a second time, 1–2 weeks later, to review, validate, and prioritize[87] needs identified from the first session and identify facilitators to caregiving. The moderator and RA will greet the participants upon arrival. Refreshments will be provided and participants given time to mingle prior to introductions. Participants will sit at a round table to encourage interaction in a room free of noise or visual distractions. To engage all participants, the moderator will initiate the focus group with the global questions followed by specific probes. Although two focus group sessions, followed by individual participant interviews, might more fully capture the depth and breadth of caregiving concerns and facilitators, a decision was made to use only the focus groups for this exploratory work in order to conserve resources, yet gather group consensus. Nominal group techniques were selected to make the best use of focus group time,[88-90] and to efficiently capture, within a short period of time, the widest range of information on concerns and their relative ranking and a list of facilitators. Focus groups will be tape recorded and transcribed for analysis. **Study procedures include:**

Phase I Focus Group session #1

1. The caregivers will be informed that the purpose of the study is to address two questions (Appendix).
2. The global questions will be posted on a flip chart. Participants will be given a sheet of paper and asked to work independently to generate words and phrases to represent their thoughts in response to the questions. Participants will be encouraged to think about the question from their personal caregiving experience and to generate as many thoughts as possible.

3. Round-robin nomination or public statement of responses will begin. Caregivers will be encouraged to follow up on other members' responses as a way to generate additional ideas. Each response will be visibly recorded on a flip chart. To conserve time for all respondents to speak, members will be requested to state their responses briefly. Round-robin format continues until there are no additional responses.

4. Each item is examined and discussed by the group to assure understanding by all. Comments are encouraged and interviewing techniques used to seek depth and breadth of caregiving issues/concerns.

Phase I Focus Group session #2

Procedures similar to the introduction phase of session #1 will welcome participants, provide summary of the first session, and state activities to occur during the second session. Each focus group reviews only their own flip chart data. Caregivers will be told the purpose of the second session is to prioritize their caregiving concerns they listed during the previous session and identify facilitators to distance caregiving (Appendix).

1. The flip charts of the responses from session 1 will be posted for review.[71, 87]

2. The moderator will summarize comments from session 1. The group will review each item on the flip chart pages to be sure that it is understood by the whole group.

3. Then, each caregiver will vote, anonymously, on a separate sheet of paper to determine the relative importance of the list of concerns/problems listed on the group flip charts, by selecting five that are personally of the greatest concern or importance to their caregiving situation.

4. Caregivers will then be asked to rank, again using the paper, the five most important concerns they have individually identified on their worksheet from 1 to 5 (1 = most important, 5 = least important).

5. Using flip charts and nominal group technique, participants will be asked a final question. The question, "What has helped or will help you to provide better care from a distance? What supports have helped you?" Round-robin format will be used as in focus group session #1, steps 2, 3, and 4, and interviewing techniques used to seek depth and breadth and clarification of understanding of the caregiving facilitators. Note: In this limited time frame the purpose is to identify the range of facilitators; therefore, caregivers will not be asked to prioritize facilitators to caregiving.

During both sessions, the moderator will use facilitation strategies to ensure each caregiver participates and to manage any overparticipation by caregivers. The research assistant, trained by the PI, will collect additional data related to schematic diagrams of seating arrangements and any pertinent data about group behavior that may influence data analysis. Face-to-face meetings of study staff (PI, RA, moderator) will occur before and after each focus group session and at intervals during the study to clarify management or interviewing issues. The research team (PI, RA, moderator, consultants) will meet via conference call prior to data collection and at set intervals to confirm data collection processes and resolve any conceptual or procedural issues.

The moderator, recruited and trained by the PI, will be an experienced nurse or therapist skilled in focus group interviewing and nominal group technique, experienced in elder care, with no prior association with the university or the Alzheimer's Association. Training will consist of a 4-hour session with the PI instructing in specific techniques and procedures for the focus group interviews, use of equipment and room set-up, and moderator role-playing under the supervision of the PI who will critique technique. The PI has previously conducted group interviews with elder patients and caregivers in the home care setting, and will consult with qualitative expert Dr. _____ to validate technique and training strategies for the moderator and RA. The PI will supervise the moderator through meetings prior to and after each interview and monitor data quality, accuracy, and completeness. IRB approval through _____ University is pending. Approval for accessing participants has been received from the university Office of Human Resources and the Alzheimer's Association and study procedures comply with federal HIPAA privacy standards.

Data Analysis: Descriptive statistics will describe the participants using the demographic data sheets. Initial analysis will identify expressed caregiving concerns from each focus group. Data from each focus group will not be combined until all focus groups have met a second time. The *concerns* identified within *each* focus group and listed on the flip charts will be tabulated (Aim 1), and the individual rank ordering scores from the participant's worksheets will be summed (Aim 2). Then data from across all the focus groups will be combined, once all focus groups have met a second time, to identify overall *ranking of concerns* (Aim 2). Differences by focus group composition (gender, culture) will be noted. Qualitative interview audiotaped data from each focus group will be transcribed verbatim by an experienced transcriptionist and entered into the Ethnograph computer software program in order to sort data by codes.[91] The PI will use content analysis to examine the narrative text of each group's interviews by word, topic, or unit of meaning and constant comparison[92] will be used after all focus groups in Phase I are concluded to compare narrative data to identify core issues and concerns prioritized by *all* the caregiver groups. The PI will use content analysis, then manually code transcripts into data segments and re-enter codes into the Ethnograph program. These raw data will focus on caregiving issues *identified by the caregivers themselves.* Using content analysis and constant comparison, the PI will independently combine the raw data into data clusters, such as caregiving support issues, care coordination issues, barriers, or facilitators. By combining and organizing these data clusters by and across groups, we will look for core categories related to caregiving needs. The coding categories cannot be predetermined since they emerge from the participants' experience with distance caregiving. The coding decisions and process related to categorizing the clusters will be recorded by the PI to provide auditability and reviewed by the study consultant at set intervals.[93] In the case of differences, the PI and consultant will meet via teleconference to gain consensus. In the event there are no similar core issues and concerns across the groups, a group composed of one predetermined representative of each focus group will be convened and the card sort technique will be used to prioritize core issues and concerns.[94] The caregiving *facilitators* (Aim 3) listed on flip charts by each focus group will be tabulated and the audiotaped data will be analyzed using content analysis and constant comparison, as described above for caregiver concerns, excluding analysis related to prioritizing.

Phase II: Identify Technology Interventions to Address Caregiving Needs (Expert Panel)

Expert Panel: The report of findings of prioritized caregiving concerns and list of facilitators (Phase I), and a list of technology-based interventions to address the concerns will be presented to a multidisciplinary panel of five experts who will estimate the feasibility of and recommend technology interventions to address priority distance caregiving needs. In order to identify and estimate the feasibility of technology-based interventions that could address identified concerns of distance caregiving, the panel will be convened for a one-day face-to-face meeting. This expert panel model is based on the NIH model of Consensus Development Conferences[77] and is purposively planned to bring experts from consumer, academic, and private sectors to the table.[95] Panelists include one distance caregiver, one nationally recognized expert each in caregiving research (Dr. _____) and aging, dementia care and technology (Dr. _____), and two experts in aging-in-place technologies and technology transfer (Mr._____ and Dr. _____); the PI and Dr. _____ co-convene the panel. The caregiver panelist will be purposively selected by the National Alliance for Caregiving. They will select from among their contacts a distance caregiver (of a CI elder living alone at home) who is able to represent the perspective of the caregiver consumer in the panel. **Data sources** for phase II include: (1) the written report of the summary of findings of the focus group interviews including caregiving concerns and facilitators, and (2) a description of selected current and/or emerging advanced technology interventions from academic and private sector sources available for addressing the top ranked concerns of this consumer group. Prior to the convened meeting, the panel members with expertise in technology (_____,_____, and_____) will be asked to review the caregiving concerns and, for those amenable to technology-based interventions, identify one or more current or emerging technology-based interventions to address top-ranked concerns. Each will prepare a one- to two-page synopsis for one, or more if necessary, technology-based interventions chosen. The synopsis will include the technology-based intervention's system components, how technology would address needs, and description of system architecture sufficient to inform other panel members about the suggested technology. Still and/or video pictures of the technology will be added to the reports and distributed to all members for review prior to convening the entire panel. **Procedures:** The PI, co-convener _____, and panel member _____ will draft format questions and strategies (brainstorming and visioning techniques, provocative probes, and psychomotor creativity stimulation) for the panel meeting to elicit innovation in creating methods of deploying technology in new ways.[96] The PI and consultant _____ will co-convene the panel. NIH Consensus Development Conference Guidelines criteria will serve to develop format questions and protocols; specific procedures to organize, plan, moderate, and evaluate the session; and recommendations,[77] with the p.m. session audiotaped and transcribed. **Data Analysis:** Prior to the meeting, all panelists will review the summary report of caregiving concerns and facilitators (from Phase I) and the list of technology-based interventions. Day one (a.m.), panelists will convene to discuss documents and receive a briefing from the technologist who prepared the synopsis on each selected technology-based intervention. During the afternoon, the panel will (1) select two or more technology-based interventions addressing top-ranked caregiver concerns and develop a matrix table matching caregiving concerns to and across technology interventions, (2) identify pros and cons of the selected technology-based interventions for use in distance caregiving, and (3) create a list of recommendations for use of technology-based interventions with distance caregivers of CI elders. Dr. _____ will lead the panel in matrix table development, using a morphology chart to examine concerns (e.g., ensure safety) matched to technology approaches to address the concerns; this allows for examining distinct functions, i.e., one function of technology that can address several caregiving concerns, that can then be melded in different configurations into various solutions.[97] The PI will use transcribed data to collate sections 1, 2, and 3 above into a written report that will be sent to and approved by each panel member. Although tele- or videoconferencing was considered for panel meeting, the face-to-face meeting is required for efficient and effective interaction among panel members. To reduce the significant costs of bringing experts together for a 2-day session, the panel process was streamlined to occur within 1 day, eliminating costs of a second night's lodging.

Phase III: Distance Caregivers' Assessment of Technology Recommendations (Caregivers' Meeting)

Sample: Focus group members from Phase I will be assembled into 2 groups to address the feasibility and usability of technology-based interventions recommended by the expert panel for use in distance caregiving (Aim 5). This enables each person to individually evaluate the suggested technology-based interventions, and makes the multiple smaller focus group format unnecessary. Caregiver attrition will be minimized by a strong introduction during the first focus group session to emphasize the importance of their involvement in assessing usefulness of technology to distance caregiving. As in Phase I, each caregiver will receive a local department store gift card and gasoline voucher at the end of the group session. Attendance will be encouraged by mailed reminder. **Instruments and Tools:** A worksheet distributed to caregivers will include questions addressing potential feasibility (privacy, acceptability, usability) of recommended technologies (ex: "For this technology, what thoughts come to mind when you consider using this in your own caregiving situation?") and experience with similar technology. Two summary questions, using a five-point Likert response scale, will be used to query an individual caregiver's (1) overall assessment of technology and (2) whether the caregiver would consider using suggested technology (Appendix). **Procedures:** The 90-minute meetings will be scheduled at a time and location convenient to the caregivers. Refreshments will be served. The moderator and PI will introduce the agenda, stating the purpose of the meeting to determine, from the caregivers' perspective, the feasibility and usefulness of the recommended technology interventions. The PI will introduce each technology by verbal description using the still and/or video pictures of suggested technology-based intervention, listing the need(s) that technology could address, and the written panel synopsis (rewritten at an 8th grade reading level) will be distributed to each caregiver with instructions for completing the worksheet. Caregivers will be encouraged to think about the question from their personal caregiving experience and to generate as many thoughts as possible in response to the questions on the worksheet. **Data Analysis:** Responses to each technology will be evaluated separately. For each open-ended question, written responses will be collated verbatim. Content analysis will be used to group the responses, using the exact language of the caregivers, into major categories. For the Likert scale response questions, frequencies and the mean will be calculated to determine overall usefulness of each intervention. **Summary of Methodology:** Results of this three-phase study will include (1) a prioritized description of clinically significant caregiving concerns specific to distance caregiving of CI elders living alone at home, (2) a description of facilitators specific to distance caregiving, (3) technology-based interventions identified and evaluated by a multidisciplinary expert panel to be helpful to caregiving, and (4) caregivers' views of the feasibility and usability of the selected technologies. It is expected that future development and testing of caregiver need-based, user-friendly, technology-based interventions will be more clinically relevant[59, 98] once the needs of distance caregiving for CI elders living alone at home are better understood. A future next step involves study of technology-based intervention(s) feasibility and acceptance, adding bioengineers to the team, and possible submission of a Small Business Innovation Research (SBIR) proposal to test the technology.

Study Limitations: The investigators acknowledge that caregiver skill and needs will change over time and the scope of this study will not address patterns of ability development.[33] The sample may be biased due to self-selection into the study. In addition, comorbidities of the caregiver and/or elder, as well as caregiver coping style and relationship with the elder, may influence caregiver concerns but will not be addressed in this study. We also acknowledge that not all caregiving needs identified by distance caregivers may be amenable to technology-based interventions.

E. HUMAN SUBJECTS

E.1 Risk to the Subjects

Human subjects involvement and characteristics. Caregivers ($N = 48$) who agree will participate in two focus groups (Phase I) and a meeting of several focus groups combined (Phase 3). Participants will consist of adult children caregivers who provide distance caregiving of elders with mild to moderate cognitive impairment living alone at home. A majority of caregivers will probably be over the age of 40 and a few under age 21. Participants will include caregivers of both genders and all racial/ethnic groups who have consented to participate in the study after a detailed explanation of the procedures. *Inclusion* criteria include (1) self-reported adult child distance caregiver of mild to moderate CI elder ≥ 60 living alone at home; (2) has provided distance care for at least three months and is currently providing caregiving; (3) ability to speak, read, and write in English; (4) access to a telephone; and (5) elder living beyond the 60-minute driving radius of the local area and residing in the United States. Caregivers whose parent is placed outside the home setting in a care facility or dies during the study will remain in the study unless they chose to withdraw. *Exclusion* criteria include distance caregivers (1) of elders who are living outside the United States, (2) who receive pay for caregiving, (3) whose parent receives full-time professional healthcare assistance in the home. Rationale for exclusion of caregivers with primary language other than English is based on a sufficiently large potential sample of Hispanics with skill in speaking, reading, and writing English, and for other exclusions, the need to eliminate other confounding variables (non-United States residency, other residential assistance to the elder) that could impact the issues and concerns of caregiving.

Sources of Materials. Materials obtained specifically for research aims include demographic information, verbal and written information obtained through group interviews, and completion of written worksheets. No existing records or data will be used in the study.

Potential Risks. Participants will have minimal risks associated with their participation. Caregivers may become tired during the interviews, or become anxious when discussing concerns related to caregiving. Because part of this study uses a group interview, total privacy cannot be guaranteed since participants will be sharing their experiences in a group. However, all group members will be asked not to talk about personal experiences shared in the group outside of the group. This is a nonintervention study, so benefits are limited to the knowledge gained for future distance caregivers. However, the benefits to future distance caregivers outweigh the minimal risk associated with the group interviews and assessment of technology-based interventions.

E.2 Adequacy of Protection Against Risks

Recruitment and Informed Consent. The PI will develop an Operations Manual detailing study procedures and all aspects of the study protocol and use it for initial and ongoing training. The manual will delineate specific procedures for participant recruitment, informed consent, appropriate interviewing techniques, and retention strategies. All team members will attend a required class on human subjects' protection. Recruitment of caregivers will be done via e-mail and hardcopy communication to all faculty/staff at the university site, and via staff announcements to staff and volunteers and hardcopy and electronic announcements in the information distributed to the audience served by the Alzheimer's Association XXXX Chapter. If the caregiver is interested in more information or wishes to participate, the caregiver will contact the researcher via telephone or e-mail. If, after the researcher explains the study, the caregiver wishes to continue to participate, the PI will obtain informed consent after explaining the purpose, risks, benefits, and the participant's right to withdraw at any time from the study. Contact information and preliminary demographic data will be collected in order to place the participant into a focus group. This information will be sent to the RA who will place participants in the focus groups. Participants will not be placed in a focus group with a supervisor or another employee from their immediate work group.

Protection Against Risk. To protect against the risk of psychological discomfort, at the beginning of each focus group meeting the moderator will explain to the participants that they do not have to answer any question and they may discontinue the interview at any time. The moderator will explain that we do not know the concerns of distance caregivers of elders with CI living alone at home, and this study will help to document and prioritize these concerns. In addition, the report of concerns will be used to identify possible technology-based interventions, and that they will help to assess the suitability of the interventions to the concerns they identified. If the participant has psychological concerns about the caregiving experience, the moderator will provide the caregiver with a list of local mental health providers and information on available resources. If severe anxiety or psychological distress is noted, the moderator will immediately refer the caregiver to a crisis hotline or mental health center.

To protect confidentiality, the participants will be asked to use only first names during the focus group's meetings and not to talk about personal experiences shared in the group outside of the group. A master list will contain the names and contact information of all the caregivers and link their names with an identifying numerical code. Only the PI and RA will have access to the master list that will remain in a locked file cabinet. Data maintenance will include measures to ensure data security and integrity. The RA may use either network computers or stand-alone personal computers and transfer data to the local area network (LAN) via zip disks. Data will be stored in an area of the LAN that only data management members of the research team (PI, RA) can access with passwords. The database will be backed-up nightly and monthly reviews will occur of all processes related to data management and security.

E.3 Potential Benefits of the Proposed Research to the Subjects and Others

While there are no direct benefits to the participants other than personal compensation for their time and travel costs, there are potential benefits to future caregivers who may be in similar circumstances. If the concerns of distance caregiving can be better understood, we can tailor technology-based interventions to specifically address the most important needs in a manner helpful to the caregiver and increase the potential success of the technology-based intervention.

E.4 Importance of the Knowledge to Be Gained

This novel approach creates a partnership[95] of experts in distance caregiving, i.e., the actual caregivers, and academic and private-sector representatives well-informed in engineering, clinical issues, aging-in-place technology, and technology transfer to investigate a clinically significant area of distance caregiving. Knowledge gained by using this innovative methodology will inform the development and application of user-friendly, clinically significant, technology-based interventions to assist distance caregiving. Next-step studies can investigate feasibility and acceptance of these advanced technology-based interventions with caregiver and CI elders, and expand the research team to include bioengineers who bring skill in adapting technology to "work" with or for the human body in an impartial way. Combining the abilities of multiple disciplines and the consumer (caregivers and CI elders) perspective will promote the success of cutting-edge technology-based intervention as modified by what is practical. Technology-based resources could provide long-distance caregivers more rapid access to information, resources, socialization and communication with the elder, and provide a sense of connectivity for caregivers and the elder. These interventions hold potential for reducing stress and role strain in caregivers who feel overloaded with adding new caregiving responsibilities to their normal duties. The use of these interventions may lead to more productive, cost-effective healthcare delivery and beneficial outcomes for distance caregivers and elders with CI living alone at home, including maintenance of independence in the environment chosen by the elder and delay in institutionalization.

Table 2   Targeted/Planned Enrollment Table

TARGETED/PLANNED ENROLLMENT: Number of Subjects			
Ethnic Category	Sex/Gender		
	Females	Males	Total
Hispanic or Latino	6	4	10
Non-Hispanic or Latino	23	15	38
Ethnic Category: Total of All Subjects *	29	19	48
Racial Categories			
American Indian/Alaska Native	0	0	0
Asian	1	1	2
Native Hawaiian or Other Pacific Islander	0	0	0
Black or African-American	7	3	10
White	20	16	36
Racial Categories: Total of All Subjects *	28	20	48

Source: Grant example with permission from Benefield, L.E. (2005). *Distance Caregiving of CI Elders Living Alone at Home*. NIH/NINR Grant 7R03NR009512-02.

INCLUSION OF WOMEN

Most caregivers (distance and on-site combined) are women (61%).[32] However, a 2004 MetLife study identified 58% of distance caregivers responding to a family life survey were male. The relatively large percentage of males is likely an artifact of the respondent pool, 2/3 of whom were male.[7] For this study, we plan inclusion of 60% females and 40% males.

INCLUSION OF MINORITIES

Participants will include women and men distance caregivers purposively recruited to match the population within the region of _____. Population characteristics for the _____ CMSA include: 69.4% White, 21.5% Hispanic or Latino,

13.8% Black or African-American, 0.6% American Indian/Alaska Native, 3.7% Asian, 0.1% Native Hawaiian/Pacific Islander, and 11.5% some other race or Multiracial.[99] By using both the university and Alzheimer's Association as recruitment sites, we anticipate being able to recruit sufficient numbers of distance caregivers within these populations groups for the focus groups. (See Table 2.)

INCLUSION OF CHILDREN

The research topic to be studied is not typically relevant to children; however, participants may include a few adult children under age 21, so children may be included in this study.

DATA MONITORING PLAN

While a data safety monitoring board (DSMB) is not required as this study is neither a clinical trial or an intervention study, the PI will meet monthly with the Research Team (RA, Moderator) to review data acquisition, trends or problems in data acquisition, and management. Trends in caregiver focus groups or meeting conditions, adverse effects of attendance at the interviews, problems with adhering to caregiver confidentiality, or factors that bias any data will be dealt with. Should any problems actually occur, they will be reported to the university IRB, and should any action result in a temporary or permanent suspension of the NIH-funded study, it will be reported to the NIH Program Director responsible for the grant.

F. VERTEBRATE ANIMALS: N/A

G. LITERATURE CITED

1. Research in Informal Caregiving: State of the Science Workgroup Meeting 2001. *National Institute of Nursing Research.* Available at: http://ninr.nih .gov/ninr/research/dea/workgroup_chronic_conditions.html. Accessed November 3, 2002.
2. Langa KM, Chernew ME, Kabeto MU, et al. National estimates of the quantity and cost of informal caregiving for the elderly with dementia. *Journal of General Internal Medicine.* 2001;16:770-778.
3. Brookmeyer R, Gray S, Kawas C. Projections of Alzheimer's disease in the United States and the public health impact of delaying disease onset. *American Journal of Public Health.* 1998;88:1337-1342.
4. Hebert LE, Scherr PA, Bienias JL, Bennett DA, Evans DA. Alzheimer disease in the U.S. population: Prevalence estimates using the 2000 Census. *Archives of Neurology.* 2003;60(8):1119-1122.
5. Koppel R. *Alzheimer's Disease: The Costs to U.S. Businesses in 2002.* Washington, DC: Alzheimer's Association; 2002.

6. Wagner DL. *Caring Across the Miles: Findings of a Survey of Long-distance Caregivers, Final Report for The National Council on the Aging*. Washington, DC: National Council for the Aging; 1997.

7. Miles Away: The MetLife Study of Long-Distance Caregiving. *Mature Market Institute, MetLife and National Alliance for Caregiving*. Available at: http://www.caregiving.org/milesaway.pdf. Accessed July 31, 2004.

8. Nearly 7 Million Long-Distance Caregivers Make Work and Personal Sacrifices. Press Release March 12, 1997. *National Council on the Aging*. Available at: http://www.ncoa.org/content.cfm?sectionID=105&detail=49. Accessed July 23, 2004.

9. Collins WL, Holt TA, Moore SE, Bledsoe LK. Long-distance caregiving: A case study of an African-American family. *American Journal of Alzheimer's Disease and Other Dementias*. 2003;18(5):309-316.

10. Baldock CV. Migrants and their parents: Caregiving from a distance. *Journal of Family Issues*. 2000;21(2):205-224.

11. Giorgianni SJ. Recognizing the word 'caregiver' is the first step in supporting caregivers. *Impact Communications, Inc*. Available at: http://www.thepfizer-journal.com/PDFs/TPJ03.pdf. Accessed August 23, 2004.

12. Brennan PF, Strombom I. Improving health care by understanding patient preferences: The role of computer technology. *Journal of the American Medical Informatics Association*. 1998;5(3):257-262.

13. The Alzheimer's Association, Intel Team Up to Expand Home Care Technology Research. *The Alzheimer's Association*. Available at: http://www.alz.org/Media/newsreleases/current/072403intelteamup.htm. Accessed August 22, 2003.

14. Schumacher K, Stewart BJ, Archbold PG, Dodd MJ, Dibble SL. Family caregiving skill: development of the concept. *Research in Nursing & Health*. 2000;23:191-203.

15. Caregiving: Ten Strategies for Long-distance Caregiving. *WebMD with AOL-Health*. Available at: http://aolsvc.health.webmd.aol.com/content/pages/5/4041_130.htm. Accessed August 18, 2004.

16. Morris M, Lundell J. Ubiquitous computing for cognitive decline: findings from Intel's proactive health research. *Intel Corporation*. Available at: http://www.alz.org/Researchers/ETAC/Intel_UbiqitousComputing.pdf. Accessed October 1, 2003.

17. Intel R. Spotlight Story: Interview with Eric Dishman. *Intel Research* [online news spotlight for Intel Research]. Available at: http://www.intel.com/research/spotlights/one_on_one_dishman.htm. Accessed November 14, 2003.

18. McClendon MJ, Bass DM, Brennan PF, McCarthy C. A computer network for Alzheimer's caregivers and use of support group services. *Journal of Mental Health & Aging*. 1998;4(4):403-420.

19. Mynatt ED, Rowan J, Jacobs A, Craighill S. Digital family portraits: Supporting peace of mind for extended family members. *CHI*. 2001;3(1):333-340.

20. Stone R. *Long-term Care for the Elderly with Disabilities: Current Policy, Emerging Trends, and Implications for the Twenty-First Century.* New York: Milbank Memorial Fund; 2000.
21. Kazdin AE. Almost clinically significant (p < .10): Current measures may only approach clinical significance. *Clinical Psychology: Science and Practice.* 2001;8(4):455-462.
22. Schulz R, O'Brien A, Czaja S, et al. Dementia caregiver intervention research: In search of clinical significance. *The Gerontologist.* 2002;42(5):589-602.
23. Pillemer K, Czaja S, Schulz R, Stahl SM. Finding the best ways to help: Opportunities and challenges of intervention research on aging. *The Gerontologist.* 2003;43 Special Issue 1:5-8.
24. Zedlewski SR, McBride TD. The changing profile of the elderly: Effects of future long-term care needs and financing. *The Milbank Quarterly.* 1992;70:247-275.
25. Greenberger H, Litwin H. Can burdened caregivers be effective facilitators of elder care-recipient health care? *Journal of Advanced Nursing.* 2003;41(4):332-341.
26. Aging Committee: Hearing Finding Summary. *Senate Special Committee on Aging.* One Hundred and Seventh Congress ed. Washington, DC: U.S. Government Printing Office; 2002.
27. Dunkle RE, Kart CS. Long-term care. In: Ferraro KF, ed. *Gerontology: Perspectives and Issues.* New York: Springer Publishing Co; 1997:221-241.
28. Kelley LS, Buckwalter KC, Maas ML. Access to health resources for family caregiving of elderly persons with dementia. *Nursing Outlook.* 1999;47(1):8-14.
29. Kuhlman G, Wilson H, Hutchinson S, Wallhagen M. Alzheimer's disease and family caregiving: Critical synthesis of the literature and research agenda. *Nursing Research.* 1991;40:331-337.
30. Schulz R, O'Brien AT, Bookwala J, Fleissner K. Psychiatric and physical morbidity effects of dementia caregiving: Prevalence, correlates, and causes. *The Gerontologist.* 1995;35:771-791.
31. Schulz R, Beach SR. Caregiving as a risk factor for mortality: The caregiver health effects study. *Journal of the American Medical Association.* 1999;262:2215-2219.
32. *Caregiving in the U.S.* Washington, DC: National Alliance for Caregiving and AARP; April 2004.
33. Schumacher KL, Stewart BJ, Archbold PG. Conceptualization and measurement of doing family caregiving well. *Image: Journal of Nursing Scholarship.* 1998;30(1):63-69.
34. Feinberg LF, Gray L, Kelly K. *Family Caregiving as a Grantsmaking Area: Current Focus and Future Trends.* San Francisco, CA: Family Caregiver Alliance, National Center on Caregiving; 2002.

35. Shyu YL. A Conceptual Framework for Understanding the Process of Family Caregiving to Frail Elders in Taiwan. *Research in Nursing & Health.* 2002;25:111-121.

36. Archbold PG, Stewart BJ, Greenlick MR, Harvath T. Mutuality and preparedness as predictors of caregiver role strain. *Research in Nursing & Health.* 1990;13:375-384.

37. Nikongho NO, Archbold PG. Working-out caregiving systems in African American families. *Applied Nursing Research.* 1996;9(3):108-114.

38. Acton G, Kang J. Interventions to reduce the burden of caregiving for an adult with dementia: A meta-analysis. *Research in Nursing & Health.* 2001;24:349-360.

39. Giogianni SJ. Employers respond to caregivers' complex needs. *Impact Communications, Inc.* Available at: http://www.thepfizerjournal.com/pdfs/TPJ03.pdf. Accessed September 20, 2004.

40. Wagner DL. *Comparative analysis of caregiver data for caregivers to the elderly: 1987 and 1997.* Bethesda, MD: National Alliance for Caregiving; 1997.

41. Lieberman F. The impact of chronic illness on the health and well-being of family members. *The Gerontologist.* 1995;35:94-102.

42. Arno PS, Levine C, Memmott MM. The economic value of informal caregiving. Data from 1987/1988 National Survey of Families and Households (NSFH). *Health Affairs.* 1999;18(2):182-188.

43. Chadiha LA, Rafferty J. The influence of caregiving stressors, social support, and caregiving appraisal on marital functioning among African American wife caregivers. *Journal of Marital and Family Therapy.* 2003;29(4):479-490.

44. Mahoney DF. Vigilance: Evolution and definition for caregivers of family members with Alzheimer's disease. *Journal of Gerontological Nursing.* Aug 2003;29(8):24-30.

45. Ory MG, Hoffman RR, III, Yee JL, Tennstedt S, Schulz R. Prevalence and impact of caregiving: A detailed comparison between dementia and nondementia caregivers. *The Gerontologist.* Apr 1999;39(2):177-185.

46. Schulz R, Williamson GM. The measurement of caregiver outcomes in Alzheimer disease research. *Alzheimer Disease and Associated Disorders.* 1997;11(Suppl 6):117-124.

47. Pearlin L, Mullan J, Semple S, Skaff M. Caregiving and the stress process: An overview of concepts and their measures. *The Gerontologist.* 1990;30:583-591.

48. Winslow BW. Effects of formal supports on stress outcomes in family caregivers of Alzheimer's patients. *Research in Nursing & Health.* 1997;20:27-37.

49. Connell C, Janevic M, Gallant M. The costs of caring: Impact of dementia on family caregivers. *Journal of Geriatric Psychiatry and Neurology.* 2001;14:179-187.

50. Acton G. Health-promoting self-care in family caregivers. *Western Journal of Nursing Research.* 2002;24(1):73-86.

51. Kahana E, Biegel DE, Wykle ML. Introduction. *Family Caregiving Across the Lifespan.* Thousand Oaks, CA: Sage Publications; 1994:xiii-xxvi.

52. Herman C. *"Doing the distance": The experience and meaning of long-distance caretaking* [Doctoral Dissertation]. Lincoln, Nebraska: Community and Human Resources, University of Nebraska; 1995.

53. Saliba D, Schnelle JF. Indicators of the quality of nursing home residential care. *Journal of the American Geriatrics Society.* 2002;50(8):1421-1430.

54. Skull DE. The multidimensional caregiver strain index (MCSI): Its measurement and structure. *Journal of Clinical Geropsychology.* 1996;2(3):175-196.

55. Long-Distance Caregiving: What to Do When Dad is in Vancouver and You are in Toronto? *Alert Newsletter,* Vol. 18, # 4 (Spring). Alzheimer's Society of Toronto. Available at: www.asmt.org/longdist.htm. Accessed July 31, 2004.

56. Gill TM, Richardson ED, Tinetti ME. Evaluating the risk of dependence in activities of daily living among community-living older adults with mild to moderate cognitive impairment. *Journal of Geronotology: Medical Sci.* 1995;50a(5):M235-241.

57. Nochajski SM, Tomita MR, Mann WC. The use and satisfaction with assistive devices by older persons with cognitive impairments: A pilot intervention study. *Topics in Geriatric Rehabilitation.* 1996;12(2):40-53.

58. Bourgeois MS, Schulz R, Burgio L. Interventions for caregivers of patients with Alzheimer's disease: A review and analysis of content, process, and outcomes. *International Journal Aging Human Development.* 1996;43:35-92.

59. Czaja SJ, Schulz R. Does the treatment make a real difference? The measurement of clinical significance. *Alzheimer's Care Quarterly.* 2003;4(3):229-240.

60. Research in informal caregiving: State of the science workshop meeting. *National Institute of Nursing Research, NIH.* Available at: http://www.nih.gov/ninr/research/dea/workshop_chronic_conditions.html. Accessed November 3, 2002.

61. Calkins M. Personal Communication, August 30, 2004.

62. Computer-based technology and caregiving for older adults. Special National Conference Report. *Public Policy and Aging Report.* Vol 14. Bethesda, MD: The Gerontological Society of America; 2003:1-32.

63. Magnusson L, Hanson E, Nolan M. Adult/elderly care nursing. Assisting carers using the ACTION model for working with family carers. *British Journal of Nursing.* 2002;11(11):759-763.

64. *Care For People With Dementia. Perspectives from Technology: A Research Planning Workshop for ETAC (Everyday Technologies for Alzheimer Care).* Philadelphia, PA, July 17, 2004.

65. Charness N, Schaie KW. *Impact of Technology on Successful Aging.* New York, NY: Springer Publishing Company, Inc; 2003.

66. Mann WC, Hurren MD, Charvat BA, Tomita MR. Changes over one year in assistive device use and home modifications by home-based older persons with Alzheimer's disease. *Topics in Geriatric Rehabilitation.* 1996;12(2):9-16.

67. Brennan PF, Moore SM, Smyth KA. The effects of a special computer network on caregivers of persons with Alzheimer's disease. *Nursing Research*. May-June 1995;44(3):166-172.

68. Czaja SJ, Rubert M. Telecommunications technology as an aid to family caregivers of persons with dementia. *Psychosomatic Medicine*. 2002;64:469-476.

69. Czaja SJ, Sharit J, Charness N, Fisk AD, Rogers W. The Center for Research and Education on Aging and Technology Enhancement (CREATE): A program to enhance technology for older adults. *Gerontechnology*. 2001;1:50-59.

70. Schumacher K. Family Caregiving Skill Measurement and Evaluation. National Institutes of Health # RO1-NR-05126-03; 1999.

71. Morgan DL, Krueger RA, eds. *The Focus Group Kit*. Thousand Oaks, CA: Sage Publishing, Inc; 1998.

72. Benefield LE. Home Health Care Nursing: A Domain Analysis. Paper presented at 3rd Annual Evidence-Based Practice Conference; December, 2001; Rochester, NY.

73. Benefield LE. A Metastructure of Home Health Care Nursing Research: Present Knowledge and Future Priorities. Paper presented at Southern Nursing Research Society 16th Annual Meeting, 2002; San Antonio, TX.

74. Benefield LE. Challenges in Evaluation: What to Evaluate, How to Decide, and Pitfalls to Avoid. Evaluation of Caregiver Education Programming. A Roundtable Discussion. Paper presented at National Council on the Aging and American Society on Aging National Conference; April, 2002; Denver, CO.

75. Benefield LE. Evaluation of the National Family Caregiver Support Program. Paper presented at National Council on Aging—American Society on Aging Annual Meeting; March, 2003; Chicago, IL.

76. Glover J, Benefield LE, Pacatte J, Schutkowski D. Just Because We Have Funding Don't Mean the Caregivers Will Come: A AAA's Experiences in Implementing the National Family Caregiver Support Program. Paper presented at: National Council on the Aging—American Society on Aging National Conference; March, 2003; Chicago, IL.

77. *Guidelines for the planning and management of NIH consensus development conferences online*. National Institutes of Health, Office of the Director, Office of Medical Applications of Research. October 2001. Available at: http://consensus.nih.gov/about/process.htm. Accessed November 17, 2003.

78. Toseland RW, Rossiter CM. Group interventions to support family caregivers: A review and summary. *The Gerontologist*. 1989;29:438-448.

79. Gwyther LP. Research on gender and family caregiving: Implications for clinical practice. In: Dwyer JW, Coward RT, eds. *Gender, Families, and Elder Care*. Newbury Park, CA: Sage; 1992:202-218.

80. Gonzalez EW. Resourcefulness, appraisals, and coping efforts of family caregivers. *Issues in Mental Health Nursing*. 1997;18:209-227.

81. Morgan DL. *The Focus Group Guidebook*. Vol 1. Thousand Oaks, CA: Sage Publications, Inc; 1998.
82. Morgan DL, Scannell AU. Planning focus groups. In: Morgan DL, Krueger RA, eds. *The Focus Group Kit*. Vol 2. Thousand Oaks, CA: Sage Publications, Inc; 1998:1-139.
83. Lee JL, Schulz R. Gender differences in psychiatric morbidity among family caregivers: A review and analysis. *The Gerontologist*. 2000;40(2):147-164.
84. Parsons K. The male experience of caregiving for a family member with Alzheimer's disease. *Qualitative Health Research*. 1997;7(3):391-407.
85. Harris PB. Listening to caregiving sons: Misunderstood realities. *The Gerontologist*. 1998;38(3):342-352.
86. Zarit SH, Todd PA, Zarit JM. Subjective burden of husbands and wives as caregivers: A longitudinal study. *The Gerontologist*. 1986;20:260-266.
87. Ruland CM, Bakken M. Developing, implementing, and evaluating decision support systems for shared decision making in patient care: A conceptual model and case illustration. *Journal of Biomedical Inform*. 2002;35(5-6):313-321.
88. Miller D, Shewchuk R, Elliot T, Richards S. Nominal group technique: A process for identifying diabetes self-care issues among patients and caregivers. *The Diabetes Educator*. 2000;26(2):305-314.
89. Elliot T, Shewchuk R. Using the nominal group technique to identify problems experienced by persons living with severe physical disabilities. *Journal of Clinical Psychology in Medical Settings*. 2002;9(2):65-75.
90. Delbecq A, Van de Ven AH, Gustafson DH. Guidelines for conducting NGT meetings. *Group Techniques for Program Planning: A Guide to Nominal Group and Delphi Processes*. Glenview, IL: Scott, Foresman; 1974:174.
91. *The Ethnograph computer program* [computer program]. Version 3.0. Littleton, CO: Qualis Research Associates; 1988.
92. Denzin NK, Lincoln YS. *Handbook of Qualitative Research*. London: Sage Publications; 1994.
93. Morse JM, Field PA. *Qualitative Research Methods for Health Professionals*. 2nd ed. London: Sage Publications, Inc; 1995.
94. Faiks A, Hyland N. Gaining user insight: A case study illustrating the card sort technique. *College and Research Libraries*. 2000;61(4):349-357.
95. NIH Roadmap: Accelerating Medical Discovery to Improve Health. Available at: http://nihroadmap.nih.gov/publicprivate/index.asp. Accessed November 18, 2003.
96. Brennan PF. Harnessing innovative technologies: What can you do with a shoe? *Nursing Outlook*. 1999;47(3):128-132.
97. Brennan PF. Personal Communication; August 3, 2004.
98. Allen RS, Burgio LD. Translating psychosocial research into practice: A methodological overview. *Alzheimer's Care Quarterly*. 2003;4(3):201-203.

99. 2000 Census of Population and Housing Summary File 1 Characteristics of Dallas-Fort Worth CMSA. Available at: http://www.census.nctcog.org/sfl.asp?Geo=Region. Accessed August 1, 2004.

H. CONSORTIUM/CONTRACTUAL ARRANGEMENTS: N/A

I. CONSULTANTS Consultants and their contribution to the study include:

- Content Expert Dementia Care Interventions

- Co-convener of Expert Panel

- Research Mentor

- Focus Group Interview Methodology & Data Management

- Content Expert in Caregiving Issues

- Focus Group Interview Data Analysis

- Expert Panel Member

- Expert Panel Member

- Expert Panel Member

- Expert Panel Member

Example of an R15 NIH Grant Application: Quantitative Methods

RESEARCH PLAN

A. Specific Aims

Each year in the United States, more than a quarter million infants are born with birth weights less than 2500 grams. Nearly 50,000 of these infants are born with very-low-birth weights (VLBW), less than 1500 grams (National Commission, 1990). These are the highest risk to survive infants. Als (1986) postulates that the persistence of subtle developmental impairments among preterm infants with essentially uncomplicated medical courses may be "the consequence of a mismatch of extrauterine environment and the capacity of the central nervous system of the fetal neonate which is adapted for an intrauterine existence" (p. 4). Characteristics of the Neonatal Intensive Care Unit (NICU), such as excessive and unpredictable **sound** levels, bright and/or continuous lighting, and repeated and painful procedures are among the "mismatched of extrauterine" environmental stimuli Als refers to. These stimuli are potential challenges to the adaptive capacity of the preterm infant's central nervous system and are potentially detrimental to preterm development.

The purpose of this repeated measures study is to assess the relationship between three sets of variables: (a) **sound** and **light** levels in the NICU, (b) **arousal** level (sleep and wake patterns) of preterm infants, and (c) **physiologic** and **behavioral responses** of preterm infants to and following a **painful stimulus**—a heelstick for necessary blood sampling. Pain research in neonates has focused primarily on **behavioral** and **physiologic responses** to brief clinical procedures in healthy, full-term infants, and in older, physiologically stable preterm infants. No studies were located that have investigated the relationship of **sound** and **light** levels in the NICU and infant **arousal** level (sleep and wake patterns) to infant responses to pain.

Therefore, this study will examine the following research questions/hypotheses:

1. What is the relationship between **sound** (as measured by a sound meter), **light** (as measured by a light meter), **arousal** levels (as measured by Als State Score) in the 2 hours preceding a heelstick procedure to:

   A. Immediate **physiological pain response** of preterm neonates to a heelstick procedure (as measured by **heart rate** and **oxygen saturation**)?

   B. Immediate **behavioral pain responses** of preterm neonates to a heelstick procedure (as measured by the Premature Infant Pain Profile [**PIPP**])?

2. Is the relationship of **sound** (as measured by a sound meter), **light** (as measured by a light meter), **arousal** levels (as measured by Als State Score) in the 2 hours preceding a heelstick procedure moderated by **gestational age**?

Source: Grant example with permission from: Walden, M. (2001). *Environment and sleep on preterm infants pain response.* 1K15NR007731-01. NIH/National Institute for Nursing Research.

3. Does variation in **sound** (as measured by a sound meter), **light** (as measured by a light meter), and **arousal** levels (as measured by Als State Score) in the 2 hours preceding a heelstick procedure predict:

    A. **Physiological disruption** from acute pain in preterm neonates (as measured by the **time for heart rate and oxygen saturation to return to baseline values).**

    B. **Behavioral disruption** from acute pain in preterm neonates following a heelstick procedure (as measured by **time for PIPP score to return to baseline value**).

4. Does **gestational age** interact with **sound** (as measured by a sound meter), **light** (as measured by a light meter), and **arousal** levels (as measured by Als State Score) in the 2 hours preceding a heelstick procedure in the prediction of:

    A. **Physiological disruption** from acute pain in preterm neonates (as measured by the **time for heart rate and oxygen saturation to return to baseline values**).

    B. **Behavioral disruption** from acute pain in preterm neonates following a heelstick procedure (as measured by **time for PIPP score to return to baseline value**).

This research will systematically address the gaps in our knowledge about the relationships between **sound, light, arousal** levels (sleep and wake patterns), and preterm neonates' **physiological** and **behavioral responses** to painful clinical procedures. The long-term aims of this program of research are to investigate nursing interventions that promote an environment that produces optimal **arousal** patterns for high-risk neonates as indicated by minimizing preterm neonates' immediate response and prolonged **disruption** following painful procedures. The research may also permit improved understanding of how these factors may influence pain assessment in critically ill preterm neonates.

B. Background and Significance

Conceptual Framework

The framework for this study is a modification of the Middle-Range Theory of Unpleasant Symptoms. This model provides the overall conceptual framework for examining the relationship between **sound** and **light, arousal** levels (sleep and wake patterns), and **pain response** of preterm neonates in this study (Lenz, Pugh, Milligan, Gift, & Suppe, 1997). This model identifies three categories of variables as potentially influencing the intensity of the **pain response: physiologic**/developmental factors (**gestational age** at birth), psychologic factors (**arousal** levels [sleep and wake patterns]), and situational factors (**sound and light**). These categories are related and may interact to influence the symptom experience (**behavioral** and **physiologic response** to pain). Data will also be collected on other potential modifiers of the infant's **pain response** including postnatal age, acuity of illness, behavioral state just before the noxious stimuli, and previous pain experiences (total number of painful procedures and time since last painful procedure). Pain may result in short-term **physiologic** and/or **behavioral disruption** as well as long-term consequences including adverse neurologic and neurobehavioral outcomes and altered pain sensation. The long-term sequelae of pain are not the focus of this study. Rather, short-term **disruption** and disorganization will be measured as **physiological** manifestations (**time for heart rate and oxygen saturation to return to baseline**) and **behavioral** manifestations (**time for pain scores on PIPP to return to baseline**). Figure 1 presents a conceptual model of the relationship between the variables identified for study in this proposal.

Franck and Gregory (1993) state that "the goals of pain management in neonates are: (1) to minimize intensity, duration, and **physiologic** cost of the pain

---

Figure 1 Model for Study

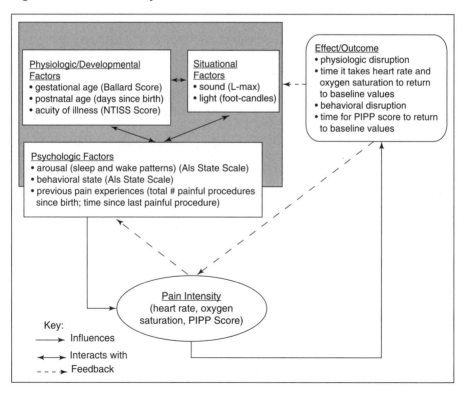

experience, and (2) to maximize neonate's ability to cope with and recover from the painful experience" (p. 522). This suggests that NICU caregivers can assist neonates to cope with and recover from painful clinical procedures by promoting a healing environment that incorporates strategies to maximize sleep and waking patterns (arousal) and optimize **sound** and **light** levels in the NICU microenvironment. While clinical observation suggests that these factors influence infant responses to pain, no studies have examined the relationship of **sound** levels, **light** levels, and infant **arousal** (sleep and wake patterns) on infant's responses to painful clinical procedures. Our understanding of how these factors affect healing and recovery from painful stimuli may help to minimize long-term consequences of painful stimuli.

Pain and the Pain Response

Painful procedures occur with relative frequency for preterm infants in the NICU. Barker and Rutter (1995) reported that preterm infants experienced an average of 61 painful procedures during their NICU stay, with increased frequency of procedures inversely related to **gestational age** and acuity of illness. One 23-week gestation, 560-gram infant had 488 procedures performed during her hospital stay. Studies have noted that neonates may be subjected to as many as three invasive procedures an hour (Pohlman & Beardslee, 1987).

Previously, preterm neonates were thought to be too immature to experience pain, but studies now confirm the preterm neonate's anatomic and functional capacity to respond to pain at birth (Anand, Phil, Grunau & Oberlander, 1997; Anand, Phil & Hickey, 1987; Fitzgerald & Anand, 1993). Acute **physiologic responses** to painful stimuli have been implicated as either causing or extending early intraventricular hemorrhage (IVH), or the development of ischemic changes leading to periventricular leukomalacia (PVL) in preterm neonates (Anand, 1998). New areas of concern suggest the cumulative effects of repeated painful medical procedures on the developing brain may be of greater biological and clinical importance than previously recognized (Anand, 1997; 1998; Anand et al., 1997). Multiple lines of evidence suggest an increased sensitivity to pain in preterm neonates as compared to term infants (Anand, 1997; 1998; Fitzgerald, Shaw & MacIntosh, 1988). Evidence suggests that acute painful stimuli may lead to the development of prolonged periods of hyperalgesia and that nonnoxious stimuli during periods of hyperalgesia may promote chronic pain in preterm neonates (Anand, 1997; 1998; Fitzgerald et al., 1988). Preliminary data suggest that repetitive painful experiences in the NICU may be associated with some of the neurobehavioral and developmental sequelae in former preterm neonates, including altered pain thresholds and abnormal pain-related behaviors during early childhood (Grunau, Whitfield & Petrie, 1994; Gruanu, Whitfield, Petrie & Fryer, 1994).

Painful procedures in the NICU may be unavoidable; however, it is vital that caregivers investigate strategies to assist infants to cope with and recover from necessary but painful clinical procedures. Pain assessment is an essential prerequisite to optimal pain management. Pain research has produced several valid and reliable pain instruments, including the CRIES (Krechel & Bildner, 1995) and the Premature Infant Pain Profile (**PIPP**) (Stevens, Johnston, Petryshen, & Taddio, 1996). While the CRIES has been validated for use in infants greater than 32 weeks **gestational age**, the **PIPP** can be used in preterm infants below 28 weeks **gestational age**. The **PIPP** is preferred over the CRIES in this study as it controls for two significant contextual factors (**gestational age** and behavioral state) known to modify pain expression in preterm neonates (Craig et al., 1993; Grunau & Craig, 1987; Johnston et al., 1999; Stevens & Johnston, 1994; Stevens, Johnston, & Horton, 1994). The **PIPP** will be used to measure acute **pain response** in this study.

Behavioral state has been shown to act as a moderator of **pain responses** in both full-term and preterm infants (Grunau & Craig; 1987; Johnston et al., 1999; Stevens & Johnston, 1994; Stevens et al., 1996). Infants in awake or alert states demonstrate a more robust reaction to painful stimuli than infants in sleep states. While clinical studies are lacking, a few laboratory studies have examined the impact of rapid eye movement (REM) sleep deprivation on pain thresholds using the rat model. Hicks, Coleman, Ferante, Sahatjian, and Hawkins (1979) and Hicks, Moore, Findley, Hirshfield, and Humphrey (1978) demonstrated that rats subjected to REM sleep deprivation showed significantly reduced pain thresholds that persisted for up to 96 hours following the termination of the REM deprivation. Another laboratory study used continuous polygraphic and behavioral recordings in freely moving cats to examine aspects of pain and sleep surrounding a persistent nociceptive stimulation (Carli, Montesano, Rapezzi, & Paluffi, 1987). These researchers demonstrated that the level of pain intensity following a formalin injection was inversely related to the duration of sleep disturbance. No clinical studies have examined the impact of **arousal** level (sleep and wake patterns) on the preterm neonate's ability to respond to and recover from painful procedures in the NICU.

Sound

Researchers have examined the immediate responses of infants to **sound** levels in the nursery. Long, Lucey, and Philips (1980) documented a repeated pattern of decreased transcutaneous oxygen tension, increased intracranial pressure, and increased heart and respiratory rates in two infants in response to sudden loud noise in the nursery. Gorski, Hale, and Leonard (1983) described mottling, apnea, and bradycardia in preterm infants exposed to sharp occurrences of **sound** such as telephone ringing, monitor alarms, and conversation during medical rounds. Both studies provide support for the notion that nursery **sound** levels are a disorganizing influence on the neurologically immature low-birth-weight infant and raise speculation regarding the energy cost to the infant that these episodes represent. Noise intensity decreased by 10 decibels resulted in longer sleep time in healthy preterm neonates (Mann, Haddow, Stokes, Goodley & Rutter, 1986). When studying the effects of noise on the sleep patterns of term infants, Gadeke, Doing, Keller, and Vogel (1969) reported that **sound** levels of greater than 70 decibels disrupted infant sleep, and **sound** levels of 55 decibels aroused an infant from light sleep. Although this study has not been replicated with LBW infants, the reported **sound** levels are similar to those present in the NICU, suggesting that **sound** may interfere with the development of sleep and rest patterns in these infants. Almost no research has been done systematically to document the relationship between **sound** levels and **pain responses** in preterm infants. Using a subjective scale to rate **sound** levels from one to nine, Walden (1997) failed to demonstrate a significant association between **sound** and **pain responses** in hospitalized preterm infants. Failure to achieve significance may have been due, in part, to the subjective nature of the measurement scale. Further research is needed using a sound meter to measure systematically the relationship between **sound** levels (Lmax) and the response pattern of preterm infants to painful clinical procedures. Again, this research may lead to improved assessment techniques for pain in critically ill preterm neonates as well as stimulate intervention research to better control **sound** levels in the NICU surrounding painful procedures.

Light

The NICU provides infants with an extremely bright environment with little diurnal variation (Lotas & Walden, 1996). Shiroiwa, Kamiya, and Uchiboi (1986) reported a significant association between lighting levels and patterns of alertness and respiratory stability in neonates. Studies exploring the effects of light/dark cycles on preterm infant **physiologic** and **behavioral** functioning have reported decreased **heart rate**, decreased respiratory rate, and improved sleep patterns and weight gain (Blackburn & Patterson, 1991; Mann et al., 1986). While continuous lighting patterns have been hypothesized to contribute to sleep disruption during the NICU stay (Holditch-Davis, 1998), little research exists that systematically documents the effects of ambient **light** levels on **pain responses** in preterm infants. Walden (1997) failed to demonstrate a significant association between ratings of **light** levels in the NICU on subjective scale and **physiologic** and **behavioral responses** of preterm infants to a heelstick procedure. Here again, failure to achieve significance may have been due, in part, to the subjective nature of the measurement scale. Further research is needed, using a more objective measure furnished by light meter recordings (foot-candles) to explore the effects of NICU **light** on **pain responses** of hospitalized preterm neonates. Again, this research may lead to improved assessment techniques for pain in critically ill preterm neonates as well as stimulate intervention research to reduce **light** levels and patterns in the NICU surrounding painful clinical procedures.

Arousal Level (Sleep and Wake Patterns)

Adequate rest is a prerequisite for optimal recovery from acute and chronic conditions. Preterm infants require more sleep than adults and, in general, spend as much as 60–70% of the day in sleep (Holditch-Davis, 1998). In the normal intrauterine environment, this amount of undisturbed time is routine; in the NICU, it is not. Nursing and medical interventions in the NICU of five times per hour have been reported (Duxbury, Henly, Broz, Armstrong, & Wachdorf, 1984). A recent study states that preterm infants are handled a mean of 113 times per 24 hours, with undisturbed rest periods of between 2 and 59 minutes (Appleton, 1997). Frequent handling has been associated with hypoxemia, tachycardia, bradycardia, tachypnea, apnea, and increased intracranial pressures in critically ill neonates (Cooper-Evans, 1991; Gorski et al., 1983; Long et al., 1980; Murdoch & Darlow, 1984; Norris, Campbell & Brenkert, 1982; Peters, 1992). Several researchers suggest that hypoxic episodes in response to handling may actually be the result of changes in sleeping and waking states (Gottfried, 1985; Holditch-Davis, 1998; Speidel, 1978). Routine caregiving may also interfere with development of normal sleep patterns, which are important for neurologic organization and growth (Appleton, 1997; Jorgensen, 1993; Wolke, 1987). Seventy-eight percent of changes in sleep-wake states in preterm neonates are associated with either nursing interventions or NICU noise (Zahr & Balian, 1995). Holditch-Davis (1990, 1998) reported that frequent nursing interventions reduce the amount of quiet sleep that preterm infants experience. In contrast, quiet periods in the NICU with reduced noise and light levels have been demonstrated to reduce stress responses in sick newborns (Slevin, Farrington, Duffy, Daly, & Murphy, 2000). No research that we could find has investigated the relationship of extended infant **arousal** levels (sleep and wake patterns) in the NICU and pain assessment in critically ill preterm neonates. In addition to improved assessment opportunities, this research may lead to the development of nursing interventions to promote optimal **arousal** (sleep and wake patterns) in the NICU. This will help preterm neonates recover from postoperative, procedural, and/or disease-related pain experiences.

Physiologic Responses

Studies of full-term as well as preterm infants provide evidence that they exhibit **physiological responses** to a heelstick procedure. Limited research suggests that preterm infants respond to noxious stimuli in patterns similar to that of full-term neonates, including increases in **heart rate** (Bozzette, 1993; Craig et al., 1993; McIntosh, Van Veen, & Brameyer, 1994; Stevens & Johnston, 1994; Stevens, Johnston, & Horton, 1993; Walden, 1997) and decreases in **oxygen saturation** (Craig et al., 1993; Stevens & Johnston, 1994; Stevens et al., 1993; Walden, 1997).

Full-term infants demonstrate slight **physiologic** distress persisting into a relatively brief recovery period following a heelstick procedure. Owens and Todt (1984) demonstrated an increased mean **heart rate** for 3.5 minutes following the heelstick procedure in full-term newborns. Beaver (1987) demonstrated a trend for increased **heart rates** for from 1 to 1.5 minutes post-heelstick in a small sample of preterm infants. Sustained elevations in **heart rate** and reduced transcutaneous oxygen levels attest to the persistent effect of the heelstick procedures on the **physiologic** stability of preterm infants (Craig et al., 1993; Stevens et al., 1993). Walden (1997) demonstrated that preterm neonates at 27 weeks postconceptional age had persistent increases in mean **heart rate** for up to 4 minutes following the heelstick itself (actual stick), while significantly elevated mean maximum **heart rates** persisted for up to 8 minutes following the heelstick procedure. Further research with longer observation of recovery intervals is needed in order to investigate more thoroughly the lasting impact of acute procedure-induced pain on the **physiologic** parameters of **heart rate** and **oxygen saturation** in preterm neonates. This study will monitor **physiologic responses** for 1 hour post-heelstick procedure to note **physiologic disruption** from acute pain in preterm neonates (as measured by **time for heart rate and oxygen saturation to return to baseline values**).

Behavioral Response

While behavioral state has been shown to act as a moderator of **behavioral pain responses** in both full-term and preterm infants (Grunau & Craig, 1987; Stevens & Johnston, 1994; Stevens et al., 1996), the research has primarily examined the immediate effects of the infant's sleep-wake state on **physiologic** and **behavioral responses** to pain. A limited number of human studies have reported that noxious procedures in neonates result in **behavioral responses** of increased sleep disruption times, particularly crying time, during and immediately following the painful event (Corff, Seideman, Venkataraman, Lutes, & Yates, 1995; Field & Goldson, 1984; Holditch-Davis & Calhoun, 1989; Van Cleve, Johnson, Andrews, Hawkins, & Newbold, 1995). We could find no studies examining the influence of disturbed sleep and wake patterns several hours preceding a clinical procedure on the preterm neonate's ability to respond to and recover from clinically needed, painful procedures experienced in the NICU.

Research examining facial and body activity has demonstrated that the magnitude of infant's **behavioral response** to pain is less vigorous and robust with decreasing postconceptional age (Craig et al., 1993; Johnston, Stevens, Yang, & Horton, 1995; Johnston et al., 1999). These observations, however, are contrary to data which suggest that more immature preterm infants have a lower threshold and are hypersensitive to painful stimuli compared to older preterm neonates (Andrews & Fitzgerald, 1994; Fitzgerald, Millard, & McIntosh, 1989). Craig et al. (1993) suggest that the less vigorous **behavioral responses** demonstrated by younger preterm infants "should be interpreted in the context of the energy resources available to respond and the relative immaturity of the musculoskeletal system" (p. 296). Stratification of infants into two groups by **gestational age** (25–27 weeks **gestational age** at birth and 34–36 weeks **gestational age** at birth) will permit systematic investigation for the presence of an interaction effect of **gestational age** on the relationships between environmental variables (**sound** and **light**) and **pain response** and **recovery**.

Furthermore, emerging evidence suggests that NICU experience may produce altered **behavioral responses** to noxious stimuli as the total number of invasive procedures that a preterm infant encounters increases with advancing postnatal age (Johnston & Stevens, 1996). More recently, Johnston et al. (1999) found that postnatal age at time of study, **gestational age** at birth, time since last painful procedure, and behavioral state predict response to a heel stick procedure in preterm neonates. Therefore, this study will systematically collect data on behavioral state just prior to the heelstick procedure. In addition, data will also be collected on the total number of painful procedures and time since last painful procedure. This information will help to describe better the previous pain experiences of the study sample. Data will also be collected within the first postnatal week in order to control for the influence of postnatal age on **pain responses** of preterm neonates.

Summary

Nurses play an important role in effectively implementing nonpharmacologic approaches to pain management. Research supports the use of hand swaddling (often referred to as "facilitated tucking," Corff et al., 1995), nonnutritive sucking (Campos, 1989; Field & Goldson, 1984; Marchette, Main, & Redick et al., 1991; Miller & Anderson, 1993; Shiao, Chang, Lannon, & Yarandi, 1997; Stevens et al., 1999), and sucrose pacifiers (Johnston, Stremler, Stevens, & Horton, 1997; Stevens & Ohlsson, 1998; Stevens, Taddio, Ohlsson, & Einarson, 1997) as nonpharmacologic therapies in newborns. However, virtually no research has been done to systematically document the effects of **sound, light,** and **arousal** levels on **pain responses** in preterm infants. Our understanding of how **sound, light,** and **arousal** levels influence the infant's ability to respond to and recover from painful procedures will provide improved assessment of pain in critically ill preterm neonates. Moreover, this improved understanding will permit caregivers to develop interventions to modify the NICU microenvironment in a manner that minimizes infant acute **physiologic** and **behavioral responses** to pain and thereby helps to decrease long-term neurobehavioral sequelae of chronic, repetitive pain experiences. Data from this study will provide the necessary information and objective clinical data methods to develop and apply for a competitive R01 grant to design and assess an intervention study.

C. Preliminary Studies

Dr. Marlene Walden, principal investigator (PI), is an Assistant Professor at the University of Texas Medical Branch (UTMB) in Galveston and a recent graduate of the University of Texas at Austin (UTA), School of Nursing. Dr. Walden's doctoral dissertation, *Changes over six weeks in multivariate responses of premature neonates to a painful stimulus* won the UTA School of Nursing Outstanding Doctoral Dissertation Award. This research also received funding support from the Foundation for Neonatal Research and Education and was awarded the Department of Nursing Research Award from Texas Children's Hospital. A database manuscript has been submitted and is included as **Appendix.**

Walden (1997) studied the **physiologic** and **behavioral responses** of preterm infants to a routinely administered **painful stimulus** (heelstick for necessary blood sampling) at weekly intervals between ages 27–32 weeks postconceptional age. The Neonatal Individualized Developmental Care Assessment Program (NIDCAP) method was used with a nonprobability convenience sample of 11 preterm infants born at 24–26 weeks postconceptional age who were admitted to one of two NICUs. Univariate **physiologic** indicators of pain included **heart rate, oxygen saturation,** and respiratory rate. These measures were collected in a time-sampling fashion in two-minute intervals. Results demonstrated that **heart rate** increased while **oxygen saturation** and respiratory rate decreased during the most invasive phase (heelstick). While the trends of these findings were in the direction demonstrated in research with other preterm populations, they failed to achieve significance across all postconceptional ages. In addition, correlations between **physiologic** indicators, **PIPP** scores, and NICU **sound** and **light** levels (as measured by subjective scales) failed to demonstrate significant associations. Further investigation of these findings is needed using a larger sample size to provide (a) the necessary power for analyses in a rigorous study, and (b) more objective measurement of **sound** and **light** levels. Such data and subsequent analyses and results are needed to examine contextual factors that may modify pain response and recovery in critically ill preterm neonates as well as to design intervention studies that may help neonates cope with painful clinical procedures. Specifically, optimizing **sound, light,** and **arousal** levels in the NICU may be found as fruitful means to alter the neonate's response to and recovery from painful procedures. Data and experiences from the PI's previous study provide preparation to conduct pain research in critically ill preterm neonates and to examine the variables of interest in this proposed research study.

Dr. Walden's research experience relates directly to the proposed project in terms of content and clinical experience and familiarity with the setting and study population. Her expertise in neonatal pain has been recognized by numerous invitations to speak on the topic at national neonatal conferences and most recently as the invited author to write the pain assessment and management guidelines for the National Association of Neonatal Nurses. She has also acquired expertise in data collection methods through a Faculty Scientist Award for Pain in Neonates from Nell Hodgson Woodruff School of Nursing, Emory University, where she consulted under Dr. Jane Evans and Dr. Terese Verklan, both currently funded by NIH. Dr. Walden gained experience in that setting for the use of data acquisition methods in neonatal research. In addition, Dr. Walden is currently serving as a data collector using **physiologic** data acquisition methods for Dr. Terese Verklan's currently funded R01 study, "Heart Rate During Transition to Extrauterine Life".

The research team for this study was carefully selected to provide the expertise necessary to conduct a rigorous scientific study. The research team members' expertise is briefly summarized below.

Carol Turnage Carrier, RN, MSN, CNS (Co-Investigator), is currently a Clinical Nurse Specialist for the Newborn Center at Texas Children's Hospital. She has conducted several quality improvement projects to analyze **sound** and **light** levels in the Newborn Center, including the design, data collection, analysis, and dissemination of findings to administration and other medical and nursing colleagues. The quality improvement projects she has conducted have used the same light meter and a similar sound meter that will be used to collect data in this study. The data from her quality improvement projects will be used to describe the environment of the Newborn Center under study setting. Ms. Carrier also has an excellent repertoire with families and the healthcare team and has familiarity and experience in site coordination for medical studies as well as collecting informed consents from parents.

Dr. Terese Verklan (Consultant) is an Associate Professor at the University of Texas-Health Science Center at Houston, School of Nursing. Dr. Verklan is a Clinical Nurse Specialist in high-risk neonatal care. Her dissertation was conducted at the University of Pennsylvania, under the direction of Dr. Barbara Medoff-Cooper, PhD, FAAN. This research investigated if a pattern of neurophysiologic maturation exists in association with increasing **gestational age**. **Heart rate** variability was examined in infants at 28-, 32-, and 40-weeks postconceptional age while controlling for behavioral state. The results demonstrated a discernible pattern of neurophysiologic growth with increasing **gestational age**. Dr. Verklan has completed two additional studies with similar aims that have built on the findings from her doctoral dissertation. Her current R01 study examines the differences/similarities in **heart rate** variability in the same individual as s/he experiences labor, delivery (fetus → neonate), immediately at birth, and the first ten hours of extrauterine life.

Dr. Steven Owen is a Professor at the University of Texas Medical Branch at Galveston, School of Nursing and Department of Preventive Medicine and Community Health. Dr. Owen is a senior biostatistician for the Office of Biostatistics and the Office for Nursing Research and Scholarship at UTMB. His current research involves aspects of social cognitive theory. In addition, Dr. Owen has extensive experience in serving on research teams and assisting faculty in developing research designs and statistical plans for data management, analysis, and interpretation.

Lester Laskowski is an Associate Professor in Health-Related Studies and currently serves as the Associate Director of the Biomedical Engineering and Electronics Department at UTMB. Mr. Laskowski is directly responsible for the day-to-day operations involving the support of patient care and laboratory equipment at UTMB, a 900-bed teaching hospital. He also provides design and fabrication services to meet various research needs at UTMB. Mr. Laskowski will be responsible for assisting in the purchase, set-up, and pilot testing of the data acquisition system required to measure the **physiological** and environmental variables within this study. He will also provide consultation regarding any troubleshooting of equipment malfunctions that may occur during the data collection period.

A research assistant will be hired to assist primarily in data collection. A currently enrolled Registered Nurse with at least two years of NICU experience will be targeted from the RN to BSN or master's student population. An experienced neonatal nurse is required due to the high-risk patient population and special knowledge and skills to handle these acutely ill neonates. The faculty-student relationship will be used to mentor the student in both research and clinical skills and will serve as a mechanism to provide encouragement and support for the student to pursue an advanced nursing degree. In addition, as an active member of the research team, the student will gain valuable experience in conducting research studies in the clinical setting. University and hospital relations between faculty, administrators, and bedside clinicians will be emphasized for the purpose of promoting clinical scholarship and research utilization projects at the bedside.

D. Research Design and Methods

Design

A repeated measures study will be employed, using a naturalistic design, to assess the relationship between **sound, light,** and **arousal** levels in the 2 hours before a noxious clinical procedure, and **physiologic** and **behavioral responses** to a routinely administered, **painful stimulus** (heelstick for blood sampling). Infants in this study will be stratified into two **gestational age** at birth groups: 25–27 weeks and 34–36 weeks. Rapid development and maturation of the nervous system occurs during the third trimester of pregnancy and is expected to be associated with systematic and substantial changes in the **physiologic** and **behavioral responses** of preterm neonates to painful clinical procedures. Stratification into two groups will determine if a moderating interaction is present when the relationship between two variables (e.g., **sound** and **pain response** or **recovery**) is different at levels of a third variable (e.g., **gestational age**).

We will observe the **physiological** and **behavioral responses** of neonates during a heelstick period during the first week of postnatal age. Heelstick observation periods will consist of the following three phases: (a) pre-heelstick observation (2 hours before the heelstick), (b) heelstick procedure (variable duration, from lance to placement of bandage), and (c) postheelstick recovery observation (1 hour). Thus, there will be systematic data collection from three observation intervals across two age-stratified groups of infants (3×2 design).

Setting and Sample

The setting for this study will be the Newborn Center at Texas Children's Hospital (TCH), a large tertiary care nursery located in the Texas Medical Center in Houston, Texas. TCH is approximately 65 miles from the UTMB School of Nursing. This site was chosen due to the large number of potentially eligible infants admitted each year. Due to the distance between UTMB and TCH, a site coordinator was selected to assist with subject enrollment and site management. PI travel to the site is not anticipated as a problem as the PI's residence is very close to TCH. Student research assistant travel similarly is not anticipated to be problematic as a large number of the RN to BSN and master's students in the UTMB program live in the Houston area.

Ms. Carrier has conducted several quality improvement projects on **sound** and **light** levels in the Newborn Center at TCH. The **sound** levels in the Newborn Center average 64.9 (Lmax). The minimum **sound** level is on average 63.3 (Lmax) with a minimum average equivalent level of 58.8 Leq. The average maximum level is 89.8 (Lmax), with occasional peaks to as high as 108.5 (Lmax).

Measurements of **light** levels have also been obtained for the Newborn Center at TCH. With overhead lighting, **light** levels range from 70.5–79.8 foot-candles (ftc). With lights on, **light** levels in an incubator with a thin blanket average 60.3 ftc and with a thick cover 19.3 ftc. In an incubator in dim lighting with no cover, the **light** levels average 4.9 ftc. When lights are turned off, **light** levels in an incubator with a thin blanket average 0.9 ftc and with thick covering 0.3 ftc.

This study uses a repeated measures, naturalistic design. No attempt will be made to manipulate the independent variables of **sound** and **light** in this study. The purpose of this study is to explore the relationships of **sound** and **light** levels in the NICU in the 2 hours preceding a heelstick procedure and **infant responses to pain.**

Participation of Children

All subjects will be children, specifically premature neonates, as the research questions are particularly pertinent to this age group. Enrollment of neonates born at **gestational age** greater than 36 weeks would not provide the data necessary to answer the specific age-related questions raised. The intensive care nursery at TCH admits approximately 185 infants per year in the respective age groups of this study. The bed capacity in the Newborn Care Center is 120 beds. This setting is expected to produce sufficient numbers for the sample based on inclusion and exclusion criteria. Total time for data collection is not expected to exceed 15 months. The PI and co-investigator have over 39 combined years of experience in working with the study population of high-risk premature infants. Because of the knowledge and expertise required to handle complex acutely ill infants, the student research assistant to be recruited will also be required to have at least two years of neonatal care experience.

Gender and Minority Inclusion

There will be no exclusion criteria related to gender; therefore an enrollment of approximately 35% females and 65% males is expected. These percentages represent the actual gender representation in the Newborn Center population at TCH in 1999. The following table provides distribution by gender and racial/ethnic categories:

Table 1

	Male	Female	Black, not of Hispanic Origin	Hispanic	White, not of Hispanic Origin	Other or Unknown	Total
25–27 weeks	45	21	20	16	29	1	66
34–36 weeks	75	44	20	38	58	3	119
Total	120	65	40	54	87	4	185

Source: Grant example with permission from: Walden, M. (2001). *Environment and sleep on preterm infants pain response.* 1K15NR007731-01. NIH/National Institute for Nursing Research.

All infants admitted to the Newborn Care Center at TCH will be considered eligible for inclusion into the study if the following criteria are met: (a) infants between 25–27 weeks or 34–36 weeks gestational age at birth and appropriate for gestational age as determined by the New Ballard Score (Ballard, Khoury, Wedig, Wang, Eilers-Walsman & Lipp, 1991); and (b) scheduled to receive a routine heelstick procedure within the first postnatal week.

Exclusion criteria include: (a) chromosomal or genetic anomalies; (b) significant central nervous system abnormality including seizures or a Grade III/IV intraventricular hemorrhage; (c) infants born to mothers with a known history of substance abuse; (d) and infants who receive paralytic, analgesic, or sedating medications within 24 hours before the heelstick procedure.

A convenience sample of consecutively admitted infants (stratified into two equal gestational age groups: 25–27 weeks and 34–36 weeks) who meet the subject criteria will be recruited for enrollment from the accessible population. Enrollment will continue until 102 infants' parents consent to participation, and the research protocol is completed on those infants. Sample size for the study was determined using PASS 2000 (Hintze, 2000) and based on the most conservative estimate of sample size to answer the research questions in this study (multiple regression power analyses = 51/group). Because no data exist to estimate effect size outcomes in this case, a medium effect size was selected (R-Squared = 0.13) for main effects and a small to medium effect size (R-Squared = 0.09) for interaction terms, i.e., gestational age group by sound, light, and arousal levels). The data gathered in this project would allow a more informed selection of an effect size in developing future study designs, for example, an intervention study to follow up on findings from this research. The following assumptions were used to perform the power analysis: (a) there will be three predictor variables (sound [mean Lmax value for preheelstick interval], light [mean foot-candles value for preheelstick interval], arousal [mean of Als states scored every two minutes during preheelstick interval]); (b) statistical power is set at .80; (c) level of significance in this study is set at $P < .05$. Under these assumptions, sample size was calculated at 51. To allow for possible differences between subgroups in the multiple regression analyses, 51 subjects will be enrolled for each subgroup (25–27 weeks and 34–36 weeks gestational age). Subject recruitment and enrollment procedures will continue until 51 infants are recruited in each gestational age group for a total sample size of 102.

Study Instruments

Three standardized instruments will be used to measure physiologic and behavioral responses to pain: the infant's bedside SpaceLabs Cardiorespiratory Monitor, Nellcor Pulse Oximeter, and the PIPP. Sound and light levels will be collected using a Quest Technologies Sound Meter and Extech Light Meter, respectively. In addition, the neonate's arousal level will be measured with Als' State Scoring System. Data from all instruments will be recorded simultaneously by an on-site study computer.

The New Ballard Score will be used to determine eligibility for inclusion in the study based on gestational age at birth. Severity of illness will be measured using the Neonatal Therapeutic Intervention Scoring System. Finally, demographic data will be collected using the Naturalistic Observation of Newborn Behavior Instrument.

Physiological Responses (Heart Rate, Oxygen Saturation): The infant's Space-Labs cardiorespiratory monitor will measure the infant's **heart rate**. Three neonatal body surface electrodes will be attached to the skin using two mid-axillary chest positions and one left lateral abdominal position. Quality ECG recording will be assured before data collection. The SpaceLabs monitor has an accuracy of $\pm$ 2 beats per minute averaged over 3 seconds.

Oxygen saturation will be recorded continuously using a Nellcor Pulse Oximeter module programmed within the SpaceLabs cardiorespiratory monitor. Reliability of the pulse oximeter reading will be verified by noting the congruence between the pulse oximeter digital reading for **heart rate** and that of the reading on the infant's cardiac monitor. In infants, the correlation between transcutaneous estimates and measured arterial saturations approaches an r-value of 0.91 using the Nellcor pulse oximeter (Fanconi, 1988).

Analog signals from **physiologic** parameters will be captured, digitized, synchronized, and stored using a desktop computer and National Instruments Data Acquisition System. All caregiving events as well as significant environmental happenings occurring during data collection for infants will be noted corresponding to an electronic event marker notation on the desktop computer.

Premature Infant Pain Profile (PIPP): Since pain is a multidimensional phenomenon, a multidimensional approach should be employed to study pain (U.S. Department of Health and Human Services, 1992). The **PIPP**, developed by Stevens and colleagues (1996) is a composite measure of pain in preterm infants < 28 weeks through 40 weeks **gestational age (see Appendix)**. The **PIPP** scores on a four-point scale the variables of **heart rate, oxygen saturation**, brow bulge, eye squeeze, nasolabial furrow, **gestational age**, and behavioral state. The sum of scores for each of the scales equals a total pain score. Internal consistency of the **PIPP** was estimated with the standardized item alpha of 0.71. Construct validity of the measure was supported using a contrasting groups approach in three samples of preterm and term infants. Ballantyne, Stevens, McAllister, Dionne, and Jack (1999) showed interrater reliability between two independent raters of 0.93–0.96 and intrarater reliability between bedside ratings and videotape ratings of 0.94–0.98. For the purposes of this study, the **PIPP** will be scored during the first 30 seconds of each 2-minute interval during data collection.

Sound Levels: Continuous **sound** levels will be measured using Quest Technologies Integrating/Datalogging Sound Level Meter (Model 2900). The accuracy of this Type 2 meter is estimated at $\pm$ 2%. The microphone will be suspended from the infant's bed (radiant warmer, incubator, or crib) and placed in direct proximity to the infant's ears. The sound level meter will be calibrated before each data collection period and set to record maximum (L-max) levels.

Light Levels: Continuous ambient **light** levels will be measured in foot-candles using Extech Heavy Duty Light Meter (Model # 407026). The recording meter will be placed in direct proximity to the infant's bed (radiant warmer, incubator, or crib), adjacent to the infant's head, and at the level of the infant's eyes. The meter will be calibrated before each data collection period. Selecting the lighting type enhances reliability of the readings: fluorescent, sodium, tungsten/daylight, or mercury. The light selection procedure will be used for data collection. The Extech Heavy Duty Light Meter has been determined to be accurate within a $\pm$ 5% error range.

Als State Scoring System: Als State Scoring System (Als et al., 1986) is a 13-state system used in the Neonatal Individualized Developmental Assessment Program (NIDCAP) specifically designed to measure sleeping and waking states of preterm infants. These sleep and wake patterns represent the **arousal** level variable. The scoring system is widely used in neonatal research (Als et al., 1986; Corff et al., 1995; Walden, 1997) and has been shown to correlate with electrophysiologic measures of brain activity (Holditch-Davis, 1998). The 13 sleep-wake state categories can be reduced into six **arousal** categories as follows: state 1 = deep sleep; state 2 = light sleep; state 3 = drowsiness; state 4 = awake, alert; state 5 = aroused, fussy; and state 6 = crying. During the time between the 2 hours preceding the heelstick to application of the bandage following the heelstick procedure, sleep-wake states will be scored every 2 minutes. Scores involve observing a 30-second interval (i.e., the last 30 seconds of every 2-minute interval) and scoring the highest behavioral state that was attained during that interval **(see Appendix)**. A synchronized nonaudible timer (Radio Shack's Big Digit Timer) will be used to indicate the two-minute intervals for the recording of sleep-wake data. The state will be immediately placed into the database by using the corresponding numbered key on the computer. For data analysis, Als sleep-wake state categories will be averaged over the 2-hour preheelstick observation period to create an **arousal** score between 1 and 6.

New Ballard Score (NBS) (Newborn Maturity Rating and Classification Assessment): The NBS will determine eligibility for enrollment in the study based on **gestational age** at birth **(see Appendix)**. The NBS is a 13-category scale designed to assess neuromuscular and physical maturity of neonates at 0 to 96 hours of life (Ballard et al., 1991). The maturity rating is evaluated on a 1 to 5 scale, with the total range of scores from –10 to 50 indicating a **gestational age** of 20 to 44 weeks, respectively. In the Ballard study, validity of the NBS was supported by correlations between **gestational age** by last menstrual period (confirmed by agreement within two weeks with **gestational age** by prenatal ultrasonography) and NBS scores. For the 530 infants studied, interrater reliability was documented by correlation between raters who rated the same infants ($r = 0.95$).

Neonatal Therapeutic Intervention Scoring System (NTISS): The NTISS (Gray, Richardson, McCormick, Workman-Daniels & Goldmann, 1992) will be used to determine the acuity of illness in preterm infants participating in the study **(see Appendix)**. The therapeutic intensity and complexity for various intensive care therapies is rated per medical record review. Eight clinical subscores are included on the NTISS and consist of respiratory, cardiovascular, drug therapy, monitoring, metabolic/nutrition, transfusion, procedural, and vascular access. The daily NTISS score is computed as the sum of therapy points received by a patient in a 24-hour period. Scores range from 0 to 47, and the higher the score, the greater the **physiologic** instability and severity of illness. Because study infants may not have certain laboratory work ordered on days that data are collected, the NTISS is more useful in determining severity of illness than other scales that depend on extensive blood/lab value calculations to determine severity of illness. In development of the NTISS instrument, internal consistency using Cronbach's alpha was estimated at 0.84. Convergent validity was supported by correlations between NTISS scores and mortality risk estimates for neonates by neonatal attending physicians ($r = 0.70, P < .0001$), and a measure of nursing acuity ($r = 0.69, P < .0001$).

Naturalistic Observation of Newborn Behavior Instrument (NONB): The
Naturalistic Observation of Newborn Behavior Instrument (Als, 1984) will be used
to collect demographic data on all participants in the study **(See Appendix)**. Data
obtained from the NONB include maternal history; infant history including complications; current status including respiratory function, medications, mode of feeding,
current medical problems; and current observation circumstances including type of
bed, facilitation devices in use, and caregiver activity. This is a commonly used
instrument in neonatal research (Als et al., 1986; Walden, 1997). Data from the
NONB will be used to describe the sample. Additional demographic information to
be obtained will include the number and type of painful procedures performed from
birth until the heelstick observation period and the time since the last painful event.
For this study, data on painful procedures will be collected using the infant's medical
record and will include heelstick, intravenous line insertion, venipuncture, lumbar
puncture, percutaneous central line insertion, percutaneous arterial puncture, chest
tube insertion/removal, central line placement/removal, endotracheal intubation, or
a surgical procedure. Time since last painful event will also be collected from the
infant's medical record and will involve the timing between any of the above procedures and the lance during heelstick data collection period.

Data Collection Procedure

The Site Coordinator will make daily rounds in the Newborn Care Center at
TCH to identify eligible subjects. After eligibility criteria have been confirmed, the
Principal Investigator or Site Coordinator will contact the parent(s) for informed
consent. Eligible infants will be assigned nonrandomly to one of two groups based on
gestational age at birth: (a) Group 1 will consist of 51 preterm infants 25–27 weeks
gestational age; (b) Group 2 will consist of 51 preterm neonates 34–36 weeks **gestational age** at birth. This grouping is for data analysis purposes only. There are no differences between the groups in the procedures used for data collection.

Data collection will occur within the first postnatal week and will begin two
hours before a scheduled heelstick procedure. Heelsticks are typically performed on a
routine schedule when a neonate has a standing order for such procedures, as is the
case in the eligible neonates, thus facilitating data collection. All measurements will
be collected during the routine laboratory collection times. Caregiving activities will
not be systematically altered in order to record the infant's routine NICU experiences surrounding the heelstick procedure. The PI has used this approach in previous
research, and it was found feasible within the NICU environment.

A standardized nonpharmacologic comfort measure will be provided throughout
the data collection period. This comfort measure will be initiated at the start of data
collection and involves maintaining the infant in the side lying position using a
Bendy Bumper (Children's Medical Ventures). The Bendy Bumper provides for
motoric containment of the infant's arms and legs in a flexed, midline position. This

type of nonpharmacologic comfort measure is now in use with preterm infants in many neonatal units across the country. It is currently the standard of care in the data collection site (TCH). While other nonpharmacologic measures will not be systematically instituted, the research assistant will record, using the on-site computer database, any other nonpharmacologic pain measure that is provided by the infant's caregiver.

During each heelstick observation period, the data signal for **physiologic** variables (**heart rate** and **oxygen saturation**) will be captured using the bedside computer and National Instruments Data Acquisition System, LabView. The data acquisition cable from the analogue-digital board will be connected to the R232 port at the back of the infant's bedside SpaceLabs cardiorespiratory monitor. The analogue-digital board will be used for the purpose of synchronization, digitization, and storage of data on the computer's zip drive. The infant's ECG wires and pulse oximeter probe will not be relocated unless an adequate signal cannot be obtained for data acquisition. At the start of data collection, the Extech Heavy Duty Light Meter (Model # 407026) will be calibrated and placed in direct proximity to the infant's bed (radiant warmer, incubator, or crib), adjacent to the infant's head, and at the level of the infant's eyes. The Quest Technologies Data Logging Sound Meter (Model 2900) microphone will be calibrated and suspended from the infant's bed (radiant warmer, incubator, or crib) and placed in direct proximity to the infant's ears. The **sound** and **light** meters will be connected to an on-site study computer via the analogue-digital board for synchronization, digitization, and storage of data. Infant **arousal** levels will be recorded during the last 30 seconds of every two minutes using the Als State Scoring System (1986). A timer (Radio Shack's Big Digit Timer) which is synchronized to correspond with continuous data collection instrumentation will be used to note the start of every two-minute interval. A **PIPP** score will be obtained during the first 30 seconds of each 2-minute interval throughout the data collection procedure.

Whenever possible, the selection of the heel will be accomplished by randomization by the research assistant by flipping a coin. The lab technician will perform the heelstick procedure according to a standard protocol. To standardize the procedure, the infant's heel will be randomly selected prior to data collection. Following the pre-heelstick observation period, the laboratory technician or research assistant will place the heel warmer on the randomized heel for two minutes. The laboratory technician will then start the heel lance procedure at the beginning of a two-minute interval by picking up the infant's foot and swabbing the heel with alcohol. The heel will be lanced using a spring-loaded incision device (Microtainer Brand Safety Flow Lancet, Becton Dickinson and Company, Rutherford, NJ) which makes a uniform incision 2.5 mm in length and 1.0 mm in depth on the lateral area of the heel. Subsequently, the technician will squeeze the heel, only repeating the lance procedure as necessary to draw sufficient blood. This process will continue until the required blood sample is collected. The heelstick procedure will end with the application of a bandage by the laboratory technician. This is the standard approach to the heelstick procedure used at TCH. The research assistant will document the start and stop times of the heelstick procedure using a time-event marker in the data acquisition system.

Throughout the duration of the data collection period, the time, duration, and characteristic of all caregiving handling and significant environmental events will be recorded in the on-site computer database, including any nonpharmacologic comfort measures that might be provided by the caregiver before or during the heelstick procedure. Furthermore, if the infant experiences significant **physiologic** distress, all interventions performed by the caregiver to stabilize the infant will be recorded.

Following the heelstick observation period, the research assistant will complete the NONB (Als, 1984) and NTISS (Gray et al., 1992) instruments using the patient's medical record. Data will also be collected on the number and types of noxious clinical procedures performed from the time of birth to the heelstick observation period using the infant's medical record. Data on time since last painful procedure will also be collected.

The diagram below illustrates the data collection procedures for the variables contained within this study:

Figure 2   Data collection protocol

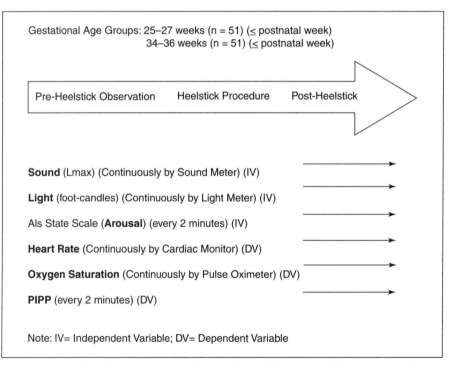

Gestational Age Groups: 25–27 weeks (n = 51) (≤ postnatal week)
34–36 weeks (n = 51) (≤ postnatal week)

Pre-Heelstick Observation   Heelstick Procedure   Post-Heelstick

Sound (Lmax) (Continuously by Sound Meter) (IV)

Light (foot-candles) (Continuously by Light Meter) (IV)

Als State Scale (**Arousal**) (every 2 minutes) (IV)

Heart Rate (Continuously by Cardiac Monitor) (DV)

Oxygen Saturation (Continuously by Pulse Oximeter) (DV)

PIPP (every 2 minutes) (DV)

Note: IV= Independent Variable; DV= Dependent Variable

Source: Grant example with permission from: Walden, M. (2001). *Environment and sleep on preterm infants pain response.* 1K15NR007731-01. NIH/National Institute for Nursing Research.

Interrater Reliability:

The reliability of the PI's and co-investigator's use of the Als State Scoring System has been estimated at greater than 0.85 with a national NIDCAP instructor (Linda Lutes, Sooner NIDCAP Training Center, Oklahoma City, Oklahoma). The PI will be responsible for ensuring that the research assistant is reliable in the Als State Scoring System before data collection.

Reliability of the PI's scoring the facial actions of the **PIPP** instrument was estimated at greater than 0.85 before data collection by an international expert in **pain responses** in infants (Bonnie Stevens, University of Toronto, Ontario, Canada). The PI will be responsible for ensuring that the co-investigator and research assistant are reliable in the **PIPP** instrument before data collection.

To further ensure reliability, 10 percent of the observations (or *n* = 10) will be randomly selected for assessment of interrater reliability between study personnel using the Als State Scoring System as well as the **PIPP** instrument. Measurements of interrater reliability will occur beginning 10 minutes before the heelstick procedure through the first 10 minutes of the postheelstick recovery observation period.

The PI received training in **physiologic** data acquisition during a Faculty Scientist Award from Emory University and is currently engaged in **physiologic** data collection and secondary analysis of **physiologic** variables during painful clinical procedures for a currently funded NIH research project entitled "Heart Rate Variability During Transition to Extrauterine Life" (Dr. M. Terese Verklan, Principal Investigator). In addition, Dr. Terese Verklan will be responsible for ensuring the reliability of the PI, co-investigator, and research assistant in **physiologic** data acquisition using the National Instruments Data Acquisition System before data collection. Furthermore, Carol Carrier will be responsible for ensuring that the PI and research assistant are reliable using the **sound** and **light** level meters before data collection.

Analysis:

Statistical analyses will be performed using the BMPD Program (Dixon, 1992). Descriptive statistics including frequencies and measures of central tendency and dispersion will be calculated for all demographic and study variables, as appropriate. For all analyses in this research, the level of significance will be $P \leq .05$. This analysis section will be organized by research questions and hypotheses.

1. What is the relationship between **sound** (as measured by a sound meter), **light** (as measured by a light meter), **arousal** levels (as measured by Als State Score) in the 2 hours preceding a heelstick procedure to:

    A. Immediate **physiological pain response** of preterm neonates to a heelstick procedure (as measured by **heart rate** and **oxygen saturation**)?

    B. Immediate **behavioral pain responses** of preterm neonates to a heelstick procedure (as measured by the **PIPP**)?

2. Is the relationship of **sound** (as measured by a sound meter), **light** (as measured by a light meter), and **arousal** levels (as measured by Als State Score) in the 2 hours preceding a heelstick procedure moderated by **gestational age**?

Mixed model general linear models (GLMs) will be arranged with between-groups independent variables of **sound, light, arousal** levels, and **gestational age**; and one within-groups independent variable, occasion. A separate GLM will be used for each of the dependent variables, **heart rate, oxygen saturation,** and **PIPP.** Instead of a full factorial design, specific design terms will be developed: for Question 1, four two-way interactions will be tested (**sound, light, arousal,** and **gestational age** X occasion). Any significant 2-way interaction will be probed with simple main effects. For Question 2, three 3-way interactions will be built (**sound, light,** and **arousal** X **gestational age** X occasion). Any significant 3-way interaction will be decomposed into 2-way interactions and simple main effects to explain the effect.

3. Does variation in **sound** (as measured by a sound meter), **light** (as measured by a light meter), and **arousal** levels (as measured by Als State Score) in the 2 hours preceding a heelstick procedure predict:

   A. **Physiological disruption** from acute pain in preterm neonates (as measured by the **time for heart rate and oxygen saturation, to return to baseline values).**

   B. **Behavioral disruption** from acute pain in preterm neonates following a heelstick procedure (as measured by **time for PIPP score to return to baseline value).**

Hierarchical regression analyses will be performed to examine the effect of **sound, light,** and **arousal** levels on **physiologic disruption** and **recovery time** of acute pain scores. The regression model will include three predictor variables (**sound** [mean Lmax value for preheelstick period], **light** [mean foot-candles value for preheelstick period], **arousal** level [mean of Als states 1–6 observed every two minutes during preheelstick period]). The dependent variables in the regression analyses are **time to return to baseline for heart rate, oxygen saturation, and PIPP scores (recovery time).**

The centered main effects (**sound, light,** and **arousal**) will be tested first, followed by a test of cross-products (**gestational age** group by **sound, light,** and **arousal** levels). In separate regression analyses, dependent variables will be regressed on the three predictor variables (**sound, light,** and **arousal**). For all regression analyses, the environmental variables of **sound** and **light** will be entered first into the regression model as they are hypothesized to affect the third predictor, **arousal.** Multicollinearity will be assessed by examining the tolerance of all predictor variables, using the statistical program, BMPD-2R. Tolerances for predictor variables that fall below .40 will be excluded from further analysis. Furthermore, residual scatterplots will be obtained and inspected for multivariate outliers and to ensure that the assumptions for multiple regression have not been violated. Significant departures from normality will be handled by transforming affected variables to stabilize their variances.

4. Does **gestational age** interact with **sound** (as measured by a sound meter), **light** (as measured by a light meter), and **arousal** levels (as measured by Als State Score) in the 2 hours preceding a heelstick procedures in the prediction of:

   A. **Physiological disruption** from acute pain in preterm neonates (as measured by the **time for heart rate and oxygen saturation to return to baseline values**).
   B. **Behavioral disruption** from acute pain in preterm neonates following a heelstick procedure (as measured by **time for PIPP score to return to baseline value**).

Using BMDP-1R, a Chow test (test for equivalency of regression slope) will examine possible differences in regression planes between **gestational age** subgroups (25–27 weeks **gestational age** vs. 34–36 weeks **gestational age**). If the Chow test is nonsignificant, the regression analyses will be completed using the entire sample ($N = 102$). If the Chow test indicates group differences, separate regression slopes will be used to analyze the data.

Limitations of the Research:

The subjects are not randomly selected for the study; rather, their inclusion depends upon the availability of the parent(s) to sign a consent form and the willingness of the parent(s) to have their infant participate in the study.

Due to the very nature of clinical research, several factors may have an impact on the way that data are collected. While the heelstick will be performed according to a standardized collection procedure, a number of different laboratory technicians may collect the blood. This, however, is a reflection of the actual practice infants experience. In addition the amount of blood to be collected may vary depending on the laboratory studies ordered and thus differences in the amount of time to collect blood are expected. Again, this is a reflection of the actual practice infants in the NICU experience. Also not all subjects will experience the same types of painful procedures or the same number of repetitions of the procedure during the first week of postnatal life. Since it would not be ethical to subject preterm infants to procedures they do not need, nor to withhold procedures they need just to ensure equivalence of experience, data will be collected on the number and type of painful procedures experienced until the heelstick is performed as well as the time since the last painful procedure.

Since infants will be cared for by different caregivers, it is possible that the infant's caregiver will provide additional nonpharmacologic comfort measures beyond the standardized comfort measure to be provided in this study. This again is a reflection of the actual practice infants experience. The research assistant will record nonpharmacologic comfort measures provided as well as a qualitative analysis of caregiving during data collection to identify caregiving factors she thinks are influencing infant responses.

Finally, one of the major problems in using data acquisition systems to collect **physiologic** measures is the voluminous amount of data that are collected. It is important to eliminate the unnecessary information coming from the analysis procedure and focus only on the pertinent information to answer the research question.

Figure 3 *Timeline*

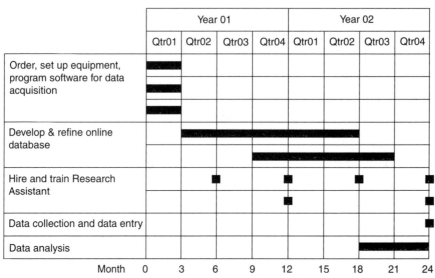

Source: Grant example with permission from: Walden, M. (2001). *Environment and sleep on preterm infants pain response.* 1K15NR007731-01. NIH/National Institute for Nursing Research.

E. Human Subjects

Sample

Every preterm infant admitted to the Newborn Care Center at TCH will be recruited for participation in a convenience sample of 102 infants who meet the following criteria: (a) infants between 25–27 weeks or 34–36 weeks **gestational age** at birth and appropriate for **gestational age** as determined by the New Ballard Score (Ballard et al., 1991); and (b) scheduled to receive a routine heelstick procedure within the first postnatal week. This subject inclusion criterion is demanded by the science of the research questions addressed.

Exclusion criteria include: (a) chromosomal or genetic anomalies; (b) significant central nervous system abnormality including seizures or a Grade III/IV intraventricular hemorrhage; (c) infants born to mothers with a known history of substance abuse; or (d) infants who receive paralytic, analgesic, or sedating medications within 24 hours before the heelstick procedure.

Recruitment of Minority Subjects

In 1999, the racial composition of neonatal patients for the respective age groups at TCH is 22% African American; 29% Hispanic; 47% Caucasian; and 2% other. The sample composition for this study is expected to be similar. Since the sample population is approximately evenly divided among minority versus nonminority groups, if more than one infant is available for inclusion in the study on any given laboratory collection day, preference will be given to infants of the youngest **gestational age**. If more than one infant meets the youngest **gestational age** criteria, preference will be given to recruitment of minority background. The rationale for choosing the youngest subjects as first preference is that there is a smaller pool of infants between 25–27 weeks **gestational age** than 34–36 weeks **gestational age**, making it more difficult to recruit this age sample. The rationale for recruiting minorities is to ensure adequate minority representation, since there will be equipment limitations. The recruitment goal for minority representation is that at least 50% of the sample will have a minority background. This percentage represents the actual minority representation at TCH. Recruitment will be reviewed monthly regarding minority inclusion.

Sources of Research Material

Once informed consent has been obtained from the parent(s), demographic data will be obtained from the medical record in order to complete the Neonatal Therapeutic Intervention Scoring System and Naturalistic Observation of Newborn Behavior Instruments. Physiologic data (heart rate, oxygen saturation) will be recorded continuously from cables connected to the infants' physiological monitor (SpaceLabs Cardiorespiratory Monitor with Nellcor Pulse Oximeter module). Sound and light levels will be collected using a Quest Technologies Sound Meter and Extech Light Meter, respectively. In addition, the research assistant will use bedside observation to measure the neonate's arousal level (Als' State Scoring System) as well as the behavioral components of the PIPP score (brow bulge, eye squeeze, nasolabial furrow). Data from all instruments will be recorded simultaneously using an on-site study computer.

Recruitment of Subjects

The Site Coordinator will make daily rounds to determine infants who meet eligibility criteria to participate in the study. Upon identification of a potential subject, the Principal Investigator or Site Coordinator will contact the parent(s) to set up an appointment to discuss the study and request informed consent. If the parent(s) agree to allow their infant to participate, they will be asked to sign a consent form. Those who sign the consent form will be given a copy to keep. A copy of the consent form will also be placed in the infant's medical record. Once 51 infants have been enrolled in each age group, subject recruitment will be halted for that respective group. To assure protection of rights of human subjects, approval to conduct the study is pending from the Institutional Review Boards of UTMB, TCH, and Baylor College of Medicine.

Potential Risks

The study proposed is repeated measures, naturalistic design; no additional procedures affecting the neonate or presenting any clinical risks are being proposed. There is, however, a potential risk of violation of confidentiality of the infant.

Protection Measures to Reduce Risks

All infants admitted into the study will be given a code number, and only the code number will appear on computer data files and data collection records. Data collection will be monitored by the principal investigator and site coordinator to ensure safety of the subjects.

Potential Benefits

The study may provide new information of how **sound, light,** and **arousal** levels influence the infant's ability to respond to and recover from painful procedures. This knowledge may improve assessment of pain in critically ill preterm neonates. Moreover, this improved understanding will permit caregivers to develop interventions to modify the NICU micro-environment in a manner that minimizes infant acute **physiologic** and **behavioral responses** to pain and thereby helps to decrease long-term neurobehavioral sequelae of chronic, repetitive pain experiences.

F. Vertebrate Animals

Not Applicable

G. Literature Cited

Als, H. (1984). *Manual for the naturalistic observation of newborn behavior (preterm and fullterm infants)*. Boston: Author.

Als, H. (1986). A synactive model of neonatal behavioral organization: Framework for the assessment of neurobehavioral development in the premature infant and for support of infants and parents in the neonatal intensive care environment. *Physical & Occupational Therapy in Pediatrics*, 6(3/4), 3-55.

Als, H., Lawhon, G., Brown, E., Gibes, R., Duffy, F., McAnulty, G., & Blickman, J. (1986). Individualized behavioral and environmental care for the very low birth weight preterm infant at high risk for bronchopulmonary dysplasia: Neonatal intensive care unit and developmental outcome. *Pediatrics, 78*, 1123-1132.

Anand, K. (1997). Long-term effects of pain in neonates and infants. In T. S. Jensen, J. A. Turner, and Z Wiesenfeld-Hallin's (Eds.), *Proceedings of the 8th World Congress on Pain, Progress in Pain Research and Management* (Vol. 8). Seattle: IASP Press.

Anand, K. (1998). Clinical importance of pain and stress in preterm neonates. *Biology of the Neonate, 73*, 1-9.

Anand, K., Phil, D., & Hickey, P. (1987). Pain and its effects in the human neonate and fetus. *New England Journal of Medicine, 317*, 1321-1329.

Anand, K., Phil, D., Grunau, R., & Oberlander, T. (1997). Developmental character and long-term consequences of pain in infants and children. *Child and Adolescent Psychiatric Clinics of North America, 6*, 703-724.

Andrews, K., & Fitzgerald, M. (1994). The cutaneous withdrawal reflex in human neonates: sensitization, receptive fields, and the effects of contralateral stimulation. *Pain, 56*, 95-101.

Appleton, S. (1997). Handle with care: An investigation of the handling received by preterm infants in intensive care. *Journal of Neonatal Nursing, 3*, 23-27.

Ballantyne, M., Stevens, B., McAllister, M., Dionne, K., & Jack, A. (1999). Validation of the premature infant pain profile in the clinical setting. *Clinical Journal of Pain, 15*(4), 297-303.

Ballard, J., Khoury, J., Wedig, K., Wang, L., Eilers-Walsman, B., & Lipp, R. (1991). New Ballard Score expanded to include extremely premature infants. *Journal of Pediatrics, 119*, 417-423.

Barker, D., & Rutter, N. (1995). Exposure to invasive procedures in newborn intensive care unit admissions. *Archives of Disease in Childhood, 72*, F47-F48.

Beaver, P. (1987). Premature infants' response to touch and pain: Can nurses make a difference? *Neonatal Network, 6*, 13-17.

Blackburn, S., & Patterson, D. (1991). Effects of cycled light on activity state and cardiorespiratory function in preterm infants. *Journal of Perinatal & Neonatal Nursing 4*(4), 47-54.

Bozzette, M. (1993). Observation of pain behavior in the NICU: An exploratory study. *Journal of Perinatal & Neonatal Nursing, 7*(1), 76-87.

Campos, R. (1989). Soothing-pain-elicited distress in infants with swaddling and pacifiers. *Child Development, 60*, 781-792.

Carli, G., Montesano, A., Rapezzi, S., & Paluffi, G. (1987). Differential effects of persistent nociceptive stimulation on sleep stages. *Behavioural Brain Research, 26,* 89-98.

Cooper-Evans, J. (1991). Incidence of hypoxaemia associated with caregiving in premature infants. *Neonatal Network, 10,* 17-24.

Corff, K., Seideman, R., Venkataraman, P., Lutes, L., & Yates, B. (1995). Facilitated tucking: A nonpharmacologic comfort measure for pain in preterm neonates. *Journal of Obstetric, Gynecologic, and Neonatal Nursing, 24,* 143-147.

Craig, K., Whitfield, M., Grunau, R., Linton, J., & Hadjistavropoulos, H. (1993). Pain in the preterm neonate: Behavioral and physiological indices. *Pain, 52,* 287-299.

Dixon, W. J. (Ed.) (1992). *BMDP statistical software manual.* Berkeley, CA: University of California Press.

Duxbury, M., Henly, S., Broz, L., Armstrong, G., & Wachdorf, C. (1984). Caregiver disruptions and sleep of high-risk infants. *Heart and Lung, 13,* 141-147.

Fanconi, S. (1988). Reliability of pulse oximetry in hypoxic infants. *Journal of Pediatrics, 112(3),* 424-427.

Field, T., & Goldson, E. (1984). Pacifying effects of nonnutritive sucking on term and preterm neonates during heelstick procedures. *Pediatrics, 74,* 1012-1015.

Fitzgerald, M., & Anand K. (1993). Developmental neuroanatomy and neurophysiology of pain. In N. Schechter, C. Berde, & M. Yaster (Eds.), *Pain in infants, children, and adolescents* (pp. 11-31). Baltimore: Williams & Wilkins.

Fitzgerald, M., Millard, C., & McIntosh, N. (1989). Cutaneous hypersensitivity following peripheral tissue damage in newborn infants and its reversal with topical anaesthesia. *Pain, 39,* 31-36.

Fitzgerald, M., Shaw, A., & MacIntosh, N. (1988). The postnatal development of the cutaneous flexor reflex: A comparative study in premature infants and newborn rat pups. *Developmental Medicine and Child Neurology, 30,* 520-526.

Franck, L., & Gregory, G. (1993). Clinical evaluation and treatment of infant pain in the neonatal intensive care unit. In N. Schechter, C. Berde, & M. Yaster (Eds.), *Pain in infants, children, and adolescents* (pp. 519-535). Baltimore: Williams & Wilkins.

Gadeke, R., Doing, B., Keller, F., & Vogel, A. (1969). The noise level in a children's hospital and the wake-up threshold in infants. *Acta Paediatrica Scandinavia, 58,* 164-170.

Gorski, P. (1983). Premature infants behavioral and physiological responses to caregiving interventions in the intensive care nursery. In J. Call, E. Gallenson, & R. Tyson (Eds.), *Frontiers of infant psychiatry* (pp. 256-263). New York: Basic Books, Inc.

Gorski, P., Hale, W., & Leonard, C. (1983). Direct computer recording of premature infants and nursing care: Distress following two interventions. *Pediatrics, 72,* 198.

Gottfried, W. (1985). Environment of newborn infants in special care units. In A. Gottfried & J. Gaiter (Eds.), *Infant stress under intensive care: Environmental neonatology* (pp. 23-54). Baltimore: University Park Press.

Gray, J., Richardson, D., McCormick, M., Workman-Daniels, K., & Goldmann, D. (1992). Neonatal therapeutic intervention scoring system: A therapy-based severity-of-illness-index. *Pediatrics, 90,* 561-567.

Grunau, R., & Craig, K. (1987). Pain expression in neonates: Facial action and cry. *Pain, 28,* 395-410.

Grunau, R., Whitfield, M., & Petrie, J. (1994). Pain sensitivity and temperament in extremely low-birth-weight premature toddlers and preterm and full-term controls. *Pain, 58,* 341-346.

Grunau, R., Whitfield, M., Petrie, J., & Fryer, E. (1994). Early pain experience, child and family factors, as precursors of somatization: A prospective study of extremely premature and full-term children. *Pain, 56,* 353-359.

Hicks, R., Coleman, D., Ferante, F., Sahatjian, M., & Hawkins, J. (1979). Pain thresholds in rats during recovery from REM sleep deprivation. *Perceptual and Motor Skills, 48,* 687-690.

Hicks, R., Moore, J., Findley, P., Hirshfield, C., & Humphrey, V. (1978). REM sleep deprivation and pain thresholds in rats. *Perceptual and Motor Skills, 47,* 848-850.

Hintze, J. (2000). *PASS 2000 User's Manual.* Kaysville, UT: NCSS, INC.

Holditch-Davis, D. & Calhoun, M. (1989). Do preterm infants show behavioral responses to painful procedures? In S. Funk, E. Tornquist, M. Champagne, et al., (Eds.), *Key aspects of comfort: Management of pain, fatigue, and nausea* (pp. 35-43). New York: Springer.

Holditch-Davis, D. (1990). The effect of hospital caregiving on preterm infants' sleeping and waking states. In S. Funk, E. Tornquist, M. Champagne, et al., (Eds.), *Key aspects of recovery: Improving nutrition, rest, and mobility* (pp. 110-122). New York: Springer.

Holditch-Davis, D., (1998). Neonatal sleep-wake states. In C. Kenner, J. Lott, & A. Flandermeyer's (Eds.), *Comprehensive neonatal nursing: A physiologic perspective* (pp. 921-938). Philadelphia: W.B. Saunders.

Johnston, C., & Stevens, B. (1996). Experience in a neonatal intensive care unit affects pain response. *Pediatrics, 98*(5), 925-930.

Johnston, C., Stevens, B., Franck, L., Jack, A., Stremler, R., & Platt, R. (1999). Factors explaining lack of response to heel stick in preterm newborns. *JOGNN, 28*(6), 587-594.

Johnston, C., Stevens, B., Yang, F., & Horton, L. (1995). Differential response to pain by very premature neonates. *Pain, 61*, 471-479.

Johnston, C., Stremler, R., Stevens, B., & Horton, L. (1997). Effectiveness of oral sucrose and simulated rocking on pain response in preterm neonates. *Pain, 72*, 193-199.

Jorgensen, K. (1993). *Developmental care of the premature infant: A concise overview.* S. Weymouth, USA: Developmental Care Division of Children's Medical Ventures.

Krechel, S., & Bildner, J. (1995). CRIES: A new neonatal post-operative pain measurement score: Initial testing of validity and reliability. *Paediatric Anaesthesia, 5*(1), 53-61.

Lenz, E., Pugh, L., Milligan, R., Gift, A., & Suppe, F. (1997). The middle-range theory of unpleasant symptoms: An update. *Advances in Nursing Science, 19*(3), 14-27.

Long, J., Lucey, J., & Philips, A. (1980). Noise and hypoxemia in the intensive care nursery. *Pediatrics, 65*, 143-145.

Lotas, M., & Walden, M. (1996). Individualized developmental care for very low-birth-weight infants: A critical review. *Journal of Obstetric, Gynecologic, and Neonatal Nursing, 25*, 681-687.

Mann, N., Haddow, R., Stokes, L., Goodley, S., & Rutter, N. (1986). Effect of night and day on preterm infants in a newborn nursery: Randomised trial. *British Medical Journal, 293*, 1265-1267.

Marchette, L., Main, R., Redick, E., et al. (1991). Pain reduction interventions during neonatal circumcision. *Nursing Research, 40*, 241-244.

McIntosh, N., Van Veen, L, & Brameyer, H. (1994). Alleviation of the pain of heel prick in preterm infants. *Archives of Disease in Childhood, 70*, F177-F181.

Miller, H., & Anderson, G. (1993). Nonnutritive sucking: Effects on crying and heart rate in intubated infants requiring assisted mechanical ventilation. *Nursing Research, 42*, 305-307.

Murdoch, D., & Darlow, B. (1984). Handling during neonatal intensive care. *Archives of Disease in Childhood, 59*, 957-961.

National Commission to Prevent Infant Mortality. (1990). *Troubling trends: The health of America's next generation.* Washington, DC.

Norris, S., Campbell, L., & Brenkert, S. (1982). Nursing procedures and alterations in transcutaneous oxygen tension in premature infants. *Nursing Research, 31*, 330-336.

Owens, M., & Todt, E. (1984). Pain in infancy: Neonatal reaction to a heel lance. *Pain, 20*, 77-86.

Peters, K. (1992). Does routine nursing care complicate the physiologic status of the premature neonate with respiratory distress syndrome? *Journal of Perinatal & Neonatal Nursing, 6*(2), 67-84.

Pohlman, S., & Beardslee, C. (1987). Contacts experienced by neonates in intensive care environments. *Maternal-Child Nursing Journal, 16*, 207-226.

Shiao, S., Chang, Y., Lannon, H., & Yarandi, H. (1997). Meta-analysis of the effects of nonnutritive sucking on heart rate and peripheral oxygenation: Research from the past 30 years. *Issues in Comprehensive Pediatric Nursing, 20*, 11-24.

Shiroiwa, Y., Kamiya, Y., & Uchiboi, S. (1986). Activity, cardiac and respiratory responses of blindfold preterm infants in a neonatal intensive care unit. *Early Human Development, 14*, 259-265.

Slevin, M., Farrington, N., Duffy, G., Daly, L., & Murphy, J. (2000). Altering the NICU and measuring infants' responses. *Acta Paediatr, 89*(5), 577-581.

Speidel, B. (1978). Adverse effects of routine procedures on preterm infants. *Lancet, 1*, 864-866.

Stevens, B., & Johnston, C. (1994). Physiological responses of premature infants to a painful stimulus. *Nursing Research, 43*, 226-231.

Stevens, B., & Ohlsson, A. (1998). Sucrose in neonates undergoing painful procedures. *Neonatal Modules of the Cochrane Data Base of Systematic Reviews*, electronic 1-13.

Stevens, B., Johnston, C., & Horton, L. (1993). Multidimensional pain assessment in premature neonates: A pilot study. *JOGNN, 22*(6), 531-541.

Stevens, B., Johnston, C., & Horton, L. (1994). Factors that influence the behavioral pain responses of premature infants. *Pain, 59*, 101-109.

Stevens, B., Johnston, C., Franck, L., Petryshen, P., Jack, A., & Foster, G. (1999). The efficacy of developmentally sensitive interventions and sucrose for relieving procedural pain in very low birth weight neonates. *Nursing Research, 48*(1), 35-43.

Stevens, B., Johnston, C., Petryshen, P., & Taddio, A. (1996). Premature infant pain profile: Development and initial validation. *Clinical Journal of Pain, 12*, 13-22.

Stevens, B., Taddio, A., Ohlsson, A., & Einarson, T. (1997). The efficacy of sucrose for relieving procedural pain in neonates: A systematic review and meta-analysis. *Acta Paediatrica, 86*, 837-842.

U.S. Department of Health and Human Services. (1992). *Acute pain management in infants, children, and adolescents: Operative and medical procedures* (AHCPR Publication. No. 92-0020). Rockville, Maryland: Author.

Van Cleve, L., Johnson, L., Andrews, S., Hawkins, S., & Newbold, J. (1995). Pain responses of hospitalized neonates to venipuncture. *Neonatal Network, 14*, 31-36.

Walden, M. (1997). *Changes over six weeks in multivariate responses of premature neonates to a painful stimulus.* Unpublished doctoral dissertation, University of Texas at Austin, School of Nursing, Austin.

Wolke, D. (1987). Environmental neonatology. *Archives of Disease in Childhood, 62,* 987-988.

Zahr, L., & Balian, S. (1995). Responses of premature infants to routine nursing interventions and noise in the NICU. *Nursing Research, 44,* 179-185.

H. Consortium/Contractual Arrangements

Subcontract to Texas Children's Hospital, Houston, Texas

Carol Carrier, RN, MSN, will serve at 5% effort as Site Coordinator for the project. She will assist the Principal Investigator in addressing staff questions related to the research project and in problem solving data collection issues as they arise. Ms. Carrier will assist the Principal Investigator in subject recruitment by making daily rounds of newly admitted infants to the Newborn Center to determine potential infants who meet study eligibility requirements. She will also assist the Principal Investigator in obtaining informed consent from parent(s). Ms. Carrier will participate as needed in data collection in conjunction with the Principal Investigator and Research Assistant. Finally, Ms. Carrier will assist the Principal Investigator in data analysis, interpretation, and dissemination, particularly as it relates to her expertise in environmental sound and light in the NICU.

This subcontract is currently under negotiation. Completed documentation of this subcontract will be forwarded as soon as it is available.

I. Consultants

Terese Verklan, PhD, RN, CCNS, is an Associate Professor at the University of Texas Health Science Center-Houston and will serve as a data acquisition consultant to the project. Dr. Verklan is an expert in the neonatal cardiovascular physiology and behavioral state. She has numerous data-based contribution in peer-reviewed professional journals and has been the principal investigator and co-investigator for several well-funded clinical studies relating to fetal and neonatal care. She is currently the principal investigator on a NIH R01 in which she uses the Physiological Data Acquisition System by National Instruments (Austin, Texas) to examine heart rate variability and state transition of the fetus to neonate through the first 10 hours of life. She will provide consultation in computerized data acquisition of the physiologic variables in this study using the National Instruments data acquisition setup. Upon completion of data collection, Dr. Verklan will assist in analysis and interpretation of the data. She will provide approximately two days of consulting services in Year 01 and four days of consultation in Year 02.

Robin D. Froman, PhD, RN, Professor and Associate Dean for Research at the University of Texas Medical Branch - Galveston will serve as a no-cost consultant for the project. She has served as a nonremunerated consultant to the principal investigator during the development of her preliminary studies leading to this study and in the development of this study. Dr. Froman brings expertise in many aspects including infant special care, research development, data management, and NIH funding. She will provide ongoing guidance and advisement during the project period on the collection and management of data as well as during data interpretation in regard to clinical relevance.

APPENDIX

A. Dissertation manuscript submitted, *Changes Over Six Weeks in Physiologic and Behavioral Responses of Extremely Preterm Neonates to a Painful Stimulus*
B. Premature Infant Pain Profile (PIPP)
C. Als State Scoring System
D. New Ballard Score
E. Neonatal Therapeutic Intervention Scoring System
F. Naturalistic Observation of Newborn Behavior Instrument (NONB)
G. Letters of Support

Protocol Worksheet

Patient's Name: _____   Medical Record #: _____

Hospital: _____

PREPARATION

_____ 1. NICU nurse identifies eligible infants on admission.
   a. Performs New Ballard Score
   b. Ensures inclusion criteria are met (at birth)
      1. 24–26 weeks PCA at birth
      2. Continuous cardiac/oximeter monitoring
      3. Parent(s) able to read and write English or Spanish
      4. Parent(s) 18 years of age or older
      5. Expected scheduled heelsticks beginning by 27 weeks PCA
   c. Ensures infant does not meet exclusion criteria (at birth)
      1. Birth weight SGA/LGA
      2. Physical or neurologic congenital anomalies
      3. Abnormal neurologic signs or a Grade III/IV IVH
      4. Known fetal exposure to drugs of addiction
      5. Systemic analgesics, including narcotic and sedative agents, within 24 hours prior to data collection with evidence of low urine output (< 1 mL/Kg/Hour)

_____ 2. Nurse seeks permission of neonatologist to approach parent(s) with letter of information.

_____ 3. Nurse reads letter of information to parent(s) and asks if they are willing to hear more about the study.

_____ 4. Nurse informs Principal Investigator if parent(s) indicate an interest in hearing more about the study.

_____ 5. Principal Investigator obtains permission of parent(s) for infant to participate in study.

_____ 6. Principal Investigator gives parent(s) a copy of consent and places a copy in the infant's medical record.

_____ 7. Principal Investigator confirms weekly eligibility criteria are met.
   a. Routine weekly heelstick scheduled
   b. Continuous cardiac/oximeter monitoring
   c. Systemic analgesics, including narcotic and sedative agents, not given within the previous 24 hours prior to data collection (also urine output > 1 mL/Kg/Hour)

_____ 8. Principal Investigator informs laboratory/nursing of data collection time day prior to observation period.

_____ 9. One hour prior to data collection, nurse performs care giving activities. The caregiver will first change the infant's diaper, while research assistant scores the infant's response using the PIPP during the first 30 seconds for each 2-minute interval. For the data observation period, the infant will be dressed only in a diaper. The infant will be placed in the right lateral position with a Bendy Bumper.

_____ 10. Principal Investigator arranges bed/infant to maximize view of infant/ monitor readings during data collection period.

_____ 11. Principal Investigator confirms with laboratory technician/nursing scheduled time of heelstick procedure.

_____ 12. Principal Investigator reminds nursery personnel that verbal communication and interruptions must be kept to a minimum during study.

_____ 13. Principal Investigator posts sign, "Study in Progress. Please do not interrupt."

_____ 14. Principal Investigator randomizes heel for heelstick procedure.

BASELINE

_____ 1. Study personnel position themselves closest to the infant's head.

_____ 2. Principal Investigator records behaviors every 2 minutes using BOS for 20 minutes.

_____ 3. At beginning of every 2-minute interval, the Principal Investigator will count the infant's respiration for 30 seconds.

_____ 4. Principal Investigator will record the heart rate and oxygen saturation at 30 seconds during each 2-minute period.

_____ 5. Research assistant will score for the presence of brow bulge, eye squeeze, and nasolabial furrow during the first 30 seconds of each 2-minute interval.

_____ 6. The research assistant will score the PIPP during the first 30 seconds of each 2-minute interval.

_____ 7. Throughout the data collection periods, the Principal Investigator will continuously record environmental conditions (activity levels, noise, lighting levels).

_____ 8. Throughout the data collection periods, the research assistant will 1) maintain the infant in the side lying position; 2) remove all extraneous stimulation such as stroking, talking, position shifts, etc., 3) provide Bendy Bumper support to keep the infant's arms and legs in a flexed, midline position.

_____ 9. If the infant experiences significant physiologic distress, the Principal Investigator will record all interventions performed by the caregiver to stabilize the infant. If the study must be halted, another observation period within the same week will be chosen.

Heelstick Procedure

_____ 1. After 20 minutes on the timer, the laboratory technician/ research assistant will apply a heel warmer to the randomized heel.

_____ 2. Data will continue to be collected as described in baseline section.

_____ 3. At 22 minutes on the timer, the laboratory technician will perform the heelstick procedure according to standard protocol (have equipment open and ready to go).

_____ 4. The Principal Investigator will document the heel used, the number of heel lances, and the start and stop times of the heelstick procedure on the BOS.

Recovery Period

_____ 1. Beginning with the time from the laboratory technician's last physical contact with the infant, Time 2 timer will be started and 20 minutes of observation will continue as described in the baseline section.

Post Data Collection Period

_____ 1. On each day heelstick observation is performed, the Principal Investigator will complete the following instruments using the patient's medical record and interviewing the neonatologists and nurses when necessary.

    a. Naturalistic Observation of Newborn Behavior Instrument.

    b. Number of heelstick procedures performed from birth to each data collection period.

    c. Neonatal Therapeutic Intervention Scoring System

_____ 2. The infant will be foot-printed for the Certificate of Appreciation to be given to the parents following data collection at 32 weeks PCA.

Data Collection Periods

_____   27 weeks (Date:_____ Time: _____)

    Technician: _____

_____   28 weeks (Date: _____ Time: _____)

    Technician: _____

_____   29 weeks (Date: _____ Time: _____)

    Technician: _____

_____   30 weeks (Date: _____ Time: _____)

    Technician: _____

_____   31 weeks (Date: _____ Time: _____)

              Technician: _____

_____   32 weeks (Date: _____ Time: _____)

              Technician: _____

Other

    1.   10% assessment of inter-rater reliability

Source: Walden, M. (1997). *Changes over Six Weeks in Multivariate Responses of Premature Neonates to a Painful Stimulus.* Unpublished doctoral dissertation, University of Texas at Austin, School of Nursing, Austin.

Example of a Final Report for an NIH Grant

Overview

FCCGP was a collaborative effort of faculty from the University of Illinois at Chicago (UIC) and Johns Hopkins University Schools of Nursing, the UIC and University of Chicago Schools of Medicine, and the University of Oklahoma, College of Nursing. The goals of the project were to (a) link personal health status with gene function, family, and the larger environment (social, culture, physical, health policy); (b) prepare learners to integrate biological knowledge of gene function with family, environment, behavior, and psychosocial, ethical, and legal knowledge; and (c) assess learner's knowledge, skills, and attitudes about genetics based on the nationally recognized core competencies developed in 2001 by the National Coalition of Health Professional Education in Genetics (NCHPEG)

An interactive, Web-based curriculum was created that integrates new genetics information into medical, nursing, and social work practice using the family as the context for care. This interdisciplinary project used a case report format to develop three modules on breast/ovarian cancer, cystic fibrosis, and bipolar affective disorder:

- **Module 1: Breast and Ovarian Cancer**
  Karen W. is a 45-year-old healthy female whose mother had breast cancer and died of ovarian cancer. Also, Karen's sister had breast cancer. This case begins with Karen W. approaching her health care professional to inquire about having a prophylactic oophorectomy.
- **Module 2: Cystic Fibrosis**
  Newborn Jason Harris has symptoms that suggest meconium ileus caused by cystic fibrosis. His elder brother was diagnosed with CF at age 8 months. Jason's parents struggle to come to terms with the realization that their second son might also have inherited the condition.
- **Bipolar Affective Disorder**
  Ruth, a 27-year-old married female with two children ages two and four, has BPAD (Bipolar Affective Disorder), Type 1. She has a significant family history of others who are similarly affected. In the past, Ruth's health care and social services, including the diagnosis, management, monitoring, and acceptance of her condition have been mostly unsuccessful.

Core competencies from the National Coalition for Health Professional Education in Genetics and other sources were used to guide case report learning objec-

Source: Family as Context for Clinical Genetics Project (FCCGP). Funded by NJH, ELSI Division: 1 R25 HG02259-01A1, Final Report.

tives, content development, and evaluation. The case reports, and their pre- and post-test questions and answers, were developed by content experts and reviewed and validated by practicing health care professionals. Throughout each module, learners have an opportunity to integrate into patient/family care genetic scientific information with family, environmental, behavioral, psychosocial, ethical, legal, and financial knowledge.

FCCG curriculum provides health care professionals (HCPs) with a step-by-step process needed to deliver basic genetic services and/or refer patients and families to genetic health care professionals. This "how-to" approach, coupled with download-able tools and continuing education credits for physicians and nurses, provides practical information to HCPs and encourages them to integrate genetics into their every-day practice. The FCCG curriculum is accessible at: http://ce.nursing.ouhsc.edu/fccg/registernew.htm.

FCCG Curriculum Evaluation

Initial evaluation data to date have been positive (See Appendix A: Module 1-3 Evaluation). Future strategies are to market the curriculum to a broader audience of health care professionals and gather additional evaluation data to make appropriate modification of the curriculum modules.

Lessons Learned

A significant challenge faced in the FCCGP was maintaining long-term stability of the project. Fostering long-term stability of a project is a challenge when there are unexpected changes in project staff and funding is limited to a relatively short period of time. Project staff changes and Web-based projects may take at least four to five years to get written, programmed, polished, pilot tested, and evaluated. A truly inter-active curriculum just from a programming standpoint is labor intensive. Critical next steps for the FCCGP is the need to market CNE and CME on UIC and OU Web sites and to expand marketing of Web-based curricula on NCHPEG and ELSI Web sites (i.e., specifying that modules can be incorporated into nursing and medical programs as well as used in in-services for practicing physicians and nurses).

Other lessons learned concerned the attempt to build in good learner evaluation patterns; however, in testing the first module the learners/pilot testers stated the module was too cumbersome, too labor intensive, and not intuitive. The tracking was dropped, and more emphasis was placed on user-friendly materials that can be easily followed. Scenarios were shortened and the family practice/genetic counselor used his expertise from other projects to test these changes with a colleague. The changes were viewed as positive. However, his experience with other projects was that physicians unless paid would not take time to use the modules.

Recommendations

Integrating genetics and genetic services into the daily practice of HCPs continues to be one of the greatest challenges of professional genetics education. From what we have learned the next steps are to assess strategies for measuring the impact of Web-based curricula on professional's behaviors, attitudes, and patient outcomes, yet there are not really strong measures. In addition, there is a need to obtain ongoing needs assessment data from health professionals regarding current genetics knowledge and its application to daily practice, yet is an area often neglected.

Publications and Presentations

Feetham, S., Knisley, M., Spreen-Parker, R. Gallo, A., & Kenner, C. (December, 2002). Families and Genetics: Bridging the Gap Between Knowledge and Practice, *Newborn and Infant Nursing Review* 2:247-253.

Bashook, P. G., Hruska, L. Spreen-Parker, R., Kenner, C., & Cummings, S. (2002). Teaching clinical genetics through the family context. A web-based curriculum. Poster presented at the International Society of Nurses in Genetics Annual Conference. Baltimore, MD. October 13, 2002.

Bashook, P.G., & Hruska, L. (2003). A metacognitive theoretical framework and instrument for constructing case-based simulations. Paper presented at the American Educational Research Association Annual Meeting, Chicago, IL. April 21-25, 2003.

Bashook, P.G., & Hruska, L. (2003). A theory-based authoring tool for constructing case-based branching simulations. Paper presentation at the Association of American Medical Colleges' Conference on Research in Medical Education, Washington, DC. November 9-13, 2003.

Kenner, C., Fineman, R., & Parker, R. Family as Context in Clinical Genetics Project. Poster for 55th Annual meeting of the Genetic Counseling and Clinical Testing, Salt Lake City, UT, September, 2005.

Kenner, C., Spreen-Parker, R., Fineman, R., Cummings, S., Michela, M., Bashook, P., Hruska, L., Swift-Scanlan, T., Olsen, S., Gallo, A., Savage, T., Knisley, M., Feetham, S., Chang, Y.T., Finkelman, A., Boyer, S., & Siow, D. Family as context in clinical genetics project (FCCP): An interactive web-based curriculum, genetics information Resource, & continuing education program for HCPs & students. 55th Annual meeting of the Genetic Counseling and Clinical Testing, Salt Lake City, UT, September 2005.

Kenner, C., Spreen-Parker, R., Fineman, R., Cummings, S., Michela, M., Bashook, P., Hruska, L., Swift-Scanlan, T., Olsen, S., Gallo, A., Savage, T., Knisley, M., Feetham, S., Chang, Y.T., Finkelman, A., Boyer, S., & Siow, D. Family as context in clinical genetics project (FCCP): An interactive web-based curriculum, genetics information Resource, & continuing education program for HCPs & students. Poster presented at the *Annual Pacific Nursing Research Conference—"Nursing Research: Defining Best Practices,"* Honolulu, HI, February 24-26, 2006.

Kenner, C., Parker, R., & Fineman, R. Family as Context in Clinical Genetics Project (FCCGP): An Interactive Web-Based Curriculum, Genetic Information Resource, and Continuing Education and Program for Health Professionals (HCPs) and Students. Poster for presentation at 10th International Nursing Research Conference, Madrid, Spain, November 2006.

Specific Aims:

1. Train 75 practicing nurses, 75 physicians, 75 nursing, and 75 medical students to integrate genetic principles into their clinical practices.

Demographics:

Module 1:   Breast and Ovarian Cancer

Status	Nurses	Nsg Students	ARNP	Nurse Midwife
Total n=8	N=4 (50%)	n=1 (12.5%)	n=1 (12.5%)	n=2 (25%)
Organization	University	Health Dept	Hospital	Missing data
Total n=8	CON N=4 (50%)	n=1 (12.5%)	n=1 (12.5%)	n=2 (25%)

Module 2:   Cystic Fibrosis

Status	CNM	Nurse	Midwife
Total n=5	N=2 (40%)	n=2 (40%)	n=1 (20%)
Organization	University CON	Missing data	
Total n=5	n=3 (60%)	n=2 (40%)	

Module 3:   Bipolar Affective Disorder

Status	CNM	Nurse
Total n=6	N=2 (33.3%)	n=2 (33.3%)
Organization	University CON	Self-employed
Total n=6	n=1 (16.6%)	n=1 (16.6%)

The first year of the grant was devoted to writing the first module then pilot testing it. During the second year we recruited and enrolled students. We had many technical difficulties and then lost a key person in the IT staff that slowed progress down. In addition we had problems with access for participants. The project director moved and assumed a new job—moved the Web server to new site and replaced the IT staff to fix the site. Well over two years into the project the second and then third modules were developed. The recruitment was a challenge as faculty stated the modules did not fit easily into the curriculum or the students were too busy to use them. The advanced practice nurses most interested in the modules (i.e., midwives) did not want to use the materials unless they could earn CMEs—the cost was prohibitive once the CME approved course status was lost with the PI's move. The modules were modified up until the end of the project based on feedback from faculty and students—primarily nursing.

2. Test the effectiveness of the Clinical Integration Model (CIM) curriculum model on the practicing nurses, physicians, nursing students, and medical students. Hypothesis: We will demonstrate that health professionals have improved their knowledge, skills, and attitudes about: (a) the importance of the role of family in genetics; and (b) the significance of the integration of the knowledge of gene function in practice.

The sample size to date is too small to do any meaningful evaluation of this aspect of the grant. However the short-term evaluations were positive. As noted by the post-test results.

3. Evaluate the project to determine: (a) learner feedback; (b) the continued accuracy and effectiveness of the CIM and curriculum; (c) the effectiveness of our method for curriculum delivery (the Web); and (d) the exportability and expandability of the curriculum to other users and settings.

As demonstrated in the appendix, the feedback to date on the content in general was positive and accurate. It was suggested by midwives that these modules be offered for CME. Other suggestions by users were to have the modules available for faculty use to drop into existing academic courses.

Final Report - Appendix A
Module 1-3 Evaluation

Module #1: Breast and Ovarian Cancer Evaluation

1. As a result of this program, I feel I have achieved the following objective: Assess hereditary susceptibility for breast and ovarian cancer using pedigrees and genetic testing information.

   To a Great Extent   63%
   To a Moderate Extent   37%

2. As a result of this program, I feel I have achieved the following objective: Interpret statistical information necessary to analyze hereditary susceptibility for BRCA1 and BRCA2.

   To a Great Extent   25%
   To a Moderate Extent   75%

3. As a result of this program, I feel I have achieved the following objective: Describe the process for identifying the signs and symptoms of breast and ovarian cancer, analyzing cancer risk with and without genetic testing, providing psychological support, and health care options available to mutation and nonmutation carriers in families.

   To a Great Extent   50%
   To a Moderate Extent   50%

4. As a result of this program, I feel I have achieved the following objective: Discuss the potential impact of genetic testing on families.

   To a Great Extent   50%
   To a Moderate Extent   38%
   Unanswered   12%

5. As a result of this program, I feel I have achieved the following objective: Recognize the ethical, legal, financial, and emotional issues that impact families when discussing genetic testing.

   To a Great Extent   50%
   To a Moderate Extent   38%
   To a Slight Extent   12%

6. As a result of this program, I feel I have achieved the following objective: Assess one's own professional expertise and knowledge of hereditary can-

cer syndromes and collaborate with appropriate health providers to obtain information, advice, and referrals.

To a Great Extent	62%
To a Moderate Extent	38%

7. Did you find that the quiz questions truly tested your knowledge of course content?

Excellent	25%
Good	62%
Fair	13%

8. Did you find that the quiz feedback augmented the content and added to learning?

Good to Excellent	100%

9. Was the organization of the content logical in sequence?

Good to Excellent	100%

10. Were you able to move around within the curriculum with ease?

Good to Excellent	75%
Fair	25%

11. Were the instructions easy to follow?

Good to Excellent	100%

12. Was presentation of the material attractive?

Good to Excellent	75%
Fair	25%

13. Did the curriculum material engage you and lure you on to the next section?

Good to Excellent	75%
Fair	25%

14. Was the curriculum informative?

Good to Excellent	100%

15. How successful was the module in helping you think about integrating genetics in a family context into your practice?

Very successful to somewhat successful	88%
Unanswered	12%

Module #2:   Cystic Fibrosis Evaluation

1. As a result of this program, I feel I have achieved the following objective: Discuss the importance of including genetic principles of autosomal recessive inheritance, and the use of family health and social history information, to diagnose and treat patients with autosomal recessive conditions like cystic fibrosis, phenylketonuria, the sickle cell anemias, etc.

To a Great Extent	20%
To a Moderate Extent	60%
To a Slight Extent	20%

2. As a result of this program, I feel I have achieved the following objective: Discuss genetic risk and risk factors as they relate to autosomal recessive inheritance and resulting clinical conditions like cystic fibrosis (CF), phenylketonuria (PKU), the sickle cell anemias (SCA), e.g., indications of a hereditary risk, genetic risk discussion, and implications for carriers, both children and adults.

To a Great Extent	40%
To a Moderate Extent	40%
To a Slight Extent	20%

3. As a result of this program, I feel I have achieved the following objective: Apply the "family as context of care" to clinical situations involving autosomal recessive inheritance, e.g., (a) encourage participation of the entire extended family for comprehensive evaluation and treatment; (b) parents feeling angry, defective, depressed, anxious, etc.; (c) blame, starting with self, and extending to other family members and to health care professionals; and (d) the changed family (a child with a significant handicap can alter relationships among members of the family for the rest of their lives, i.e., a crisis that can split families).

To a Great Extent	60%
To a Moderate Extent	40%

4. As a result of this program, I feel I have achieved the following objective: Identify, in their role as health care and social services professionals, key financial, ethical, legal, and social issues regarding genetics, genetic testing, and genetic counseling, and referral to genetic services in clinical situations involving autosomal recessive inheritance, including utilization of genetic testing and its impact on patient/family health

care management, e.g., (a) discrimination, insurance issues, informed consent, privacy, confidentiality, patient autonomy; (b) the obligation of a health care professional to manage the immediate and extended family; (c) the professional's role in the referral to genetic services or the provision, follow-up, and quality review of genetic services; and (d) religious, ethnic, and cultural factors/issues that can affect decision making, especially in terminating a pregnancy or using birth control, etc.

To a Great Extent	60%
To a Moderate Extent	40%

5. As a result of this program, I feel I have achieved the following objective: Identify high-quality resources available to help health professionals when caring for families with autosomal recessive conditions, i.e., know what credible resources exist and where to find them, e.g., the Internet, government and private nonprofit sources, and professional organizations.

To a Great Extent	40%
To a Moderate Extent	40%
Unanswered	20%

6. Did you find that the post-test questions truly tested your knowledge of course content?

Good to excellent	80%
Fair	20%

7. Was the organization of the content logical in sequence?

Good to Excellent	100%

8. Were you able to move around within the curriculum with ease?

Good to Excellent	80%
Fair	20%

9. Were the instructions easy to follow?

Good to Excellent	100%

10. Was presentation of the material attractive?		
Good to Excellent		100%

11. Did the curriculum material engage you and lure you on to the next section?		
Good to Excellent		100%

12. Was the curriculum informative?		
Good to Excellent		80%
Fair		20%

13. How successful was the module in helping you think about integrating genetics in a family context into your practice?		
Very successful		60%
Somewhat successful		40%

Module #3:   Bipolar Affective Disorder Evaluation

1. As a result of this program, I feel I have achieved the following objective: Identify genetic, environmental, and other BPAD risk and protective factors, including their influence on phenotypic expression.		
To a Great Extent		20%
To a Moderate Extent		80%

2. As a result of this program, I feel I have achieved the following objective: Distinguish the prevalence and lifetime risk of BPAD and recurrent major depression in the general population and in families with a first-degree relative(s) with BPAD.		
To a Great Extent		40%
To a Moderate Extent		60%

3. As a result of this program, I feel I have achieved the following objective: Identify a process for obtaining a comprehensive psychiatric genetic history, for constructing a pedigree and/or genogram, and for utilizing reliable and valid clinical assessment tools.		

To a Great Extent	20%
To a Moderate Extent	60%
Slight Extent	20%

4. As a result of this program, I feel I have achieved the following objective: Identify appropriate ways of diagnosing and the pharmacological and nonpharmacological methods of treating BPAD and recurrent major depression, within a family context.

| Moderate Extent | 100% |

5. As a result of this program, I feel I have achieved the following objective: Recognize the impact of the suspected or confirmed diagnosis and treatment of individuals with BPAD on family and communal dynamics including, but not limited to, financial, ethical, legal/policy, and psychosocial issues.

| To a Great Extent | 80% |
| Slight Extent | 20% |

6. As a result of this program, I feel I have achieved the following objective: Evaluate one's (i.e., a professional's) expertise in regard to obtaining a psychiatric family history, health assessment, and management of BPAD; knowing about the genetic underpinnings of BPAD; and determining when it is appropriate to refer patients and families to other health care, social services, and/or other professionals.

To a Great Extent	40%
To a Moderate Extent	40%
Slight Extent	20%

7. As a result of this program, I feel I have achieved the following objective: Identify information and resources available to help health care and other professionals in working with patients and families with BPAD including, for example, participation in research projects.

To a Great Extent	40%
To a Moderate Extent	40%
Slight Extent	20%

8. Did you find that the post-test questions truly tested your knowledge of course content?

Good to Excellent	100%

9. Was the organization of the content logical in sequence?

Good to Excellent	100%

10. Were you able to move around within the curriculum with ease?

Good to Excellent	100%

11. Were the instructions easy to follow?

Good to Excellent	100%

12. Was presentation of the material attractive?

Good to Excellent	60%
Fair	20%
Unanswered	20%

13. Did the curriculum material engage you and lure you on to the next section?

Good to Excellent	80%
Fair	20%

14. Was the curriculum informative?

Good to Excellent	80%
Fair	20%

15. How successful was the module in helping you think about integrating genetics in a family context into your practice?

Very successful	40%
Somewhat successful	60%

SAMPLES FROM NIH GRANT APPLICATION FORM SF242

Cover Sheet

Senior/Key Person Profile

Research & Related Budget—Section A & B, Budget Period 1

Research & Related Budget—Cumulative Budget

R&R Subaward Budget Attachment(s) Form

PORTION OF A GRANT SUMMARY STATEMENT (FORMERLY KNOWN AS THE PINK SHEET)

SUMMARY STATEMENT

Principal Investigator: Dr. Marlene Walden

Project Title: "Modulation of Neonatal Pain by Intensive Care Unit Environment and Sleep State"

This study is a partial replication of a previous study (Walden, 1997) that measured premature infant responses to heelsticks using the PIPP and several physiological measures similar to those proposed in this pilot. The investigator wishes to repeat the study using better measures of NICU sound and light. The relationship between quality of sleep, environmental factors, and infant's responses to pain are clinical relevant. Knowledge concerning these relationships in adults cannot be automatically transposed on premature infants.

(Reviewer #1): The background, theoretical basis, and review of literature (including prior work by the investigators) are nicely presented, extensive, and relevant. The lack of significant findings in the 1997 study was attributed to a sample size (N=11) that was too small; yet the sample size proposed for this study is the same (N=13-2 lost to attrition=11). The title of this pilot is somewhat misleading in that this study will not test cause-effect relationships between environment and sleep upon pain. Instead, this study proposes to examine relationships among behavioral and physiological responses to acute procedural pain with light and noise in the ICU and the infant's sleep stages 24 hours prior to the painful procedure. There are no comparisons between infants with different light/dark experiences or with different levels of environmental sound. Rather, a naturalistic design will be used wherein any differences in lighting or noise that occur in the natural course of events during each infant's stay in the NICU will be recorded and examined together with ongoing recordings of infant physiology, REM, and state variables to see if any relationships exist. The instruments are clearly described and their validity and reliability (stability) are addressed. The table that describes all variables and the time line for repeated measures is valuable. This table shows that five physiological measures and REM State, NICU noise, and NICU light, will be measured for the 24 hours prior to 4 heelsticks occurring at 28, 30, 32, and 34 weeks of postconceptional age. Some variables will be measured continuously, some at specified intervals. For a total of 20 minutes that include time prior to, during, and after each heelstick, ten PIPP scores of the infant will be recorded.

This will produce rather "dense" quantitative data for eleven infants. Given this information, the methods for data analysis are unclear. Relationships between physiological measures and state will be examined using correlational methods. This is reasonable, except that plans for treating the continuously measured physiological variables are not delineated, except to say that they would be categorized somehow.

Furthermore, it is unclear whether these contingency tables would be constructed intraindividually or interindividually.

Since each infant will have data collected for the 24 hours prior to several heel-stick episodes, pooling all data together for the contingency tables means that each infant would be counted four times. For the second and third research questions, all the biobehavioral infant measures and all the measures of NICU noise and light levels that were obtained in the preceding 24 hours will be compared to the PIPP scores per heelstick episode per infant. It is difficult to envision how this would be accomplished. The PIPP scores change over time before, during, and after the heelstick. Ten PIPP scores will be obtained per infant per heelstick episode. The data analysis description speaks of a single PIPP score as the dependent variable. It is unclear which of the ten PIPP scores would be chosen as the single dependent variable for these RMANOVAs.

Furthermore, it is difficult to visualize a two-level (age, PIPP) RMANOVA involving several hundred measures of a single ICU (noise, light) or infant (physiological or sleep or state) variable for eleven infants. If some type of times series analysis, using RMANOVA, is planned, it is not described as such. If some sort of data reduction is planned for the measurements obtained for 24 hours, this is not clearly described either. Finally, there is not provision made for correcting the alphas given that at least nine RMANOVAs will be run. This project will use consulting services from both the biobehavioral and data management and analysis cores.

(Reviewer #2): The significance of the study is well documented in the literature review and the study is relevant to the Center. The design is appropriate. The sample size calculation is based on the literature described and validity and reliability of the instruments addressed with the exception of the physiological measures. Several of these measures appear to be clinical measures such as the NONB, NBS, the NTISS, and the Als State Scoring System. Are these tools sensitive enough to detect differences in change over time so that they might be used in an intervention study? If, as the author describes, these neonates have frequent invasive procedures, how will the investigators be able to observe "normal" sleep wake patterns in the 24 hours prior to the heelstick? A data collection protocol is provided and helpful. Will the assumptions of the ANOVA be met with the quasi-experimental design?

Investigators: The Principal and Co-Investigators appear well qualified, by virtue of previous research experience, to conduct this study. Dr. Walden has done previous research involving the same variables and research questions as this pilot.

Human Subjects: Issues are not addressed for this Pilot. Presumably, the cover statement for the entire grant proposal that all proposals will obtain IRB approval and minorities will be included applies here.

Gender/Minorities/Children: Since this study deals with premature infants, the exclusion of older subjects is scientifically acceptable. Provisions for equal representation by gender and ethnic minority are not described.

Budget: Expenses seem reasonable. The budget is recommended as requested.
Action: The pilot is scored in the good to very good range.

Source: Summary Statement prepared by the Scientific Review Administrator of the Initial Review Group for National Institute of Nursing Research (NINR). The comments refer to an evaluation of one of the three pilot/feasibility studies within a Center Grant application submitted May, 1999.

Note on next step after scientific review—An R15 (AREA) grant was submitted to NINR in September 2000 using recommendations provided in this Summary Statement. Specific changes included title, increased sample size, and description of plans for inclusion of gender and ethnic minorities. Additionally, extensive revisions were made in the data analyses section to address reviewer concerns.

Grant Application Process Planning Tool (GAPPT)

Preliminary Development

Event/Action	Suggested Deadline
• Decide on problem of interest. • Define/specify variables of concern. • Start literature search and retrieval. Contract staff to set up research and retrieval services. • Meet with staff to arrange funding search if necessary.	6 to 8 months prior
• PI (and coinvestigators, if appropriate) to meet with Associate Dean/Director and staff to plan grant application process and support to be provided.	6 months prior
• Complete literature search and retrieval.	5 to 6 months prior

• Meet with staff to identify and schedule (add to Process Planning Tool):
  • external and internal proposal reviews,
  • availability/appropriateness of templates, boilerplates, and forms and
  • **deadlines** for application development/ assembly.	

• Write 1 to 2 page precis (an abbreviated version) outlining project significance, long-term goals, specific aims (if possible), population(s), human subject involvement, and tentative time line. • Begin process of identifying 3 to 4 well-known experts in content and methods areas as (1) potential proposal reviewers, and/or (2) consultants.	5 months prior

• Use precis as basis for meetings with clinical agencies, community groups agencies, etc. in arranging access to subjects/support. If appropriate/relevant:
  • Offer template letter of support.
  • Collect information to describe performance site: resources and services to be available.	

Proposal Development and Review

Event/Action	Suggested Deadline
• Change precis to preliminary version of the research plan that includes background and significance, subject access, time line changes, methods summary. • Contact funding agency representative if not already done. Send proposal/precis if requested.	3 to 4 months prior

• Contact external reviewer(s): Obtain agreement and schedule review.
• Select, contact, and obtain agreement from consultants.
  • Discuss roles/responsibilities, periods/methods of contact/support, and reimbursement.
  • Solicit letter of support and modular budget style biosketch, or information to construct one.
• Revise preliminary proposal to full Research Plan (A–D + G at least).
	3 months prior

• Send Research Plan to expert reviewer. • Work with staff and staff who collect specific costs for projected budget items. • Collect letters of support/agreement from agencies and consultants and own school, if appropriate. • Meetings with Director and staff about budget. Complete budget worksheet for staff, who will begin preparing the detailed budget. • Discuss faculty buyout(s) with chairperson(s).	2 to 3 months prior

• Staff follow-up (if necessary) to collect biosketch information for all key personnel. **Deadline for all CVs that need to be converted to biosketch format/template.** • Revise Research Plan on the basis of external reviewer comment. Add sections E, H, and I. • Revise Research Plan to internal reviews (2 to 3 weeks prior to review).	2 months prior
• **Deadline for creation of budget spreadsheet (capped budget).** • **Deadline for graphics, complex tables to be created, or instruments to be formatted.** • Internal review of proposal. • See template to prepare budget narrative.	1 month prior
• Finalize title and final changes to personnel. • Finalize Research Plan (A–I) on basis of Internal Review feedback. • Consortial/subcontractual agreements: get required forms and documents from consortial/subcontractual agencies. • Work with staff to finalize budget and budget narrative. Staff will check budget documents with designated school/college and university research office personnel. • Collect appendix material→staff for assembly and copying.	2 weeks to 1 month prior
• Add agency/other site information to Resources boilerplate document and tailor to fit project. • Schedule transmittal signatures of chairperson and deans. • Write abstract→staff for "fit" and revision, if necessary. • Begin work on Institution Review Board protocol, if human subjects are involved.	2 weeks prior

• Deadline for Face Page Information. • Deadline for Final version abstract (Form BB). • Deadline for Resources document. • Deadline for final Research Plan (A–I) to be formatted by staff. • Deadline for Budget Justification.	1 week prior
• Deadline for Transmittal Form information. • Deadline for Checklist information. • Deadline for appendix materials. • Deadline for Personal Data Form information.	Deadline: 1 week prior
• Final PIs check for all application components, if not previously approved. • Write cover letter on letterhead → staff. • Obtain necessary signatures on Transmittal Form. • Staff will copy the application, and assemble and deliver all materials to the University Research Office.	Deadline: 1 week prior

Source: Used with permission from Crain, H.C., & Broome, M.E. 2000. Tool for planning the grant application process. *Nursing Outlook* 48(6): 288–293.

APPLICATION FOR FEDERAL ASSISTANCE

SF 424 (R&R)

2. DATE SUBMITTED	Applicant Identifier
3. DATE RECEIVED BY STATE	State Application Identifier

1. * TYPE OF SUBMISSION

☐ Pre-application ☐ Application
☐ Changed/Corrected Application

4. Federal Identifier

5. APPLICANT INFORMATION   * Organizational DUNS:

* Legal Name:

Department: Division:

* Street1:   Street2:

* City: County: * State: * ZIP Code:

* Country: USA

Person to be contacted on matters involving this application

Prefix: * First Name: Middle Name: * Last Name: Suffix:

* Phone Number: Fax Number: Email:

6. * EMPLOYER IDENTIFICATION (EIN) or (TIN):

7. * TYPE OF APPLICANT:

Please select one of the following

8. * TYPE OF APPLICATION: ☐ New

☐ Resubmission ☐ Renewal ☐ Continuation ☐ Revision

Other (Specify):

Small Business Organization Type

☐ Women Owned   ☐ Socially and Economically Disadvantaged

If Revision, mark appropriate box(es).

☐ A. Increase Award ☐ B. Decrease Award ☐ C. Increase Duration

☐ D. Decrease Duration ☐ E. Other (specify)

9. * NAME OF FEDERAL AGENCY:

Department of Health and Human Services   Defaults based on
application package
10. CATALOG OF FEDERAL DOMESTIC ASSISTANCE NU downloaded

* Is this application being submitted to other agencies? Yes ☐ No ☐

10.001

What other Agencies?

TITLE: Program Title

11. * DESCRIPTIVE TITLE OF APPLICANT'S PROJECT:
PROJECT TITLE

12. * AREAS AFFECTED BY PROJECT (cities, counties, states, etc.)

13. PROPOSED PROJECT:

* Start Date   * Ending Date

14. CONGRESSIONAL DISTRICTS OF:

a. * Applicant   b. * Project

15. PROJECT DIRECTOR/PRINCIPAL INVESTIGATOR CONTACT INFORMATION

Prefix: * First Name: Middle Name: * Last Name: Suffix:

Position/Title: * Organization Name:

Department: Division:

* Street1:   Street2:

* City: County: * State: * ZIP Code:

* Country: USA

* Phone Number: Fax Number: * Email:

OMB Number: 4040-0001
Expiration Date: 04/30/2008

Source: NIH/National Institute for Nursing Research.

SF 424 (R&R) APPLICATION FOR FEDERAL ASSISTANCE **Page 2**

16. ESTIMATED PROJECT FUNDING	17. * IS APPLICATION SUBJECT TO REVIEW BY STATE EXECUTIVE ORDER 12372 PROCESS?

16. ESTIMATED PROJECT FUNDING

a. * Total Estimated Project Funding

b. * Total Federal & Non-Federal Funds

c. * Estimated Program Income

17. * IS APPLICATION SUBJECT TO REVIEW BY STATE EXECUTIVE ORDER 12372 PROCESS?

a. YES ☐ THIS PREAPPLICATION/APPLICATION WAS MADE AVAILABLE TO THE STATE EXECUTIVE ORDER 12372 PROCESS FOR REVIEW ON:

DATE:

b. NO ☐ PROGRAM IS NOT COVERED BY E.O. 12372; OR

☐ PROGRAM HAS NOT BEEN SELECTED BY STATE FOR REVIEW

18. By signing this application, I certify (1) to the statements contained in the list of certifications* and (2) that the statements herein are true, complete and accurate to the best of my knowledge. I also provide the required assurances * and agree to comply with any resulting terms if I accept an award. I am aware that any false, fictitious, or fraudulent statements or claims may subject me to criminal, civil, or administrative penalties. (U.S. Code, Title 18, Section 1001)

X ☐ * I agree

* The list of certifications and assurances, or an Internet site where you may obtain this list, is contained in the announcement or agency specific instructions.

19. Authorized Representative

Prefix: * First Name: Middle Name: * Last Name: Suffix:

* Position/Title:

* Organization:

Department:

Division:

* Street1:

Street2:

* City:

County:

* State:

* ZIP Code:

* Country: USA

* Phone Number:

Fax Number:

* Email:

* Signature of Authorized Representative

Completed on submission to Grants.gov

* Date Signed

Completed on submission to Grants.gov

20. Pre-application

Add Attachment   Delete Attachment   View Attachment

OMB Number: 4040-0001

Expiration Date: 04/30/2008

Source: NIH/National Institute for Nursing Research.

RESEARCH & RELATED Other Project Information

1. * Are Human Subjects Involved?   ☐ Yes   ☐ No

1.a   If YES to Human Subjects

Is the IRB review Pending?   ☐ Yes   ☐ No

IRB Approval Date: ☐

Exemption Number: ☐1 ☐2 ☐3 ☐4 ☐5 ☐6

Human Subject Assurance Number: ☐

2. * Are Vertebrate Animals Used?   ☐ Yes   ☐ No

2.a.   If YES to Vertebrate Animals

Is the IACUC review Pending?   ☐ Yes   ☐ No

IACUC Approval Date: ☐

Animal Welfare Assurance Number ☐

3. * Is proprietary/privileged information included in the application?   ☐ Yes   ☐ No

4.a. * Does this project have an actual or potential impact on the environment?   ☐ Yes   ☐ No

4.b. If yes, please explain: ☐

4.c. If this project has an actual or potential impact on the environment, has an exemption been authorized or an environmental assessment (EA) or environmental impact statement (EIS) been performed?   ☐ Yes   ☐ No

4.d. If yes, please explain: ☐

5.a. * Does this project involve activities outside the U.S. or partnership with International Collaborators?   ☐ Yes   ☐ No

5.b. If yes, identify countries: ☐

5.c. Optional Explanation: ☐

6. * Project Summary/Abstract ☐   [Add Attachment] [Delete Attachment] [View Attachment]

7. * Project Narrative ☐   [Add Attachment] [Delete Attachment] [View Attachment]

8. Bibliography & References Cited ☐   [Add Attachment] [Delete Attachment] [View Attachment]

9. Facilities & Other Resources ☐   [Add Attachment] [Delete Attachment] [View Attachment]

10. Equipment ☐   [Add Attachment] [Delete Attachment] [View Attachment]

11. Other Attachments   [Add Attachments] [Delete Attachments] [View Attachments] ☐

OMB Number: 4040-0001
Expiration Date: 04/30/2008

Source: NIH/National Institute for Nursing Research.

RESEARCH & RELATED Senior/Key Person Profile

PROFILE - Project Director/Principal Investigator

Prefix	* First Name	Middle Name	* Last Name	Suffix

Position/Title: Department:

Organization Name: Division:

* Street1:   Street2:

* City: County: * State: * Zip Code: * Country:

* Phone Number	Fax Number	* E-Mail

Credential, e.g., agency login:

* Project Role: PD/PI   **Other Project Role Category:**

*Attach Biographical Sketch		Add Attachment	Delete Attachment	View Attachment
Attach Current & Pending Support		Add Attachment	Delete Attachment	View Attachment

PROFILE - Senior/Key Person 1

Prefix	* First Name	Middle Name	* Last Name	Suffix

Position/Title: Department:

Organization Name: Division:

* Street1:   Street2:

* City: County: * State: * Zip Code: * Country: USA

* Phone Number	Fax Number	* E-Mail

Credential, e.g., agency login:

* Project Role: **Other Project Role Category:**

*Attach Biographical Sketch		Add Attachment	Delete Attachment	View Attachment
Attach Current & Pending Support		Add Attachment	Delete Attachment	View Attachment

Reset Entry   Next Person

ADDITIONAL SENIOR/KEY PERSON PROFILE(S) | Add Attachment | Delete Attachment | View Attachment

Additional Biographical Sketch(es) (Senior/Key Person) | Add Attachment | Delete Attachment | View Attachment

Additional Current and Pending Support(s) | Add Attachment | Delete Attachment | View Attachment

OMB Number: 4040-0001

Expiration Date: 04/30/2008

Source: NIH/National Institute for Nursing Research.

RESEARCH & RELATED Project/Performance Site Location(s)

Project/Performance Site Primary Location

Organization Name:

* Street1:   Street2:

* City: County: * State: * ZIP Code: * Country:

Project/Performance Site Location   1

Organization Name:

* Street1:   Street2:

* City: County: * State: * ZIP Code: * Country:

Reset Entry   Next Site

Additional Location(s)   Add Attachment   Delete Attachment   View Attachment

OMB Number: 4040-0001
Expiration Date: 04/30/2008

Source: NIH/National Institute for Nursing Research.

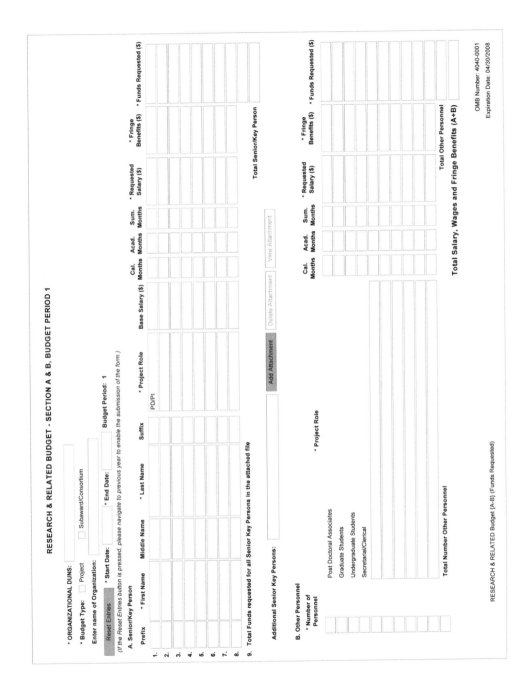

Source: NIH/National Institute for Nursing Research.

RESEARCH & RELATED BUDGET - SECTION C, D, & E, BUDGET PERIOD 1

* ORGANIZATIONAL DUNS:

* Budget Type: ☐ Project   ☐ Subaward/Consortium

Enter name of Organization:

[Reset Entries]   * Start Date: * End Date: Budget Period: 1

(If the Reset Entries button is pressed, please navigate to previous year to enable the submission of the

C. Equipment Description

List items and dollar amount for each item exceeding $5,000

Equipment item	* Funds Requested ($)
1.	
2.	
3.	
4.	
5.	
6.	
7.	
8.	
9.	
10.	

11. Total funds requested for all equipment listed in the attached file

Total Equipment

Additional Equipment: [Add Attachment] [Delete Attachment] [View Attachment]

D. Travel   Funds Requested ($)

1. Domestic Travel Costs (Incl. Canada, Mexico and U.S. Possessions)

2. Foreign Travel Costs

Total Travel Cost

E. Participant/Trainee Support Costs   Funds Requested ($)

1. Tuition/Fees/Health Insurance

2. Stipends

3. Travel

4. Subsistence

5. Other

Number of Participants/Trainees   Total Participant/Trainee Support Costs

RESEARCH & RELATED Budget {C-E} (Funds Requested)

OMB Number: 4040-0001
Expiration Date: 04/30/2008

Source: NIH/National Institute for Nursing Research.

RESEARCH & RELATED BUDGET - SECTION F-K, BUDGET PERIOD 1   Next Period

* ORGANIZATIONAL DUNS:

* Budget Type: ☐ Project   ☐ Subaward/Consortium

Enter name of Organization:

Reset Entries   * Start Date: * End Date: Budget Period: 1

(If the Reset Entries button is pressed, please navigate to previous year to enable the submission of the

F. Other Direct Costs	Funds Requested ($)
1. Materials and Supplies	
2. Publication Costs	
3. Consultant Services	
4. ADP/Computer Services	
5. Subawards/Consortium/Contractual Costs	
6. Equipment or Facility Rental/User Fees	
7. Alterations and Renovations	
8.	
9.	
10.	
Total Other Direct Costs	

G. Direct Costs   Funds Requested ($)

Total Direct Costs (A thru F)

H. Indirect Costs

Indirect Cost Type	Indirect Cost Rate (%)	Indirect Cost Base ($)	* Funds Requested ($)
1.			
2.			
3.			
4.			
Total Indirect Costs			

Cognizant Federal Agency
(Agency Name, POC Name, and POC Phone Number)

I. Total Direct and Indirect Costs   Funds Requested ($)

Total Direct and Indirect Institutional Costs (G + H)

J. Fee   Funds Requested ($)

K. * Budget Justification   Add Attachment   Delete Attachment   View Attachment
(Only attach one file.)

OMB Number: 4040-0001
Expiration Date: 04/30/2008

RESEARCH & RELATED Budget {F-K} (Funds Requested)

Source: NIH/National Institute for Nursing Research.

RESEARCH & RELATED BUDGET - Cumulative Budget

Totals ($)

Section A, Senior/Key Person

Section B, Other Personnel

Total Number Other Personnel

Total Salary, Wages and Fringe Benefits (A+B)

Section C, Equipment

Section D, Travel

1. Domestic

2. Foreign

Section E, Participant/Trainee Support Costs

1. Tuition/Fees/Health Insurance

2. Stipends

3. Travel

4. Subsistence

5. Other

6. Number of Participants/Trainees

Section F, Other Direct Costs

1. Materials and Supplies

2. Publication Costs

3. Consultant Services

4. ADP/Computer Services

5. Subawards/Consortium/Contractual Costs

6. Equipment or Facility Rental/User Fees

7. Alterations and Renovations

8. Other 1

9. Other 2

10. Other 3

Section G, Direct Costs (A thru F)

Section H, Indirect Costs

Section I, Total Direct and Indirect Costs (G + H)

Section J, Fee

OMB Number: 4040-0001
Expiration Date: 04/30/2008

Source: NIH/National Institute for Nursing Research.

R&R SUBAWARD BUDGET ATTACHMENT(S) FORM

Instructions: On this form, you will attach the R&R Subaward Budget files for your grant application. Complete the subawardee budget(s) in accordance with the R&R budget instructions. Please remember that any files you attach must be a Pure Edge document.

Click here to extract the R&R Subaward Budget Attachment

Important: Please attach your subawardee budget file(s) with the file name of the subawardee organization. Each file name must be unique.

1) Please attach Attachment 1 — Add Attachment | Delete Attachment | View Attachment
2) Please attach Attachment 2 — Add Attachment | Delete Attachment | View Attachment
3) Please attach Attachment 3 — Add Attachment | Delete Attachment | View Attachment
4) Please attach Attachment 4 — Add Attachment | Delete Attachment | View Attachment
5) Please attach Attachment 5 — Add Attachment | Delete Attachment | View Attachment
6) Please attach Attachment 6 — Add Attachment | Delete Attachment | View Attachment
7) Please attach Attachment 7 — Add Attachment | Delete Attachment | View Attachment
8) Please attach Attachment 8 — Add Attachment | Delete Attachment | View Attachment
9) Please attach Attachment 9 — Add Attachment | Delete Attachment | View Attachment
10) Please attach Attachment 10 — Add Attachment | Delete Attachment | View Attachment

OMB Number: 4040-0001
Expiration Date: 04/30/2008

Source: NIH/National Institute for Nursing Research.

Biographical Sketch Form SF424

BIOGRAPHICAL SKETCH

Provide the following information for the key personnel and other significant contributors.

NAME	POSITION TITLE
eRA COMMONS USER NAME	

EDUCATION/TRAINING (*Begin with baccalaureate or other initial professional education, such as nursing, and include postdoctoral training.*)

INSTITUTION AND LOCATION	DEGREE (*if applicable*)	YEAR(s)	FIELD OF STUDY

Please refer to the application instructions in order to complete sections A, B, and C of the Biographical Sketch.

Source: NIH/National Institute for Nursing Research.

Index

Note: Page numbers followed by f denote figures; those followed by t denote tables; and those followed by *f* denote forms.

SUMMARY

Why We Sleep

Matthew Walker

Unlocking the Power of Sleep and Dreams

Speed-Summary

TABLE OF CONTENTS

INTRODUCTION

Thank you for purchasing *"Why We Sleep: Unlocking the Power of Sleep and Dreams"* book summary! If you like the summarized content, please purchase and read the original book for full content!

"Why We Sleep" is a book written by Matthew Walker. In this book, the author writes about what he learned about understanding sleep. Why sleep is important, what causes bad sleep and how the modern world affects our everyday night sleep- all this and much more can be found in this book.

The truth is that great number of people do not sleep well and that there are many things that contribute to bad sleep. Some of the most common contributors to a bad night's sleep are alcohol, caffeine, blue light from smartphones or computers, and others. When we become sleep deprived, we suffer. This means that our entire being suffers. Not just our bodies, but our minds also suffer. Our physical, emotional, and mental capabilities decline drastically. Therefore, Walker writes what we can do in order to eliminate such sleep disruptors in order to enjoy good quality sleep.

SUMMARY

PART 1: THIS THING CALLED SLEEP

CHAPTER 1: INTRODUCTION TO SLEEP

In the first chapter of the book, the author writes that not getting eight hours of sleep can have devastating consequences on our bodies. Moreover, he explains that we no longer value a good night's sleep as we should and that this needs to change. All this causes what the author calls as "sleep-deprivation epidemic."

According to the author, if we consistently fail to get six or seven hours of sleep per day, our immune system will be considerably weakened. Moreover, less than six hours of sleep per day greatly increases our chances of getting cancer, it can increase our blood pressure and can cause the blockage of coronary arteries. Insufficient sleep is also one of the greatest contributors to anxiety and depression. Moreover, if we do not get enough sleep, our bodies will start to release more of the hunger hormone. This will cause us to eat more and thus to gain more weight. Regardless of the fact that in the most Western nations the most preferred solution for the sleep epidemic is sleeping pills, the author disagrees with this as the best solution.

After the first part, the author writes how the lack of sleep can harm us so much, that it can kill us. There are two potential ways a person can die because of lack of sleep. The first way is a rare genetic disease that starts as insomnia. This disease causes a person to stop sleeping completely. The second way is drowsy driving. According to the author, the death of one person per hour is caused by traffic accidents, which are caused by fatigue.

People believe sleep only serves one function, we now know this to be incorrect. It is true that sleep benefits our bodies in numerous ways, such as conserving our energy and recovery. However, according to the author, sleep has many more benefits than just that. Sleep optimizes our learning capacity, our memory, and our emotional composure. Good sleep also improves our immunity, it inspires creativity, prevents infections, controls our appetite, lowers our blood pressure, and much more. The author also discusses that one night of poor sleep is worse than starvation or lack of exercise.

CHAPTER 2: SLEEPING SIGNALS

The author opens this chapter by explaining that humans and plants function in a similar way when it comes to control of their sleep rhythm. Moreover, the author writes that in order for us to get enough sleep, our internal clock needs to know when to send sleep and wake signals. There are two big factors, which influence and maintain sleep-wake cycles of our bodies. These are the circadian clock and the adenosine chemical. The bad thing about our biological clock is that it can be impaired by things like caffeine, jet lag, and melatonin.

After this, the author writes about the meaning of the circadian rhythm. He writes that this is a twenty-four hour rhythm, which determines the sleep-wake cycle of every living creature on this planet. Moreover, this sleep-wake cycle also determines when is it time for eating, what is our core body temperature, our hormones, and our metabolic rate.

The next part of the chapter is about the length of the circadian rhythm. Here Walker writes that without the sunlight, the circadian rhythm is longer than twenty-four hours. This was proven when Professor Kleitman and his assistant Richardson performed an experiment back in 1938. The experiment involved thirty-two days in a Kentucky cave in absolute darkness. During that time spent in the caves, they discovered that their sleep-wake cycle was much longer that they previously thought it was.

One of the conclusions when it comes to sleep-wake cycles was that our internal clock has an average cycle of twenty-four hours and fifteen minutes. However, most of us do not live in complete darkness. Since we are regularly exposed to sunlight, our internal clock resets this every day. This means that our circadian clock will run exactly twenty-four hours.

However, regardless of the fact that our circadian rhythm is twenty-four hours, the peak, and trough of the sleep-wake cycle will vary from person to person. This is why some people are morning types, other are the "night owls" and the third group is somewhere in between. Another thing the author deduces is that the society's working structure tends to favor morning types of people. This is why those who don't go to sleep until very late are considered lazy. However, these people are not lazy. They simply respond to their DNA hardwiring.

The next part of the chapter is where the author explains the connection between sleep and adenosine.

Adenosine is a chemical that triggers our brain to fall asleep. When this hormone builds up in our brain, it will create sleep pressure and we will begin to feel drowsy. Adenosine will normally increase after we stay awake between twelve and sixteen hours. However, the effect of adenosine can be blocked by consuming drinks that contain caffeine. Thus, the author argues that too much caffeine (especially seven hours before sleep) will drastically decrease the quality of our sleep and leave our brains tired.

CHAPTER 3: WHAT IS SLEEP?

Here in this chapter, the author writes an elaborate expose on how to identify what the sleep really is. Walker describes the NREM and REM phases of sleep. We also read here how each of these phases serves a special function. According to the author, we are more likely to dream when we are in the latter phases of REM sleep, which means right before we wake up.

How can we tell if someone is asleep? According to Walker, there are five signals, which tell us when a person is sleeping. The first signal a person is sleeping is their body posture. Most of people sleep horizontally. The second sign is a reduction of muscle tone. When we sleep, our skeletal muscles will be relaxed. The third signal is lack of overt response to the external environment. The fourth signal is that we can wake a person. The fifth and final signal is that people who sleep have a reliable sleeping schedule and that they stick to it.

The next part of the chapter is a part in which the author writes about two signals, which prove that we have been asleep. The first signal that a person was sleeping is a loss of external consciousness. This means that if we sleep, we become unaware of things and situations revolving around us. The second sign is that we feel distorted when it comes to time. After we wake up, the first thing we usually do is checking the time to see how long we were sleeping. This proves the fact that when we sleep we lose track of time. However, at the same time, our brains unconsciously catalog time. This is the main reason why people tend to wake up several minutes after their alarm starts ringing.

The next important thing the author discusses is two phases of sleep. The first phase is called NREM and the second is REM. The author explains here that human beings normally cycle between these two phases of sleep several times during the night sleep and that the cycle is characterized by restful eyes and calmness and slow work of brainwaves.

The NREM phase of sleep is mostly dominant in the early stages of sleep (this happens usually between 11 pm and 3 am). The REM phase of sleep is characterized by rapid eye movement and extreme active brain activity. This phase usually happens during the latter stages of sleep (which is typically between 3 am and 7 am). When we do not get enough sleep, we do not allow our brains to clean out old and unnecessary neural connections. Moreover, lack of sleep also prevents our brains from strengthening useful neural connections. In other words, lack of sleep (especially if it is prolonged) causes numerous mental and physical problems.

CHAPTER 4: SLEEP ACROSS SPECIES

The first thing the author tries to explain in this chapter is when exactly sleep emerged in animals. Besides that, the author also tries to explain specific factors why different animals sleep differently. The author deduced that sleep was so important for some animals that when they sleep, they shut down one part of their brains, while other part remains active.

According to Walker, sleep first emerged when life was created on Earth. Studies showed that even worms also sleep.

Even though every living creature on this planet sleeps, not everyone sleeps for the same amount of time. The example of that is elephant, which sleep only four hours per day, while lions sleep for fifteen hours daily. In comparison to that, bats sleep nineteen hours per day. Therefore, the author deduces that the variation in sleep cannot be attributed to body size, predator or prey status or any type of activities living creatures do.

The next part of the chapter is a part where the author explains that every species experiences NREM sleep. However, contrary to that only birds and mammals have REM phase of sleep. The only mammals that do not experience REM are aquatic mammals.

Some of the animals that sleep with their brains half-awake are, for example, dolphins. After one part of their brain had enough sleep, the "awakened" half gets its share of NREM sleep. Birds also sleep with only half of their brains and one eye open to watch out for possible predators.

After this, the author writes that under specific conditions, some animals can even endure sleep deprivation. For example, a mother killer whale will stay awake until they rejoin the rest of the pod. Birds during their migration also stay awake for thousands of miles, only sleeping for a few seconds at a time.

When it comes to humans, the author writes that we are created and designed so that we need to sleep twice per day. This means that we should have a good night sleep and thirty to sixty minutes of sleep in the afternoon. Elimination of afternoon naps increases the possibility of getting cardiovascular diseases and overall shortening of our lifespan.

CHAPTER 5: CHANGES IN SLEEP ACROSS THE LIFESPAN

In chapter 5, the author tries to explain the big differences when it comes to sleep of different age groups. Moreover, the author describes how REM sleep affects the lives of fetuses, adolescents, middle-aged people, and the elderly. The conclusion of this chapter is that anything that interferes with REM phase of sleep will have severe consequences on a person's health.

When it comes to pregnant women, every time a fetus kicks and punches, a logical assumption will be that a fetus is awake. However, the truth is that fetuses spend most of their time sleeping. Every time a woman feels a fetus kick or punch is actually the random arm and leg flick. Those punches and kicks are caused by brain activity, which occurs typically during the REM phase of sleep. The only time a fetus spends two to three hours awake is in the third trimester.

According to some studies, an infant whose REM phase is disturbed will suffer from numerous brain problems. The main reason for this is that infants require REM phases of sleep in order to develop the roof of their cerebral cortex. Moreover, there is evidence of connection between autism and the lack of REM sleep.

The author writes that numerous new parents argue that their children are often sleeping and waking. This happens because during the first three years the circadian rhythm is still not developed. However, when a child turns the age of four, it experiences daytime naps and a nighttime bout of sleep. During their late childhood, children have one long sleep session at night.

The next point the author writes about is why adolescents often behave irrationally. The main reason for this is that their brain is not still fully formed. According to what the author states, when human beings reach the adolescent stage of their life they begin experiencing less REM and more NREM sleep. Moreover, teenagers need longer bouts of NREM sleep to transition into adulthood. Another thing with NREM sleep and teenagers is that the first thing NREM sleep does is that it grows the back of the brain first. This means that the frontal lobe of the brain (the part responsible for rational thinking) matures later.

Contrary to this, elderly people often struggle to sleep. The main reason for this is that their medical conditions worsen and because of this, they need to take medication. The author discovered that by the time a person reaches seventy years of life, he or she will have lost almost ninety percent of her (or his) deep sleep ability. The result of this is further deterioration of health.

PART 2: WHY SHOULD YOU SLEEP?

CHAPTER 6: BENEFITS OF SLEEP

This chapter begins with the author's statement that many people are ignorant of the great benefits that sleep has on our health. One of the reasons for our ignorance is poor public education. As result of this, people become proud when they have very little sleep. However, the importance of good sleep is more than evident. Furthermore, sleep is crucial for all forms of learning, memorizing, and creativity. One of the most commonly ignored functions of sleep is to help us forget specific memories.

When we are awake, our brains learn by collecting and storing information. Our hippocampus acts as a short-term memory reservoir. One thing about the hippocampus is that it has a limited storage capacity. This means that we cannot add more information. The only thing we can do is to overwrite old information. After this, the author explains how sleep gives our brains the ability to transfer our memories from hippocampus to the cortex. The cortex is something like the hard disk of our bodies – it has the ability to storage information for a long time. When our information is stored in our cortex, our hippocampus becomes free, thus has more room for creating new memories. This means that taking a nap before learning something will give us the edge over those who do not want to sleep before learning.

One of the most important functions of sleep is storing information we have recently learned. Every time we sleep, our brains further enhance our memory by up to forty percent, regardless of the type of information we just learned.

Research shows that sleep can improve many types of motor skills, regardless of what those skills actually are. The author explains that the spinal cord and patients suffering from stroke can gradually recover their motor functions by getting enough sleep.

CHAPTER 7: IMPACTS OF SLEEP DEPRIVATION

Here Walker provides evidence on how dangerous sleep deprivation can be to our health. Not getting enough sleep can (and will) have devastating and severe effects on our brains and bodies.

The first thing that happens when sleep deprivation takes effect is that we quickly lose brain function. One of the most dangerous consequences is drowsy driving. This is why accidents in traffic occur. When a person starts sleeping for several seconds, thus losing all motor functions, he or she loses all connection to the conscious world. These several seconds are more than enough to drift into the wrong lane or to cause a crash with severe consequences.

Another thing about sleep deprivation is that we can never know what level of our sleep deprivation is. When we are sleep deprived for months or even years, we gradually accept the consequences of this as something normal. Not long after that, people become accustomed to energy loss, lower alertness, and worse physical performance.

When it comes to the media and sleep, the media constantly pushes that a twenty-minute power nap is enough to make up for sleep insufficiency. The author says that is not true. The fact is that a power nap can help us boost our concentration for a few hours when we are fatigued. However, it will not help us when it comes to decision-making, learning, and reasoning capacity.

One more thing sleep deprivation can cause is emotional irritability. Infants who do not sleep well often scream more than they usually would if they had enough sleep. When we are sleep deprived, our amygdala becomes reactive. This means that we become unable to balance our positive and negative emotions. Not getting enough sleep is also connected with aggression, pleasure seeking, doing risky activities, depression, and many types of addictions.

CHAPTER 8: WHAT ARE LONG-TERM CONSEQUENCES?

The author believes that if we want to have a healthy life we need to have good sleep. Moreover, the author argues that good sleep is more important than a good diet and exercise. This means that if we focus on exercise and diet but we are sleep deprived, we will not be able to achieve the desired results. Some test results proved that sleep deprivation is so powerful that it can change our DNA.

Some studies even confirm that sleep deprivation causes a shorter lifespan. Sleep shorter than six hours per day drastically increases the risk of cardiac failure up to forty-five percent. The author also deduces that the effect of sleep deprivation becomes bigger as we approach mid-life.

The second part of this chapter is about the connection between diabetes and sleep deprivation. The author states that sleep deprived people have blood cells that refuse to follow the instructions issued by insulin. This means that instead of cleaning up the excess glucose the cells actually repel it. Moreover, chronic sleep deprivation can put a person in a pre-diabetic state and can contribute to Type 2 diabetes.

Another thing sleep deprivation is connected to, is weight gain.

People gain weight when there is an imbalance in the function of leptin and ghrelin hormones. According to studies, sleep deprived people have decreased levels of leptin (the hormone that tells our bodies we are not hungry) while at the same time levels of ghrelin drastically increase.

Sleep deprivation can also cause lower virility and fertility. When a male person sleeps less than seven or eight hours per day for a prolonged period, his testosterone level will drop significantly. The same goes for women.

The strength of our immune system also depends on how much we sleep. Every time we are sick, our bodies are trying to get us to go to sleep. The author states that one night of sleep loss will take the immunity from our bodies. The less sleep we get the more chance of getting common infections such as pneumonia and influenza we have.

PART 3: HOW AND WHY WE DREAM

CHAPTER 9: ROUTIUNELY PSYCHOTIC

Chapter 9 opens with the author's description of dreams. Walker describes dreams as some forms of psychotic episodes, which involve hallucinations, delusions, disorientation, even mood swings and amnesia. Dreaming mostly happens during REM phase of sleep.

Thanks to MRI scans, scientists have succeeded in figuring out that there are four main regions that experience intense activity during dreaming. Those regions are responsible for visual-spatial perceptions, movement, memory, and emotions. However, one thing that tends to be switched off when we dream is the logical prefrontal cortex.

Later in this chapter, the author argues that is scientifically possible to determine the content of our dreams. This can presumably be accomplished thanks to MRI scans.

Studies have proven that dreams are actually not replays of experiences we went through during our awake stage. Instead, our emotions play huge role in predicting our dreams.

CHAPTER 10: DREAM THERAPY

Here in this chapter, the author tries to decipher dreams by investigating their true purpose. However, in order to understand this, we need to understand the functions that REM sleep serves.

According to what the author writes, REM sleep can heal our emotional wounds. This means the more time we spend dreaming, the more we will be healed of our emotional wounds. Walker believes that dreaming acts as our emotional therapy. The main reason for this is that during our sleeping, our brains stop producing noradrenaline, which is anxiety hormone.

Another benefit of REM sleep is that it will help us to read people's emotions and facial expressions. This is crucial when we want to form relationships and even survive in a social setting. When we sleep, our brains become re-calibrated. This improves our abilities of precisely recognizing very small facial expressions of another people. Not experiencing REM during sleep means we will not be able to discern a friend from foe. Furthermore, this leads to fear bias and the main reason why everyone around us suddenly start looking very dangerous and threatening to us.

CHAPTER 11: DREAM CREATIVITY AND DREAM CONTROL

When it comes to the REM phase, it does not just protect our well-being. The REM phase of sleep also serves our creativity and problem-solving abilities. When we lack REM sleep, we have a significantly higher chance of failing tests. Studies showed that the participants of tests that were awakened during NREM phase had more problems than those who were awakened during REM phase.

Another benefit of REM is that it helps our brains to connect things and dots between seemingly unrelated concepts. Research showed that REM sleep helps us greatly to see hidden patterns, which connect different concepts of problems. This is where a daytime nap can be of great help for us. Every time we want to solve a certain problem and it seems we are stuck, take a nap between sixty and ninety minutes. After we awake, we will discover we have gained new wisdom, perceptions and ideas, and knowledge for solving that specific problem.

PART 4: FROM SLEEPING PILLS TO SOCIETY TRANSFORMED

CHAPTER 12: SLEEPING DISORDERS

According to the author, there are more than one hundred disorders that can happen within the human population and that can be related to sleep. Walker here writes a short summary of four sleep disorders so that we can have better understanding why both sleeping and dreaming are crucial for us. These disorders include somnambulism, insomnia, narcolepsy, and fatal familiar insomnia. Although some of these disorders are treatable, others have no cure.

The first disorder the author talks about is somnambulism. This disorder involves making some kind of movement while we sleep. Common symptoms involve sleepwalking, sleep sex, sleep eating, and even sleep homicide. The author argues that this disorder is caused by a sudden spike in activity within the nervous system.

Insomnia is the second disorder. The main difference between insomnia and sleep disorder is that insomnia prevents people from falling asleep regardless of how they try. There are two groups of insomniac people. The first group has problems staying asleep, while other group cannot fall asleep.

Narcolepsy is a neurological problem with three main symptoms. The first is extreme daytime drowsiness. The second is sleep paralysis and the third is cataplexy (or random loss of muscle control, triggered whenever a person experiences strong positive or negative emotions).

The author states that fatal familial insomnia is a disease without known cure or treatment. The disease is caused by a genetic anomaly that attacks the thalamus thus preventing it from falling asleep.

CHAPTER 13: SLEEP DISRUPTORS

According to Walker, there are several main sleep disruptors. These are electricity, alcohol, temperature, and early work schedules. Each of these, so-called "technological areas" affects the quality of sleep in one way or another.

Oil lamps, LED lights, and light bulbs drastically influenced our 24-hour brain clock. Moreover, every artificial source of light can force our brain to think that it is daytime. This inhibits REM sleep.

When it comes to alcohol, it also suppresses REM sleep and induces non-continuous sleep, which makes us feel very tired when we wake up.

Another thing that influences when we will go to sleep is our body core temperature. Evening causes temperature drops and the production of melatonin, which then makes us feel sleepy. However, thanks to blankets, central heating and other types of artificial keepers of temperature, our bodies have troubles dropping their temperatures. This leads to hot ambient temperature, which then prevents our brains from falling asleep.

After the Industrial Revolution, people began to wake up early in the morning to the sound of their alarms. This artificial termination of sleep leads to a state of shock. Every time we hear an alarm buzzing, our bodies enter a stage of shock, which leads to a surge in blood pressure and increase in heart rate.

CHAPTER 14: HURTING AND HELPING YOUR SLEEP

A great number of people rely on sleeping pills as a primary helping "tool" for sleeping. However, not only that the author says the sleeping pills are bad for us, but he also provides an alternative way of encouraging better night sleep.

The main reason why sleeping pills are ineffective in the long run is that they only sedate our brain's cortex and knock us unconscious. However, our brainwaves still behave as if we are awake. Some of the side effects this can have on us are grogginess, addiction, and weakened memory capacity. The best alternative the author offers for this is CBT or cognitive behavioral therapy. Two other very beneficial things for a good night's sleep are proper diet and exercise. A moderate level of exercise during the day help us boost our level of NREM sleep. In addition, good sleep will also improve our ability to exercise.

When it comes to diet, we should both avoid starvation and the consumption of high-carb, high-sugar, and low-fat diet, since these reduce deep NREM sleep. Moreover, we should not go to sleep when we are too hungry or too full.

CHAPTER 15: SLEEP AND SOCIETY

According to the author, four main areas can be used to show how damaging sleep deprivation can be for society in general. These are employment, torture, education, and healthcare.

Nowadays in great number of modern companies, employees who sleep less are considered role models and are glorified. Companies love to equate longer working hours with greater productivity. However, studies showed that sleep deprivation often leads to less productivity.

Sleep deprivation is also used as a military torture tactic. However, this is a barbaric technique for at least two reasons. First, sleep deprivation interferes with the logic of our brain, which can induce memory loss and emotional instability. As a result, the prisoner can be dishonest and can confess something he did not even do.

Second, sleep deprivation leads to mental and physical damage.

Public schools in the U.S. begin at 8.15 a.m. numerous school buses pick up kids by 6.45 a.m. This means that kids need to get up as early as 5.15 a.m. This can (and often does) lead to many health problems.

Moreover, chronic sleep deprivation can lead to chronic health problems, such as suicide, ADHD, depression, anxiety, substance abuse, and more.

The next part of the chapter is where the author writes about the fact that many doctors also do not get enough sleep. A great number of doctors and nurses spend numerous sleepless nights during their residency trainings. After they officially become doctors, they spend their careers working thirty-hour shifts. According to research, doctors who work thirty hours straight without sleep make around 460% more medical mistakes in the ICU than those that get enough sleep.

CHAPTER 16: A NEW VISION FOR SLEEP IN THE TWENTY-FIRST CENTURY

Here in this chapter, the author explains a roadmap that tackles the sleep deprivation issue on many fronts.

There are some technological methods, which can be used in order to improve the quality and longevity of sleep. Here the author envisions a future where people will wear sleep trackers, which will then chart their circadian rhythm.

When it comes to schools, Walker argues that students also need to be better educated about the overall importance of sleep. This can be achieved through simple modules that every school can adopt.

Organizations can also do more boost sleep quantity and quality. For example, there are companies that pay their employees a $25 bonus for every night that an employee sleeps for longer than seven hours. In the medical field, patients need to be allowed to sleep in rooms that do not have noisy equipment. When it comes to society as a whole, the author says that we all should have better, deeper, and broader understanding about the importance of sleep and its benefits for us.

ANALYSIS

Why We Sleep is compelling, self-help, professional guide in which the author explains why good, quality sleep is crucial for us. The book begins with one simple thesis: the importance of seven (eight hours max) hours of sleep. As we read the book, we find advice and solutions on how to improve our overall quality of sleep, what causes poor sleep quality, what sleep deprivation is and its devastating effects on human health, and more.

Sleep is very important for our health. The author of the book argues that a good night's sleep (the importance of night sleep is especially emphasized) is even more important that exercise or proper diet. However, thanks to influences of modern world, people tend either to reduce their night sleep or to completely skip it. As a result, our physical and mental health deteriorates over time, which becomes visible in many ways. In order to prevent this from happening (or to salvage what can be salvaged), the author offers his practical solutions on the problem.

Why We Sleep is a detailed, fun to read, logical and professional book where its readers can learn everything they ever wanted to learn about the importance of sleep. Therefore, it is highly recommended for readers to purchase and read the original book for a full content experience.

QUIZ

Welcome to our short quiz! Here in this quiz you can test your knowledge about the *Why We Sleep* book summary! Questions are simple to answer, with quiz answers section on the next page. Let's get started!

QUESTION 1

"When it comes to control of the sleep rhythm, plants and animals function in a similar way."

FALSE   TRUE

QUESTION 2

"According to the author, _____ main areas can be used   to   show   how   damaging   sleep _____ can be for the society in general. These are employment, torture, _____, and _____."

QUESTION 3

According to the author of this book how many hours per night is sufficient for good night sleep?

  A. Seven hours is what the author recommends as sufficient.
  B. Six hours is sufficient.
  C. Five or less hours are more than enough.
  D. This depends on people and their age.

QUESTION 4

What are two phases of sleep? What do they stand for?

  A. These are REM and AREM. They stand for "Rapid Eye Movability" and "Active Rapid Eye Movability."
  B. Two phases of sleep are called REM and NREM. They stand for "Rapid Eye Movement" and "Non-Rapid Eye Movement."
  C. The author does not mention any sleep phase.
  D. There are more than two phases of sleep mentioned in the book.

QUESTION 5

"Sleep deprivation is bad for our health because it can cause irritability (even in infants), it can affect the hormones, and it can eventually lead to numerous health problems and disorders."

TRUE   FALSE

QUIZ ANSWERS

QUESTION 1 – FALSE

QUESTION 2 – "four, deprivation, education, healthcare."

QUESTION 3 – A

QUESTION 4 – B

QUESTION 5 – TRUE

CONCLUSION

Sleep plays a crucial role in the lives of numerous living creatures that live on this planet. Humans are no exceptions. However, more often we tend do diminish the importance sleep has on us. Modern day life, (especially among Western societies), even glorify and proclaim the benefits of sleeping less. This leads to people sleeping less and less, which then leads to numerous mental and physical health problems.

"Why We Sleep: Unlocking the Power of Sleep and Dreams" is a book about the importance of sleep. The fact there are not many books that talk about the importance of sleep further emphasize the quality of this book. Why we need to sleep, the difference between REM and NREM phases, the importance of afternoon naps, the connection between diet, food, exercise, and health- all this and much more can be read in this book. *"Why We Sleep"* is a book for everyone. Its reader-friendly manner will attract many readers and its content will make you return to it long after you finish it.

Thank You and more...

Thank you for taking your time to read this book, I hope now you hold a greater knowledge about *Why We Sleep.*

Before you go, would you mind leaving us a review where you purchased your book?

It will mean a lot to us, and help us continue making more summaries for you and for others.

Thank you once again!

Yours warmly,

FURTHER READINGS

If you are interested in other self-help summary books. Click the link below.

1- Summary of Atomic Habits by Speed-Summary

   https://www.amazon.com/dp/B07RBT6ZBG/

2- Summary of Dr. Gundry Diet Evolution by Speed-Summary

   https://www.amazon.com/dp/B07RL831SC/

3-   Summary of The Obesity Code by Speed-Summary

   https://www.amazon.com/dp/B07RSN3ZJP/

You can click the link below or just search Speed-Summary on Amazon.

   https://www.amazon.com/s?i=digital-text&rh=p_27%3ASpeed-Summary&s=relevancerank&text=Speed-Summary&ref=dp_byline_sr_ebooks_1

Made in the USA
Monee, IL
06 January 2020